Diabetic Nephropathy

Diabetes

dp

in Practice

Other titles in the Wiley *Diabetes in Practice* Series

Prediction, Prevention and Genetic Counselling in IDDM
Jerry P. Palmer (Editor)

Diabetes in Pregnancy: An International Approach to Diagnosis and Management
Anne Dornhorst and David R Hadden (Editors)

Diabetic Complications
Ken Shaw (Editor)

Childhood and Adolescent Diabetes
Simon Court and Bill Lamb (Editors)

Hypoglycaemia in Clinical Diabetes
Brian M. Frier and B. Miles Fisher (Editors)

Exercise and Sport in Diabetes
Bill Burr and Dinesh Nagi (Editors)

Psychology of Diabetes Care
Frank Snoek and T. Chas Skinner (Editors)

Diabetic Nephropathy

Edited by
Christoph Hasslacher

St Josefskrankenhaus, Heidelberg, Germany

JOHN WILEY & SONS, LTD
Chichester · New York · Weinheim · Brisbane · Singapore · Toronto

Other Wiley Editorial Offices

John Wiley & Sons, Inc., 605 Third Avenue,
New York, NY 10158–0012, USA

WILEY-VCH Verlag GmbH, Pappelallee 3,
D-69469 Weinheim, Germany

John Wiley & Sons Australia Ltd., 33 Park Road, Milton,
Queensland 4064, Australia

John Wiley & Sons (Asia) Pte, Ltd., 2 Clementi Loop #02–01,
Jin Xing Distripark, Singapore 129809

John Wiley & Sons (Canada), Ltd., 22 Worcester Road,
Rexdale, Ontario M9W 1L1, Canada

Library of Congress Cataloging-in-Publication Data

Diabetic nephropathy / edited by C. Hasslacher.
    p. ; cm. — (Diabetes in practice)
    Includes bibliographical references and index.
    ISBN 0-471-48992-1 (cased : alk. paper)
    1. Diabetic nephropathies. I. Hasslacher, C. II. Series.
    [DNLM: 1. Diabetic Nephropathies. 2. Diabetes Mellitus—complications. 3. Kidney
Diseases—etiology. WK 835 D53567 2001]
    RC918.D53 D528 2001
    616.6'1071—dc21

2001024253

British Library Cataloguing in Publication Data

A catalogue record for this book is available from the British Library

ISBN 0-471-48992-1

Typeset in 10/12pt Palatino from the author's disks by Kolam
Printed and bound in Great Britain by Biddles Ltd, Guildford and King's Lynn
This book is printed on acid-free paper responsibly manufactured from sustainable forestry,
in which at least two trees are planted for each one used for paper production.

Contents

Contributors

Birgit Adam *Diabetesberaterin an der Inneren Abteilung des St Josefskranken-haus, Landhausstrasse 25, 69115 Heidelberg, Germany*

Georg Biesenbach MD Dozent *2nd Department of Medicine, General Hospital, Krankenhausstrasse 9, A 4020 Linz, Austria*

Henk J. G. Bilo MD, *Isalaklinieken, Locatie Weezenlanden, Postbus 10500, 8000GM Zwolle, The Netherlands*

Rudy Bilous MD, FRCP, Professor *University of Newcastle upon Tyne, New-castle, and South Tees Acute NHS Trust, Middlesbrough TS4 3BW, UK*

Béatrice Bouhanick MD *Unite de Diabetologie, Service de Medecine B, Centre Hospitalier Universitaire, 49033 Angers, France*

Anette E. Buyken MD *German Diabetes Research Institute at the Heinrich-Heine-University, Clinical Department, Auf'm Hennekamp 65, 40225 Düssel-dorf, Germany*

Daniel Cordonnier MD, Professor *Centre Hospitalier Universitaire, BP 217 X, 38043 Grenoble, France*

Thomas Danne MD, Priv. Dozent *KinderKrankenhaus auf der Bult, Jannst-Kovctok-Allee, 12, 30173, Hannover, Germany*

Elisabeth Engelmann MD *Klinik fur Allgemeine Padiatrie, Charite, Campus Virchow-Klinikum, Humboldt-Universität Berlin, Augustenburger Platz 1, 13353 Berlin, Germany*

Rijk O. B. Gans MD, Professor *Free University Hospital, Amsterdam, The Netherlands*

Manfred Ganz MD *Roche Diagnostics GmbH, Sandhofes Strasse 116, 68305 Mannheim, Germany*

Samy Hadjadj MD *Unite de Diabetolgie, Service de Medecine B, Centre Hospi-talier Universitaire, 49033 Angers, France*

Serge Halimi MD *Centre Hospitalier Universitaire, BP 217 X, 38043 Grenoble, France*

Christoph Hasslacher MD, Professor *Chefarzt der Inneren Abteilung des St Josefskrankenhaus, Landhausstrasse 25, 69115 Heidelberg, Germany*

Olga Kordonouri MD *Klinik fur Allgemeine Padiatrie, Charite, Campus Virchow-Klinikum, Humboldt-Universität Berlin, Augustenburger Platz 1, 13353 Berlin, Germany*

Peter Lütkes MD *Universitatsklinikum Essen, Zentrum fur Innere Medizin, Abteilung fur Nieren- und Hochdruckkrankheiten, Hufelandstrasse 55, 45122 Essen, Germany*

Alisdair Mackie MD *Department of Diabetes and Endocrinology, Northern General Hospital, Sheffield S5 7AU, UK*

Ruggero Mangili MD, Professor *Divisione Medicina I, Istituto Scientifico San Raffaele, Via Olgettina 60, 20132 Milano, Italy*

Michel Marre MD, Professor *Service d'Endocrinologie Hopital Bichat, 46 rue Henri Huchard, 75877 Paris cedex 18, France*

Claire Maynard MD *Centre Hospitalier Universitaire, BP 217 X, 38043 Grenoble, France*

Thomas Philipp MD, Professor *Universitatsklinilum Essen, Zentrum fur Innere Medizin, Abteilung fur Nieren- und Hochdruckkrankheiten, Hufelandstrasse 55, 45122 Essen, Germany*

Nicole Pinel MD *Centre Hospitalier Universitaire, BP 217 X, 38043 Grenoble, France*

Massimo Porta MD, Professor *Department of Internal Medicine, University of Turin, Corso AM Dogliotti 14, I-10126 Torino, Italy*

Rainer Proetzsch MD *Roche Diagnostics GmbH, Sandhofes Strasse 116, 68305 Mannheim, Germany*

Thomas Quaschning MD *Department of Medicine, Division of Nephrology, University Hospital Würzburg, Josef-Schneidstrasse 2, 97080 Würzburg, Germany*

Eberhard Ritz MD, Professor *Klinikum der Universitat Heidelberg, Sektion Nephrologie, Bergheimer Strasse 56a, 69115 Heidelberg, Germany*

Ivan Rychlík MD *1st Department Medicine, 3rd Faculty Medicine, Charles University, Srobarova 50, 100 34 Prague 10, Czech Republic*

Peter T. Sawicki MD, Professor *Department of Internal Medicine, St. Franziskus Hospital, 50825 Cologne, Germany*

Rafael F. Schäfers MD Priv. Dozent *Universitätskinikum Essen, Zentrum fur Innere Medizin, Abteilung fur Nieren- und Hochdruckkrankheiten, Hufeland-strasse 55, 45122 Essen, Germany*

Piet M. ter Wee MD *University Hospital Groningen, The Netherlands*

Monika Toeller MD *German Diabetes Research Institute at the Heinrich-Heine-University, Clinical Department, Auf'm Hennekamp 65, 40225 Düsseldorf, Germany*

Fokko J. van der Woude MD, Professor *Vth Medical University Clinic (Nephrology/Endocrinology), Klinikum Mannheim, University Heidelberg, Theodor Kutzer Ufer 1–3, 68135 Mannheim, Germany*

Nicole F. van Det MD *Vth University Clinic (Nephrology/Endocrinology), Klinikum Mannheim, University of Heidelberg, Theodor Kutzer Ufer 1–3, 68135 Mannheim, Germany*

Christoph Wanner MD, Professor *Department of Medicine, Division of Nephrology, University Hospital Würzburg, Josef-Schneidstrasse 2, 97080 Würzburg, Germany*

Benito A. Yard MD *Vth Medical University Clinic (Nephrology/Endocrinology), Klinikum Mannheim, University of Heidelberg, Theodor Kutzer Ufer 1–3, 68135 Mannheim, Germany*

Martin Zeier MD, Professor *Department of Medicine/Nephrology, University of Heidelberg, Bergheimerstrasse 56a, 69115 Heidelberg, Germany*

Josef Zimmermann MD *Department of Medicine, Division of Nephrology, University Hospital Würzburg, Josef-Schneidstrasse 2, 97080 Würzburg, Germany*

Preface

In many countries in the world, diabetic nephropathy is the most frequent reason for renal replacement therapy today. The majority of dialysis-dependent patients are not type 1 but type 2 diabetics. Extrapolations suggest that the number of patients with type 2 diabetes will multiply in coming years. It is feared that the number of patients with terminal renal insufficiency will rise accordingly unless the means of early diagnosis and treatment of diabetic nephropathy available today are used to the full.

In the last two decades, our knowledge on the clinical course of diabetic nephropathy, the factors influencing it and the possibilities of treatment have substantially improved. In numerous centres, both the occurrence and the progression of diabetic nephropathy can be prevented or at least slowed down markedly, even in advanced stages of kidney diseases. Consequently, it may be hoped that the number of diabetics with renal insufficiency can be reduced if the available methods of diagnosis and treatment are consistently applied on a broad scale.

The primary objective of this book is to present a synopsis of important practical aspects in diagnosis, differential diagnosis and treatment of diabetic nephropathy based on present-day knowledge. However, specific aspects of pathogenesis and clinical features, e.g. pregnancy, diabetic nephropathy in adolescents, cardiovascular complications, disorders of lipid metabolism, etc, are also considered. The chapters were written by colleagues who have been treating diabetic patients with these complications and have also worked scientifically in the field for years. We all hope that this book will not only attract interest in, and improve comprehension of, diabetic nephropathy, but will above all contribute to a wide-scale implementation of modern methods of treatment.

C. Hasslacher
March 2001

Part I

Natural Course, Pathogenesis, Morphology And Genetics

1

Diabetic Nephropathy—the Size of the Problem

EBERHARD RITZ[1] AND IVAN RYCHLÍK[2]

[1]Department of Internal Medicine, Ruperto Carola University, Heidelberg, Germany [2]Department Medicine, Charles University, Prague, Czech Republic

TRENDS IN THE INCIDENCE AND PREVALENCE OF ENDSTAGE RENAL FAILURE OF PATIENTS WITH DIABETES IN THE WESTERN WORLD

In the late 1970s and early 1980s, American authors (1) reported on what then appeared to most European nephrologists to be an implausibly high incidence and prevalence of diabetes in patients admitted for renal replacement therapy. With a lag of approximately one-and-a-half decades, the incidence of diabetes amongst patients admitted for renal replacement therapy began to rise in Europe as well (2). Raine (3) drew attention to the "flood" of patients to be expected. This assessment was based upon the increasing number of patients with diabetes, particularly type 2 diabetes, admitted for renal replacement therapy in Europe, according to the data of the EDTA Registry (Figure 1.1). These early observations have been impressively confirmed by more recent data from the registry of The Netherlands (Figure 1.2) which illustrates that the prevalence of diabetic patients on treatment of endstage renal disease (ESRD) increased both for type 1 and type 2 diabetes (4). A similar increase is now seen worldwide. Table 1.1 shows data from the ANZDATA registry that illustrate a continuous and substantial increase, although in Australia and New Zealand the

Diabetic Nephropathy. Edited by C. Hasslacher.
© 2001 John Wiley & Sons, Ltd.

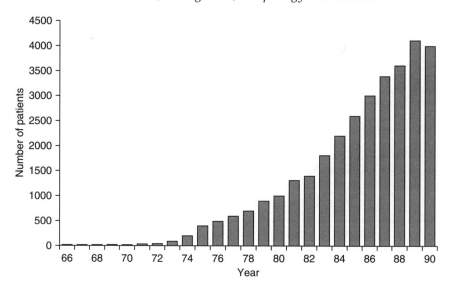

Figure 1.1 Patients with endstage renal failure due to diabetic nephropathy commencing renal replacement therapy in Europe in 1966–1990, according to EDTA registry. From (2), © 1993 Springer-Verlag, with permission

Table 1.1 Incidence of diabetic patients admitted for renal replacement therapy in Australia and New Zealand. Comparison of the years 1986 and 1996

	Year	Number of diabetic patients		Diabetics as percentage of total incident ESRD patient
		(*n*)	(pmp)	(%)
Auxstralia	1986	69	4	9.7
	1996	260	14	18.5
New Zealand	1986	20	6	16.1
	1996	102	29	35.8

After (5) by permission of ANZDATA. pmp, per millian population.

prevalence of diabetes type 2 and diabetic nephropathy is still comparatively low (5).

We compared the overall incidence of patients with ESRD requiring renal replacement therapy and the admission rate of diabetic patients in the lower Neckar, a region of Germany (6) and Lombardy, a north Italian province (7). Table 1.2 shows that the number of diabetic patients admitted for renal replacement therapy in south-west Germany has reached an order of magnitude in line with that reported for Caucasian US citizens (8). It is also

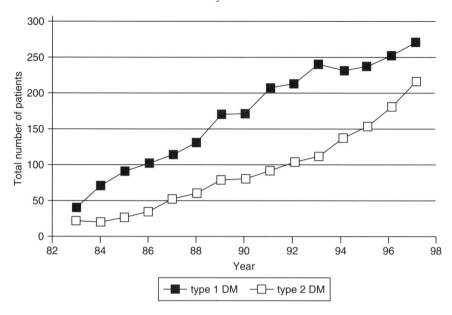

Figure 1.2 The evolution of admissions for renal replacement therapy of patients with type 1 and type 2 diabetes in The Netherlands. From (4), with permission

Table 1.2 Admission of diabetic patients for renal replacement therapy—comparison of Lombardy (Italy) [after (7)] and Lower Neckar (Germany) [after (6)]

	Incidence overall	Incidence diabetes	Type 2 diabetes	Incidence (pmp/year)	
	(pmp/ year)	(pmp/ year)	(% of diabetics)	Type 1	Type 2
Lombardy (1992)	95.2	10.4	48	5.4	5.0
Lower Neckar (1993)	125.0	52.0	90	5.0	47.0

obvious that the great majority of patients admitted suffered from type 2 diabetes. Indeed, the incidence of ESRD in patients with type 1 diabetes was almost similar in south-west Germany and Lombardy.

A continuous increase in admission rate of diabetic patients, most of them of type 2 (with the exception of the Northern European countries) is documented by Table 1.3, based on the EDTA registry data. Analysis was restricted to countries with a > 50% response rate. The table confirms that large differences exist between European countries. The magnitude of the problem worldwide is illustrated by Table 1.4, which gives the annual incidence of all patients with ESRF and diabetic patients with ESRF per

Table 1.3   Diabetic patients on renal replacement therapy—evolution during the last decade according to country

		1984/85	1986/87	1988/89	1990/91	1992/93
Austria	Incidence	8.9	15.4	16.4	20.4	20.7
	Prevalence	16.5	31.9	44.2	57.9	69.2
Cyprus	Incidence	4.2	3.3	12.4	12.2	8.6
	Prevalence	18.3	18.3	30.7	37.2	48.6
Czechoslovakia	Incidence	1.1	2.4	3.5	5.1	10.5
	Prevalence	1.6	3.6	7.0	11.6	20.8
Denmark	Incidence	7.1	8.1	9.1	12.5	17.8
	Prevalence	18.0	24.5	33.3	49.2	66.5
Finland	Incidence	11.1	11.9	14.2	14.8	20.6
	Prevalence	37.9	48.0	60.2	70.5	87.3
France	Incidence	4.3	5.1	6.3	8.3	9.3
	Prevalence	13.4	17.5	23.7	31.6	40.3
Iceland	Incidence	0.0	2.5	12.5	5.0	7.5
	Prevalence	0.0	2.5	22.5	30.0	37.5
Israel	Incidence	8.0	12.0	11.3	21.4	17.3
	Prevalence	19.3	22.2	32.2	49.9	56.9
Italy	Incidence	5.0	5.6	6.7	7.6	9.1
	Prevalence	13.8	18.2	24.0	29.7	35.4
Luxembourg	Incidence	5.0	10.0	21.7	14.6	22.5
	Prevalence	18.8	38.4	58.4	52.1	52.5
The Netherlands	Incidence	4.4	6.2	8.1	10.0	10.7
	Prevalence	12.3	18.3	26.2	32.9	37.1
Spain	Incidence	5.2	6.9	8.4	8.7	8.8
	Prevalence	13.1	19.5	27.2	35.0	44.6
Sweden	Incidence	14.8	15.5	17.3	21.3	22.8
	Prevalence	44.7	56.5	68.3	85.1	109.2
Switzerland	Incidence	6.4	8.6	8.6	9.6	9.8
	Prevalence	18.2	27.3	34.4	43.1	49.6
UK	Incidence	4.1	4.9	4.8	5.3	–
	Prevalence	9.9	15.2	19.8	25.1	–

Data from the EDTA Registry; courtesy of Dr E. Jones, London. Data as patients per million population per year for all countries with > 50% response rate

million population in different European countries compared to some Asian countries and the USA (4–9, 11, 12). The epidemiology in some countries in Western Europe has become similar to what is observed in the USA. Based on data from the US Renal Data System (8), Table 1.5 gives the incidence of diabetic patients with ESRD in the period 1991–1995 according to age, gender and race. Although there is almost certainly misclassification of the types of diabetes, it is immediately apparent that the main problem is ESRD in patients with type 2 diabetes. This is particularly true in the elderly, in females and in non-Caucasoids. ESRD in patients with type 2 diabetes is largely a disease of the elderly. The age distribution is remarkably similar in the USA, in the European registry, in Australia and in individual European countries.

Table 1.4 Annual incidence of patients overall, and of diabetic patients, admitted for renal replacement therapy (RRT)

Country	Year	Patients overall (PMP)	Diabetic patients (PMP)	Reference
European Union	1995	120*	11.5**	–
Denmark	1996	95.3	21.3	9
France	1995	112.0	17.6	A
Lombardy (Italy)	1996	–	10.1	B
Catalonia (Spain)	1994	111.1	19.8	11
Lower Neckar (Germany)	1993	125.0	52.0	6
The Netherlands	1996	85.4	13.3	4
Taiwan	1995	223.0	59.0	C
Australia	1996	77.0	14.0	5
New Zealand	1996	78.0	28.0	5
Japan	1995	210.0	66.0	12
USA	1995	262.0	107.0	8

Annual incidence of patients admitted for RRT

Data per million population (pmp).
*According to Annual Report on management of renal failure in Europe, XXVIII, 1997.
**Data of the EDTA Registry for 1994; courtesy of Dr E. Jones, London.
A, personal communication; Dr S. Halimi, Grenogle.
B, personal communication; Dr F. Locatelli, Lecco.
C, personal communication; Dr D.-C. Tarng, Taipei.

In interpreting the results, one must be aware of certain shortcomings in the epidemiological analysis. On the one hand, many data are flawed by misclassification of patients. A particularly frequent error is that patients with type 2 diabetes who use insulin are reported as patients with type 1 diabetes. This source of error is carefully excluded in some of the smaller regional registries and reports (4, 9). Another confounder is the fact that approximately 25% of patients with type 2 diabetes admitted for RRT suffer from standard primary chronic renal disease, e.g. ischemic nephropathy, glomerulonephritis, autosomal dominant polycystic kidney disease, analgesic nephropathy, etc. (10). This was noted by us and by others. Since the frequency of diabetic patients with primary renal disease reaching endstage renal failure apparently exceeds what is anticipated by multiplying the expected frequencies of diabetes and primary renal disease in the general population, the interesting possibility is raised that superimposition of diabetes upon primary renal disease accelerates progression.

Conversely, one potential source of error results in underreporting, i.e. the known disappearance of hyperglycaemia when patients with type 2 diabetes reach endstage renal failure. This leads to the paradox of normoglycaemic patients having advanced diabetic glomerulosclerosis as the persisting sequelae of past hyperglycaemia (10).

Table 1.5 Incidence of diabetic patients with endstage renal disease (ESRD) in USA in the period 1991–1995

	Total number (and percentage of all ESRD)	Age group (Percentage of all ESRD)			Gender (Percentage of all ESRD)		Race (Percentage of total number of admissions)			
		< 20	20–40	> 64	M	F	White	Black	Asian	Native American
All ESRD	305 876	4 767	156 572	144 537	162 420	143 456	197 741	89 261	8 626	4 337
Diabetes total	115 938(37.4)	17.6	42.7	33.9	33.5	42.8	38.0	36.4	39.9	63.4
DM type 1 (juvenile type, ketosis prone)	47 836 (15.4)	0.9	20.3	11.0	14.4	17.1	16.9	13.3	12.2	17.7
DM type 2 (adult onset or unspecified type)	68 099(22.0)	0.7	22.3	22.9	19.2	25.7	21.1	23.1	27.7	45.7

After (8). The data reported here have been supplied by the United States Renal Data System (USRDS). The interpretation and reporting of these data are the responsibility of the author(s) and in no way should be seen as an official policy or interpretation of the US Government.

A final source of potential underreporting may be failure of admission of elderly patients with type 2 diabetes and ESRF to the nephrologist, a practice which was certainly prevalent in Eastern Europe (13) and is still seen, even in some Western European countries.

DIFFERENCES BETWEEN EUROPEAN COUNTRIES

It is of interest that the prevalence of patients with diabetes on dialysis in Germany is much lower than anticipated from the incidence figures. The German registry (Quasi-Niere) (14) reported that 6% of patients on dialysis had type 1 and 14% type 2 diabetes. The discrepancy with the incidence figures reported in Table 1.2 can be easily explained by the poor survival of diabetic patients on dialysis (see below).

It is apparent from Tables 1.2 and 1.3 that large differences exist between European countries and even regions within European countries (15) with respect to the annual number of diabetic patients reaching endstage renal failure (incidence) and the proportion of diabetic patients on renal replacement therapy (prevalence).

Large regional differences exist, e.g. in France, a country with notoriously low prevalence of diabetic patients in the dialysis population (10). The frequency is particularly low in the Departements bordering Italy and Spain (countries with known low frequency of renal failure in diabetics) and high in the Departements bordering Belgium and Germany (countries with known high frequency of renal failure in diabetics). As of 1995, in a study conducted by S. Halimi (personal communication), the proportion of diabetic patients on maintenance haemodialysis had risen from 6.9% (in 1989) to 13.02% in mainland France. The proportion of type 2 diabetes increased from 80% to 86%. In the north and east of France, 25% of patients admitted had diabetes and in Strassburg the proportion exceeded 40% (16). Of particular interest is the observation that in the overseas territories of France, type 2 diabetes is much more prevalent in the dialysis population. Albitar found in La Reunion (17) that in this Departement, with an incidence of ESRD of 188 pmp, 33.6% of incident patients suffered from type 2 diabetes.

In other Southern European countries with historically low incidence and prevalence of diabetic nephropathy, the incidence of ESRD in patients with type 2 diabetes is also on the rise. In Catalonia (Spain), a region of 6 million inhabitants, admission of patients with type 2 diabetes and ESRD increased from 3 pmp in 1984 to 26.6 pmp in 1994 (11). This trend is worldwide. Figure 1.3 shows data from Kikkawa (Shiga University), according to which in Japan ESRD in diabetic patients (more than 90% of whom have diabetes type 2) will become the single most frequent cause of ESRF by the year 2000 (12). This development is similar to what has already occurred in the

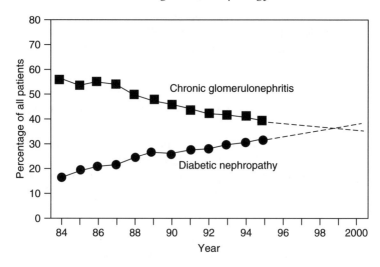

Figure 1.3   Annual change of number of patients starting dialysis therapy in Japan. From (12), with permission

USA (8) and Germany (6). If the above trends (Table 1.3) continue, one can expect that the same will be seen in many other countries as well.

POTENTIAL CAUSES FOR THE CURRENT EPIDEMIOLOGICAL TREND

Several factors may account for the current apparently relentless increase of the incidence of ESRD in patients with type 2 diabetes. Some factors are listed in Table 1.6.

In former communist East Germany, the prevalence of diabetes increased by a factor of 4 within two decades (18). A similar trend for increasing prevalence of type 2 diabetes has been noted in many other countries as well (19).

Based on extrapolation from retinopathy data, it has been estimated that in Germany the diagnosis of type 2 diabetes is made on average only 4–5 years after onset of hyperglycaemia (20). There are numerous reports indicating that glycaemic control and control of hypertension is suboptimal, thus enhancing the risk of diabetic nephropathy (21). The average HbA_{1c} of type 2 diabetic patients seen by general practicioners in Germany is 8.5%. The proportion of patients with type 2 diabetes who are normotensive

Table 1.6 Potential causes for rising incidence of endstage renal disease (ESRD) in patients with type 2 diabetes

---

- Higher prevalence of type 2 diabetes in the population (partly due to ageing of the population)
- Late diagnosis of diabetes
- Suboptimal correction of hyperglycaemia and hypertension
- Better survival of patients, particularly of proteinuric patients, because of reduced cardiovascular mortality
- Higher rates of referral to nephrologists

---

according to JNC VI criteria (22) is below 20% (23). Interestingly, it has been argued that the low incidence of ESRD in type 2 diabetic patients in Australia is due to the tradition of very careful blood pressure control in this country (Cooper, Melbourne; personal communication).

Undoubtedly, however, the major factor for the increasing incidence of ESRF in patients with type 2 diabetes is the progressively decreasing cardiovascular mortality in this high-risk population. In the Department Internal Medicine at Heidelberg (24), the 5 year mortality in type 2 diabetic patients with proteinuria decreased in the course of one decade from 65% to 25%, and this has been confirmed by several other authors. As a result, patients today live long enough to be exposed to the risk of developing diabetic nephropathy and endstage renal failure. There is no doubt that recently a higher proportion of type 2 diabetic patients with ESRD are also referred to the nephrologist. Unfortunately, however, today most of these patients are treated by GPs (25) and referral is usually extremely late. This is illustrated by the observations of Pommer (26) in Berlin and by our group in Heidelberg (23). In a recent series from Strassbourg, no less than 18% of the patients with type 2 diabetes and ESRD had to be dialysed on an emergency basis immediately after referral (16).

SURVIVAL AND QUALITY OF LIFE IN PATIENTS WITH TYPE 2 DIABETES ON RENAL REPLACEMENT THERAPY

The 5 year survival on renal replacement therapy is very poor in Germany (27) as well as in other countries, as indicated by Table 1.7. This is mainly the result of high cardiovascular mortality (28), as was noted in our study (Table 1.8) and is confirmed by the US Renal Data System (8). We emphasize that the survival of a patient with type 2 diabetes on haemodialysis is currently comparable to that of patients with advanced gastrointestinal carcinoma (Figure 1.4). Quality of life on renal replacement therapy is much poorer in

Table 1.7 Comparison of actuarial 5 year survival of non-diabetic and diabetic patients on renal replacement therapy (% surviving patients)

Country	Non-DM	DM	Reference
Australia	60	42/27*	5
Japan	–	47	12
Taiwan	65	37	A
Hong Kong	70	20	B
Lombardy (Italy)	61	28	7
Catalonia (Spain)	65	30	11
Germany	–	38/5*	27
USA	44.6	28.1	8

* Reported as diabetes type 1/type 2.
A, personal communication, Dr D.-C. Tarng, Taipei.
B, personal communication, Dr K. N. Lai, Hong Kong.

diabetic patients compared to non-diabetic patients, as illustrated by the results of the ANZDATA report (5) from Australia and New Zealand (Table 1.9). This fact is also reflected by the observation that withdrawal from dialysis is much more common in diabetic than in non-diabetic patients (Table 1.10).

Currently, only a negligible minority of patients with type 2 diabetes undergo renal transplantation. In the Catalonia registry (M. Clèries, Barcelona, personal communication), of 2211 patients alive with functioning grafts, 66 have type 1 diabetes but only eight have type 2 diabetes (compared to 338 patients with type 2 diabetes on haemodialysis or CAPD). On the other hand, Hirschl et al (29) showed that, in patients with type 2 diabetes, the results of transplantation are remarkably good if macroangiopathy

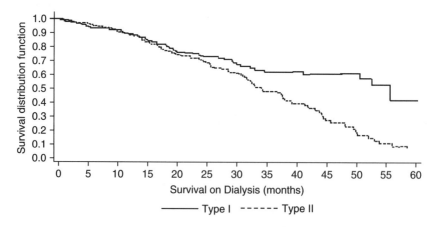

Figure 1.4 Actuarial 5 years survival in type 1 ($n = 181$) and type 2 ($n = 231$) diabetic patients with end-stage renal disease in prospective multicenter study in Germany. From (27), with permission

is excluded, particularly coronary heart disease (29). This is also illustrated by the actuarial patient survival figures, kindly provided by Professor Opelz, Heidelberg (Figure 1.5). According to Port (30), the gain in survival after transplantation, relative to survival on dialysis, is greater in the diabetic than the non-diabetic patient (Figure 1.6). In other words, the

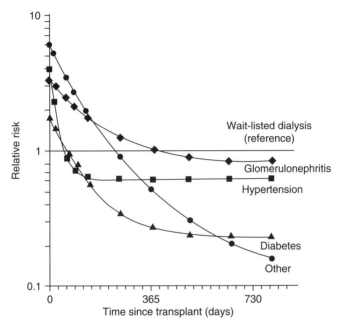

Figure 1.5 Relative risk of mortality for cadaveric transplant recipients by cause of end-stage renal disease (ESRD) vs. dialysis patients of same cause of ESRD. The reference line is specific for each cause of ESRD. From (30), with permission of American Medical Association

Table 1.8 Causes of death in diabetic patients followed for 57 months after start of dialysis

	Type 1 diabetes ($n = 67$)	Type 2 diabetes ($n = 129$)
Dead [n (%)]	29 (43)	80 (62)
Total cardiovascular deaths [n (%)]	18 (62)	48 (60)
Myocardial infarction	8	12
Sudden death	7	13
Cardiac other	3	17
Stroke	0	6
Septicaemia [n (%)]	7 (24)	11 (14)
Withdrawal from treatment	2	8
Other	2	13

After (28).

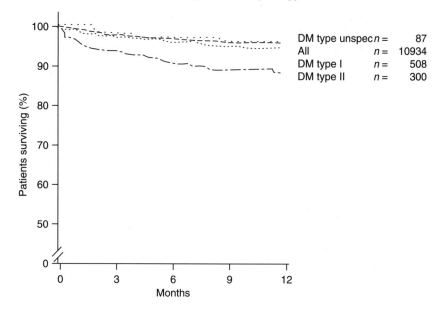

Figure 1.6 Actuarial patient survival in diabetic patients receiving kidney grafts (Collaboration Transplant Study, 1996, Professor G. Opelz, Heidelberg)

Table 1.9 Quality of life. Comparison of non-diabetic vs. diabetic patients

Age group	Australia		New Zealand	
	Non-DM	DM	Non-DM	DM
25–44 years (*n*)	880	145	180	42
Self-care (%)	9	21	11	29
Disabled (%)	2	12	3	7
45–64 years (*n*)	1549	372	275	208
Self-care (%)	14	28	14	21
Disabled (%)	5	12	4	10

After (5).

Table 1.10 Withdrawal from dialysis by age and diabetes status, USA 1993–1995

Age	Number of deaths/100 dialysis patient-years	
	DM	non-DM
20–44	2.1	0.7
45–64	3.1	1.7
> 65	7.0	6.6

Note: withdrawal = 19% of all deaths.
After (8).

diabetic patient can expect more survival benefit from renal transplantation than the non-diabetic patient. In view of the scarcity of organs, it is uncertain whether this consideration will lead to increased transplantation activity.

CONCLUSIONS

It emerges from the above that the rising tide of type 2 diabetes with endstage renal failure (6) represents an enormous public health problem in Europe. Not only will the immensely costly renal replacement therapy with unsatisfactory outcome strain the health budget, it is also sobering that a disease that is preventable, at least in principle, has become the single most common cause of endstage renal failure in many countries of the Western world.

The epidemiology of this condition calls for intense efforts to improve diabetes care (10, 33). Prevention must include measures: (a) to stem the tide of type 2 diabetes in the population; (b) to screen type 2 diabetic patients for microalbuminuria in order to detect high-risk patients; (c) to improve glycaemic control by earlier administration of insulin; (d) to educate patients in self-control of glycaemia and blood pressure; (e) to spread in the medical community information about the possibility of prevention of diabetic nephropathy (including the benefit of ACE inhibitors and possibly ANG II receptor antagonists); and (f) to integrate nephrologists early into the medical care of these patients in order to implement effective renal prevention. Today the nephrologist is usually reduced to the function of a caretaker who, at the end of a futile journey, receives the patients with type 2 diabetes in endstage renal failure on an emergency basis to perform belatedly a form of treatment with bleak outlook (10, 16).

ACKNOWLEDGEMENT

I.R. was supported by a training grant from the International Society of Nephrology.

REFERENCES

1. Friedmann EA Diabetes with kidney failure. *Lancet* 1986; **2**: 1285.
2. Raine AEG (on behalf of the EDTA Registry). Epidemiology, development and treatment of end stage renal failure in non-insulin dependent diabetics in Europe. *Diabetologia* 1993; **36**: 1099–104.

3. Raine AEG. The rising tide of diabetic nephropathy. The warning before the flood? (Editorial Comments). *Nephrol Dial Transplant*, 1995; **10**: 460–61.
4. Ramsteijn PG, de Charro FTh, Geerling W et al. *Registratie nierfunctievervanging Nederland. Statistisch Verslag 1998.* Stichting Renine: Rotterdam, 1998.
5. Australia and New Zealand Dialysis and Transplant Registry (ANZDATA) (1998). Disney APS, Russ GR, Walker R, Sheil AGR (eds). Adelaide, South Anzdata: Australia, 1998.
6. Lippert J, Ritz E, Schwarzbeck A, Schneider P. The rising tide of endstage renal failure from diabetic nephropathy type II—An epidemiological analysis. *Nephrol Dial Transplant* 1995; **10**: 462–7.
7. Marcelli D, Spotti D, Conte F et al. Prognosis of diabetic patients on dialysis: analysis of Lombardy Registry data. *Nephrol Dial Transplant* 1995; **10**: 1895–1901.
8. US Renal Data System (USRDS). *Annual Data Report 1997.* National Institutes of Health, National Institute of Diabetes and Digestive and Kidney Diseases: Bethesda, MD, 1997.
9. Danish Society of Nephrology. *Danish National Registry Report on Dialysis and Transplantation in Denmark, 1997.*
10. Ritz E, Stefanski A Diabetic nephropathy in type II diabetes. *Am J Kidney Dis* 1996; **27**: 167–94.
11. Rodriguez JA, Clèries M, Vela E, Renal Registry Committee. Diabetic patients on renal replacement therapy: analysis of Catalan. *Nephrol Dial Transplant* 1997; **12**: 2501–9.
12. Kikkawa R, Kida Y, Haneda M Nephropathy in Type II Diabetes – Epidemiological issues as viewed from Japan. *Nephrol Dial Transplant* 1998; **13**: 2743–5.
13. Thieler H, Achenbach H, Bischoff J et al. Evolution of renal replacement therapy in East Germany from 1989 to 1992. *Nephrol Dial Transplant* 1994; **9**: 238–41.
14. Nierenersatztherapie in Deutschland. Bericht über Dialysebehandlung und Nierentransplantation in Deutschland 1998. *Nephrol Dial Transplant* 1999; **14**: 1085–90.
15. Zmirou, Benhamou PY, Cordonnier D et al. Diabetes mellitus prevalence among dialysed patients in France (UREMIDIAB study). *Nephrol Dial Transplant* 1992; **7**: 1092–7.
16. Chantrel F, Enache M, Bouiller M et al. T. Abysmal prognosis of type type 2 diabetes patient entering dialysis. *Nephrol Dial Transplant* 1999; **14**: 129–36.
17. Albitar S, Bourgeon B, Genin R et al. on behalf of the Indian Ocean Society of Nephrology. Epidemiology of end-stage renal failure in Reunion Island (results form the registry of the Indian Ocean Society of Nephrology). *Nephrol Dial Transplant* 1998; **13**: 1143–5.
18. Michaelis D, Jutzi E. Epidemiologie des Diabetes mellitus in der Bevölkerung der ehemaligen DDR. Alters und geschlechtsspezifische Inzidenz- und Prävalenztrends im Zeitraum 1960–1987. *Z Klin Med* 1991; **89**: 147–50.
19. Harris MI. Diabetes in the United States: epidemiology, scope and impact. In *Diabetic Renal–Retinal Syndrome* Friedman EA, L'Esperance FA Jr (eds). Kluwer Academic: Dordrech, 1998; 1–11.
20. Standl E, Stiegler H. Microalbuminuria in a random cohort of recently diagnosed type 2 (non-insulin-dependent) diabetic patients living in the greater Munich area. *Diabetologia* 1993; **36**: 1017–20.
21. Ritz E, Fliser D. Nephropathy in NIDDM—an update. In *Diabetic Renal–Retinal Syndrome*, Friedman EA, L'Esperance FA Jr (eds). Kluwer Academic: Dordrecht, 1998; 27–39.

22. Joint National Committee. The sixth report of the Joint National Committee on detection, evaluation and treatment of high blood pressure. *Arch Intern Med* 1998; **57**: 2413–46.
23. Keller C, Ritz E, Pommer W, Stein G, Frank J, Schwarzbeck A. Behandlungsqualität niereninsuffizienter Diabetiker in Deutschland. *Dtsch Med Wschr* 2000; **125**: 240–4.
24. Hasslacher C, Borgholte G, Panradl U, Wahl P. Verbesserte Prognose von Typ-I- und Typ-II-Diabetikern mit Nephropathie. *Med Klin* 1990; **85**: 643–6.
25. Passa P. Diabetic nephropathy in the NIDDM patients on the interface between diabetology and nephrology. What do we have to improve? *Nephrol Dial Transplant* 1997; **12**: 1316–17.
26. Pommer W, Bressel F, Chen F, Molzahn M. There is room for improvement of preterminal care in diabetic patients with endstage renal failure. The epidemiological evidence in Germany. *Nephrol Dial Transplant* 1997; **12**: 1318–20.
27. Koch M, Kutkuhn B, Grabensee B, Ritz E. Apolipoprotein A, fibrinogen, age, and history of stroke are predictors of death in dialysed diabetic patients: a prospective study in 412 subjects. *Nephrol Dial Transplant* 1997; **12**: 2603–11.
28. Koch M, Thomas B, Tschöpe W, Ritz E. Survival and predictors of death in dialysed diabetic patients. *Diabetologia* 1993; **36**: 1113–17.
29. Hirschl MM. The patient with type II diabetes and uremia—to transplant or not to transplant? *Nephrol Dial Transplant* 1995; **10**: 1515–16.
30. Port FK, Wolfe RA, Mauger EA et al. Comparison of survival probabilities for dialysis patients vs. cadaveric renal transplant recipients. *J Am Med Assoc* 1993; **270**: 1339–43.
31. Disney APS. Some trends in chronic renal replacement therapy in Australia and New Zealand, 1997. *Nephrol Dial Transplant* 1998; **13**: 854–9.
32. Excerpts from the USRDS 1997 Annual Data Report. Executive Summary. *Am J Kidney Dis* 1997; **30** (suppl 1): S10–S20.
33. Ismail N, Becker BN, Strzelczyk P, Ritz E. Renal disease and hypertension in non-insulin-dependent diabetes mellitus (editorial). *Kidney Int* 1999; **5**: 1–28.

2

Natural Course of Diabetic Nephropathy

CHRISTOPH HASSLACHER

St Josefskrankenhaus, Heidelberg, Germany

The course of diabetic nephropathy is mainly characterized by changes of urinary albumin excretion and glomerular filtration rate. In type 1 diabetic patients the course is well defined and progresses through five stages, according to Mogensen (1). The characteristics of these stages are described in Table 2.1. In type 2 diabetes the course of diabetic nephropathy is less well characterized, due to the often unknown date of onset of disease or other factors influencing progression of nephropathy, such as hypertension, age or race. Patients with diabetic nephropathy, especially with type 2 diabetes, have a high cardiovascular risk. Thus, the development of nephropathy can be stopped through premature death without having reached the stage of renal insufficiency.

URINARY ALBUMIN EXCRETION

Patients with type 1 diabetes usually show an elevated urinary albumin excretion rate (AER) at the time of diabetes diagnosis (stage 1). In response to effective metabolic control by insulin treatment, AER decreases in most patients within 3–6 months. During the next years AER usually stays in normal range (stage 2). During phases of poor metabolic control or with the development of other diseases, AER can rise temporarily.

Diabetic Nephropathy. Edited by C. Hasslacher.
© 2001 John Wiley & Sons, Ltd.

Table 2.1 Stages of diabetic nephropathy

Stage	Designation	Glomerular filtration rate	Urinary albumin excretion	Blood pressure	Main structural changes
I	Hyperfunction/ hypertrophy	May be increased	May be increased	Usually normal	Hypertrophy, increased kidney volume
II	Norm-albuminuria	Normal/ increased	Normal	Normal	Increasing basement membrane thickness and mesangium expansion
III	Incipient diabetic nephropathy	Normal/ increased	20–200 µg/min (micro-albuminuria)	Increasing ≈ 3 mmHg/ year	
IV	Overt diabetic nephropathy	Decreasing	> 200 µg/min (macro-albuminuria)	Usually frank	Increasing glomerular occlusion and severe mesangial expansion
V	Endstage renal failure	< 20 ml/min	Macroalbuminuria, often decreasing due to glomerular occlusion	hyper-tension	

After (1).

In a wide range of time after diabetes diagnosis (5–15 years) AER starts raising in some patients. AER of 20–200 µg/min is called microalbuminuria; AER over 200 µg/min it is called macroalbuminuria.

The appearance of microalbuminuria is the first laboratory finding of a glomerular damage. This stage is called incipient nephropathy (stage 3). Since AER shows a high day-to-day variation and is influenced by several extrarenal factors, diagnosis of incipient nephropathy demands "persistent" microalbuminuria, i.e. presence of microalbuminuria during a 3 month period (see Chapter 8). It must be emphasized that special tests must be used for detection of microalbuminuria. The usual urine dipstick tests for protein will be negative and and 24 hour urine protein excretion are in the normal range.

The onset of microalbuminuria has a high predictive power for further progression: under standard treatment, AER increases by mean of 20% year (2). About 80% of the patients with persistent microalbuminuria will develop overt nephropathy within the next 10 years (3). The rate of increase in AER is clearly related to glycaemic control and blood pressure status, as indicated later. Patients who develop microalbuminuria after a longer duration of diabetes (> 15 years) usually show a slower rate of progression (4).

Macroalbuminuria or persistent proteinuria usually develops 15–25 years after the diagnoses of diabetes. It is the characteristic sign of overt nephro-pathy (stage 4). In contrast to the microalbuminuric stage, proteinuria is now not selective, i.e. apart from albumin, a lot of different proteins are excreted. The entire protein excretion, however, is mostly not in the nephrotic range. If a nephrotic syndrome is diagnosed in these patients, further prognosis is usually poor (5).

The course of AER in type 2 diabetic patients is similar to type 1 diabetes but shows some characteristic differences. At the time of diagnosis, 15–30% of these patients show microalbuminuria and 2–8% already macroalbuminuria (6–8). In response to metabolic normalization by diet or oral hypoglycaemic agent, elevated AER declines during weeks and months. In contrast to type 1 diabetes, elevated AER persists in a significant proportion (10–48%) of the patients (9,10). This can be an expression of underlying renal damage due to a considerable preceding time of undetected hyperglycaemia. As in type 1 diabetes, persistent microalbuminuria predicts the further progression of nephropathy. Under standard treatment, 32–42% of microalbuminuric type 2 diabetes patients will develop overt nephropathy within 4–5 years (11, 12). However, considerable individual variation in the rate of changes of AER has been reported (13). Macroalbuminuria usually develops around 16 years after the diagnosis of diabetes. The shorter range of time compared to type 1 diabetes probably reflects the fact that the point of diabetes diagnosis can not be determined exactly in type 2 diabetic patients. In endstgage renal failure AER may decrease in both type 1 and type 2 diabetic patients, due to occlusion of the glomeruli.

GLOMERULAR FILTRATION RATE

The glomerular filtration rate (GFR) and the renal plasma flow (RPF) are increased in patients diagnosed with type 1 diabetes (stage 1). Sonographic investigations of the kidneys usually reveals increased volumes. GFR and RPF can in many cases be normalized again over weeks or months by insulin treatment. However, the GFR remains raised compared to non-diabetic controls in 25–40% of cases (14,15). Increased kidney size is partially reversed by better metabolic control. The GFR remains constant during nephropathy stages 2 and 3. After manifestation of macroalbuminuria (sometimes even in more severe microalbuminuria), kidney function begins to decline. According to studies conducted in the 1960s and 1970s, in which intensified treatment measures were not possible, the mean GFR loss is an average of 10–12 ml/year. The renal and life prognosis in this stage was very poor in the past: 6–10 years after onset of macroalbuminuria about half the patients reached endstage renal failure or died (16). However, advances in the treatment modalities during the last two decades has substantially improved prognosis. The rate of decline in GFR and the excess mortality could be at least halved by intensive treatment of these patients (16; see Chapter 21).

In type 2 diabetic patients, GFR is also raised at time of diagnoses of diabetes compared to non-diabetic controls (17,18). However, hyperfiltration with GFR values in excess of 140 ml/min tends to be rare. A decrease of the raised GFR can likewise be demonstrated after weeks or months in this group of patients as a result of better glycaemic control. Similar to the situation in type 1 diabetes, the GFR decreases continuously after the manifestation of advanced microalbuminuria or macroalbuminuria without appropriate intervention. According to earlier studies, i.e. without intensive treatment, the annual decrease of GFR was around 10–12 ml/min/year and is thus similar to that in type 1 diabetes (19,20). About half of these patients reached endstage renal failure within 7 years after the onset of microalbuminuria, or died (16). Under better metabolic and antihypertensive treatment, the prognosis of proteinuric type 2 diabetic patients also improved. Two studies from the last decade (21, 22) found an average rate of decline of GFR of 5.3 and 5.7 ml/min/year, respectively. However, as in type 2 diabetes, the rate of progression is very variable; this was also the case in proteinuric type 2 diabetic patients.

INCIDENCE/PREVALENCE OF DIABETIC NEPHROPATHY

Studies on the incidence or prevalence of the various stages have sometimes led to very divergent results. This is due to various factors: patient population investigated (clinical-based, primary care supervision, population-based; ethnic influences); methods and criteria of diagnosis used; socioeconomic status of the population investigated. Most data on the incidence and prevalence are available from Europe and the USA.

Microalbuminuria

In type 1 diabetes, a prevalence of microalbuminuria of 21% was found in the Euro-Diab Study, the cross-sectional study comprising the largest number of cases ($n = 3250$) (23). Similar figures were observed in a population-based study in Wisconsin, USA (21.2%) (24). Lower prevalences were reported, for example, from Norway (population-based study, 12.5%) (25) and the UK (clinic cohort-based study, 6.7%) (26). The prevalence data are in a similar range for patients with type 2 diabetes, at least for the European population. For other ethnic groups, e.g. Pima indians or Pacific islanders, the prevalence is markedly higher.

The incidence of microalbuminuria was investigated in two studies on type 1 diabetic patients. They revealed an annual incidence of persistent microalbuminuria of 1.6–2% (27,28). The DCCT Study show for the first time the effect of better metabolic control on the incidence of microalbuminuria. In the primary prevention group (= patients without retinopathy and duration of diabetes < 5 years) the annual incidence was 0.9% per year under conventional treatment and 0.4% per year under intensified therapy. The corresponding figures for the secondary prevention group (= patients with retinopathy and duration of diabetes < 15 years) were higher: 2.53% and 1.1%, respectively (29).

Macroalbuminuria

The prevalence of macroalbuminuria or persistent proteinuria varies between 5% and 30% in type 1 and type 2 diabetics. In these cross-sectional studies, only a spot urine sample was investigated; this is subject to a high rate of false-positive results. The cumulative incidence is hence a better indicator for the clinical importance of overt diabetic nephropathy.

For patients with type 1 diabetes, studies in Europe and the USA revealed a cumulative incidence of around 20% after a duration of diabetes of 20 years (19,30,31). In patients with type 2 diabetes, there were similar cumulative incidences; in an American study of 1131 patients, it was 24.6% after a diabetes duration of 20 years (7) and the corresponding figure was 27% in a German investigation (19) (Figure 2.1). Thus, the development of diabetic nephropathy is very similar in type 1 and type 2 diabetes, at least in Europoid patients. A high incidence of persistent proteinuria has been recently reported in early-onset Japanese type 2 diabetic patients (32). In some ethnic groups, higher cumulative incidences were described in some cases, e.g. in Pima Indians it was 50% after a duration of diabetes of 20 years.

The annual incidence of overt nephropathy is in the range 0.4–3.6% depending on diabetes duration. As shown in Figure 2.2 there are two peaks of annual incidence, one after 16 years and a smaller one after 32 years (30). The incidence rate declines to about 1% in patients who have suffered from diabetes for 40 years or more. That means that patients surviving 35 years of diabetes seem to be at very low risk for development of overt diabetic nephropathy. Studies of the cumulative incidence of overt diabetic nephropathy in long-term diabetes clearly indicate that only about 45–50% of type 1 and type 2 diabetic patients will ever develop nephropathy (19,30,33).

Recent studies suggest that the incidence of diabetic nephropathy declines, at least in type 1 diabetic patients. Swedish patients who developed type 1 diabetes during 1961–1965 exhibited a cumulative incidence of persistent proteinuria of 38% after a diabetes duration of 20 years.

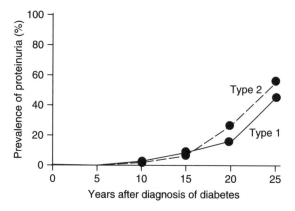

Figure 2.1 Cumulative incidence of persistent proteinuria in type 1 and type 2 diabetic patients from a single clinic in Germany (19). Reproduced by permission of Oxford University Press

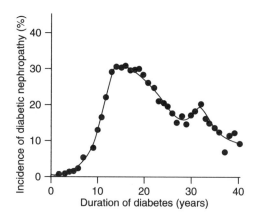

Figure 2.2 Annual incidence of diabetic nephropathy in relation to duration of diabetes in type 1 diabetic patients (30). Reproduced by permission of Springer-Verlag

However, patients with onset of diabetes during 1971–1975 developed persistent proteinuria in only 9% of cases (34). Similar results were reported in a study from the UK (35) and Japan (33). This positive trend has been interpreted as a consequence of better management of type 1 diabetic patients. However, there are no corresponding findings with respect to type 2 diabetic patients (33).

Renal Failure

Data on the incidence of ESRF have mostly been obtained from the Register of Renal Replacement Therapy. However, besides the factors that influence the epidemiological investigations mentioned at the beginning, differences in referral for renal replacement therapy must be considered. Thus, reports from these registers only partially represent the natural course of diabetic nephropathy. The figures available today are shown in detail in Chapter 1. Irrespective of the country investigated, they show the great importance of diabetic nephropathy in type 2 diabetes for the number of patients receiving renal replacement therapy.

There are few investigations on the incidence of ESRF that are not register-based. In type 1 diabetes, estimates of the cumulative incidence of renal insufficiency varied markedly: 8% after 25 years of diabetes in a population-based study in Rochester (36), 21% over a 35 year period of a clinical-based cohort from the Joslin Clinic (37), 18% in a Copenhagen cohort followed for 15 years (38). The newest report from the Wisconsin study revealed a 10 year incidence of renal insufficiency of 14.4% (39). It varied from 5.6% in those with 5–9 years of diabetes to 33.5% in those with > 35 years of diabetes. However, comparisons among studies are difficult due to the different definition of renal insufficiency, the different time periods in which the groups were studied and the different treatment modalities, i.e. quality of glycaemic and blood pressure control.

In type 2 diabetes there is now abundant evidence that the risk of renal insufficiency or endstage renal failure is similar to type 1 diabetes. Figure 2.3

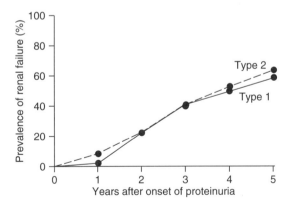

Figure 2.3 Cumulative prevalence of renal failure among patients with type 1 and type 2 diabetes from a single clinic in Germany (19). A serum creatinine concentration of more than 1.4 mg/dl was considered to indicate renal failure. Reproduced by permission of Oxford University Press

shows the cumulative prevalence of renal insufficiency among patients with type 1 and type 2 diabetes according to the duration of proteinuria. It is obvious that the clinical course from the occurrence of proteinuria up to the beginning of kidney failure (i.e. serum creatinine > 1.5 mg/dl) was the same. Similar results were obtained in the population-based study from Rochester (36). These findings have major significance for public health, as the incidence of type 2 diabetes is rapidly growing world-wide.

DETERMINANTS OF NATURAL COURSE OF DIABETIC NEPHROPATHY

The development and progression of diabetic nephropathy is influenced or modulated by several factors, which are listed in Table 2.2. It is obvious that most of these can be influenced by therapeutic procedures.

Susceptibility to Nephropathy

As shown previously, about 30–50% of patients with long-standing diabetes will develop diabetic nephropathy. The annual incidence of proteinuria in type 1 diabetic patients shows a strong increase over the first 15–20 years of diabetes and than declines sharply (30). Furthermore, there are reports that some apparently well-controlled patients will develop proteinuria, whereas other poorly-controlled patients will not. These findings lead to the assumption that there is a variable individual susceptibility to develop renal complications, which is partly independent of metabolic control or other influencing factors.

These assumption has been supported by several studies in type 1 and type 2 diabetic patients. In Chapter 1 is has been shown that there are considerable inter population differences in the prevalence of diabetic nephropathy. Furthermore, Seaquist (40) reported familiar clustering of

Table 2.2   Influencing or modulating factors of natural course of diabetic nephropathy

Age, gender
Duration of diabetes
Genetic (familial and racial) factors
Metabolic control
Blood pressure
Smoking
Protein intake
Hyperlipidaemia
Proteinuria

albuminuria and/or endstage renal failure among diabetic siblings of diabetic probands; 83% of siblings of probands with diabetic nephropathy also suffered from renal disease, compared with 17% of siblings of probands without nephropathy. These findings have been confirmed by a Danish study (41). In type 2 diabetes an inherited predisposition to diabetic nephropathy was studied in Pima Indian families with diabetes in two generations (42). Proteinuria was detected in 14% of diabetic offsprings of diabetic patients without proteinuria, in 23% if one parent had proteinuria and in 46% if both parents had diabetes and proteinuria. These studies are consistent with a genetic influence on the susceptibility to diabetic nephropathy. However, they can not completely exclude shared environmental effects.

Further studies assume that susceptibility to diabetic nephropathy is associated to hypertension and/or cardiovascular disease. Thus, it has been shown that the risk of nephropathy in type 1 diabetic patients was three times higher in those who had parents with a history of hypertension than in those without hypertensive parents (43). Earle et al (44) reported that a family history of cardiovascular complications increased the risk of diabetic nephropathy, compared with patients with a negative family history (odds ratio 3.2). Furthermore, cardiovascular events were considerable higher in proteinuric patients with a positive family history (odds ratio 6.2). Knowledge of individual susceptibility to renal desease would be of great benefit for treatment modalities, since intensive therapy may be most beneficial in patients identified as being at risk. Therefore, an intensive research interest exists in this field (see Chapter 7).

Glycaemic Control

The occurrence of hyperglycaemia is an absolute condition for the development of diabetic nephropathy, as shown by numerous experimental and histological progress investigations in humans. *A priori*, the quality of the glycaemic control is thus of crucial importance for the development of nephropathy. These correlations were already shown in appropriate progress studies conducted in the past. As an example, Table 2.3 shows the relationship between blood glucose values during the pre-proteinuric stage and the time interval between diagnosis of diabetes and onset of persistent proteinuria (= macroalbuminuria) in a group of type 1 and type 2 diabetic patients treated during 1965–1985 in Heidelberg, Germany (45,46). The time till onset of proteinuria increased with better metabolic control in both type 1 and type 2 diabetic patients. The progression to renal insufficiency is, furthermore, influenced by metabolic control, as illustrated in Figure 2.4. In the 1990s, the correlation between glycaemic control and the development and progression of nephropathy was convincingly confirmed by further

Table 2.3   Postprandial blood glucose during the preproteinuric phase and onset of persistent proteinuria

Blood glucose (mg/dl) (annual median)	Time interval between diagnosis of diabetes and persistent proteinuria (years)	
	Type 1 diabetes	Type 2 diabetes
Persistent < 200	23	18
Intermittent > 200	19	17
Persistent > 200	14	14

After (45, 46).

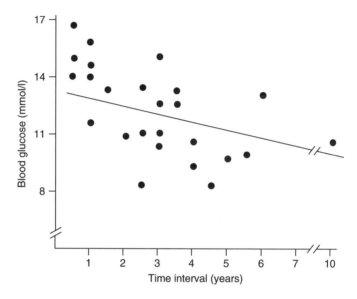

Figure 2.4   Correlation between metabolic control and onset of renal failure type 1 diabetic patients. Median post-prandial blood glucose at time of persistent proteinuria and the time interval between onset of persistent proteinuria and elevation of serum creatinine are shown ($r = 0.53$; $p < 0.01$) (45). Reproduced by permission of Springer-Verlag

prospective progression studies (47,48,49) and by large-scale intervention studies in type 1 and type 2 diabetics (DCCT, UKPDS). A dose–effect correlation between HbA$_{1c}$ as a parameter of glycaemic control and the occurrence of microalbuminuria or macroalbuminuria could be demonstrated for the first time (50). These results will be examined in detail in Chapter 15.

Hypertension

Hypertension is one of the most important influencing factors for onset and progression of diabetic nephropathy in both type 1 and type 2 diabetes. Blood pressure shows an characteristic course during the development of diabetic nepropathy, which differs greatly in type 1 and type 2 diabetic patients. Table 2.4 shows the prevalence of hypertension in the different stages of nephropathy according to WHO and JNCV-criteria (51). In type 1 diabetics with normal albumin excretion, the prevalence of hypertension is usually just as high as in the general population. With the onset of micro-albuminuria, blood pressure usually begins to rise but initially it remains in the "normotensive" range. With the occurrence of macroalbuminuria, hypertension is present in 60–70% of these patients, whereas practically all patients are hypertensive in the stage of renal failure.

In contrast to type 1 diabetes, patients with type 2 diabetes demonstrated hypertension in a high percentage of cases at the time of diagnosis of diabetes (Table 2.4). With onset of micro-or macroalbuminuria the prevalence increases further and in the stage of renal failure all patients are hypertensive.

Table 2.4   Prevalence of arterial hypertension in diabetic patients with and without nephropathy

Stage of nephropathy	Patients (n)	Prevalence of antihypertensive treatment (%)	World Health Organization †	JNCV †
Type 1 diabetes				
Normoalbuminuria	562	8	15 (12–18)	42 (38–46)
Microalbuminuria	215	12	26 (20–33)	52 (45–59)
Macroalbuminuria	180	48	61 (53–68)	79 (72–85)
Type 2 diabetes				
Normoalbuminuria	323	30	51 (45–57)	71 (66–76)
Microalbuminuria	151	39	73 (65–81)	90 (84–95)
Macroalbuminuria	75	65	82 (72–90)	93 (85–98)

After (51).
† Data are given as mean (range).

Numerous progress studies were able to show that the occurrence of microalbuminuria or macroalbuminuria in type 2 diabetics is predicted and promoted by an already pre-existing arterial hypertension. For example, Table 2.5 gives the blood pressure status of type 2 diabetic patients who will develop overt nephropathy and those who will not. These patients were treated during 1965–1985 in Heidelberg. Median systolic blood pressure and prevalence of hypertension are significantly higher during the pre-proteinuric stage in patients who will develop nephropathy. In this patient group, higher blood pressure was associated with a shorter time interval

Table 2.5   Hypertension as a predictor of nephropathy in type 2 diabetic patients during the preproteinuric phase

Patients	Median blood pressure (mmHg)	Prevalence of Hypertension n (%)
Developing persistent proteinuria ($n=63$)	164 (105–215) 87 (70–106)	44/63 (70%)
Not developing persistent proteinuria ($n=63$)	149 (122–183) 84 (68–97)	27/63 (43%)

After (46).

Table 2.6   Median systolic blood pressure during the preproteinuric phase and onset of persistent proteinuria in 63 type 2 diabetic patients

Systolic blood pressure (annual median) (mmHg)	Time interval between diagnosis of diabetes and persistent proteinuria (years)
Persistent < 160	21
Intermittent > 160	17
Persistent > 160	13

After (46).

between the diagnosis of diabetes and the onset of persistent proteinuria (Table 2.6). In more recent studies, besides glycaemic control the systolic blood pressure could be identified as the pre-eminent factor influencing the development of nephropathy (48,49,52).

After the manifestation of proteinuria, the blood pressure is the most important progression factor in type 1 and type 2 diabetic patients, as shown by numerous progress and intervention studies (see Chapter 16). Figure 2.5 gives an example for the typical relationship between the loss of kidney function and blood pressure in proteinuric diabetics.

However, hypertension is a crucial determinant not only for the loss of kidney function but also for the prospects of survival of diabetics with nephropathy. The WHO Multinational Study of Vascular Disease in Diabetes stated that patients with both hypertension and proteinuria experienced a strikingly high mortality risk: in type 1 diabetes, 11-fold for men and 18-fold for women; and in type 2 diabetes, five-fold for men and eight-fold for women (53).

In the meantime, several intervention studies have clearly shown the great importance of treating hypertension in patients with diabetes (see Chapter 16). These results should be put into practice as a matter of urgency. Table 2.4 shows the prevalence of antihypertensive therapy in hypertensive patients with microalbuminuria or macroalbuminuria. It becomes evident that only about half of the hypertensive patients were treated with medication.

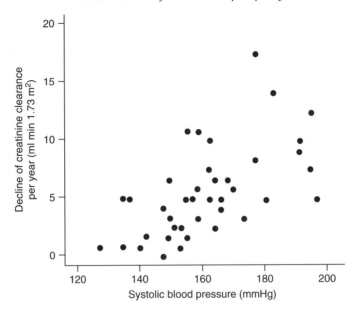

Figure 2.5 Correlation between mean systolic blood pressure during the observation period and annual decline of creatinine clearance in proteinuric type 2 diabetic patients (22). Reproduced by permission of Springer-Verlag

Protein Intake

An unequivocal correlation could be found between the intake of dietary protein and the excretion of albumin in a large-scale study (54). As a rule, a higher protein intake correlated with a greater excretion of albumin in the urine. Epidemiological studies provided further indications for an effect of dietary protein intake and the occurrence of kidney diseases. It is known that the incidence of nephropathy is higher, for example, in northern countries with a higher proportion of animal protein in the food than in the western countries of Europe, in which the diet contains more fat or carbohydrates. Furthermore, some intervention studies suggest that reduction of protein intake promotes the loss of kidney function (see Chapter 18).

Dyslipoproteinemia

Dyslipoproteinemia occurs with the appearance of microalbuminuria or macroalbuminuria, especially in type 2 diabetes. This is characterized by a rise of triglycerides and LDL-cholesterol as well as a decrease of HDL-cholesterol. In animal experiments, an effect on the progression of nephropathy could be shown. Early investigations in humans point in a similar direction. In proteinuric type 2 diabetic patients, a significant correlation between mean serum triglyceride levels and the decline of kidney function was described (22). A regression analysis with decrease of kidney function as the dependent variable showed that, aside from systolic blood pressure and metabolic control, the mean triglyceride level is to be regarded as an independent factor affecting the decline in kidney function. Further studies and their relevance for cardiovascular mortality in patients are described in detail in Chapter 12.

Smoking

Cigarette smoking is a relevant factor in the clinical course of diabetic nephropathy in both type 1 and type 2 diabetes. In cross-sectional studies, for instance, Telmer et al (55) found a higher prevalence of persistent proteinuria in type 1 diabetic patients who were, or had been, smokers compared with non-smokers (19% vs. 12%). There was a clear correlation between cigarette consumption and the prevalence of nephropathy. These findings have been confirmed by other studies (56,57). In type 2 diabetes, Olivarius et al found that albuminuria was more prevalent in smokers (8.2%) and former smokers (7.3%) than in non-smokers (2.1%) (58).

Prospective studies showed further an association of smoking and progression of nephropathy. Chase et al (59) found, in young diabetic patients with microalbuminuria over a follow-up period of 2–3.5 years, a faster progression of albuminuria and retinopathy in smokers. Sawicki et al (60) studied the progression of diabetic nephropathy in 92 type 1 diabetic patients who where under intensified insulin and antihypertensive treatment. Progression of nephropathy, i.e. increase in proteinuria or serum creatinine, was found in 53% of smokers as compared with 11% of non-smokers. There was a dose-dependent increase in risk for progression with the number of smoked cigarettes.

In the Wisconsin study, the risk of developing proteinuria has been analysed in a great number of type 2 diabetic patients who had normal protein excretion of time of recruitment (61). During a follow-up of 4 years, the relative risk of developing gross proteinuria was 2–2.5 for heavy smokers compared with non-smokers. Biesenbach et al (20) noted that the rate of progression to endstage renal failure was about twice as high in smoking than in non-smoking patients. These studies showed that smoking is an important risk factor for the development of diabetic nephropathy. Furthermore, it is known that smoking diabetic patients have an approximately two-fold increase in cardiovascular mortality (62,63). This risk is excessively increased in patients with persistent proteinuria (64,65).

Proteinuria

Proteinuria is generally regarded as a marker of glomerular demage. Recent experimental studies, however, suggest that proteinuria itself may be harmful (66). Danish authors evaluated the impact of albuminuria and other factors on the progression of nephropathy in type 1 diabetic patients with persistent albuminuria (67). They found a significant correlation between the rates of decline in the glomerular filtration rate and diastolic blood pressure on one side and albuminuria on the other side. Stepwise multiple linear regression analysis, however, only showed a significant correlation between the rate of decline in glomerular filtration rate and diastolic blood pressure. However, in patients with normal blood pressure, statistical analysis showed that albuminuria but not blood pressure was correlated significantly with the decline in glomerular filtration rate. Similar results have also been obtained by other study groups in diabetic and non-diabetic kidney disease (68,69). In line with these findings is the observation of Rossing et al (70), that a reduction of albuminuria during antihypertensive treatment predicts a beneficial effect on diminishing the progression of nephropathy.

From the pathophysiologic point of view, it is assumed that in cases of albuminuria the proximal tubular cells increase their protein absorption rate. As a consequence of increase protein absorption and digestion, local production of cytokines and chemokines rises. These processes lead to an interstitial inflammation and finally to an interstitial fibroses.

REFERENCES

1. Mogensen CE, Christensen CK, Vittinghus E. The stages in diabetic renal disease with emphasis on the stage of oncipient diabetic nephropathy. *Diabetes* 1983; **28**: 6–11.
2. Christensen CK, Mogensen CE. The course of incipient diabetic nephropathy: studies of albumin excretion and blood pressure. *Diabet Med* 1985; **2**: 97–102.
3. Mogensen CE, Christensen CK. Predicting diabetic nephropathy in insulin dependent patients. *N Engl J Med* 1984; **311**: 89–93.
4. Mackin P, MacLeod JM, New JP, Marshall SM. Renal function in long-duration type 1 diabetes. *Diabet Care* 1996; **19**: 249–51.
5. Watkins PJ, Blainey JD, Brewer DB et al. The natural history of diabetic renal disease. *Q J Med* 1972; **164**: 437–56.
6. Uusitupa M, Sitonen O, Penttila I, Aro A, Pyorala K. Proteinuria in newly diagnosed type II diabetic patients. *Diabet Care* 1987; **10**: 191–4.
7. Ballard DJ, Humphrey LL, Melton LJ III et al. Epidemiology of persistent proteinuria in type II diabetes mellitus. Population-based study in Rochester, Minnesota. *Diabetes* 1988; **37**: 405–12.
8. Keller CK, Bergis KH, Fliser D, Ritz E. Renal findings in patients with short term type 2 diabetes. *J Am Soc Nephrol* 1996; **7**: 2627–35.

9. Schmitz A, Hansen HH, Christensen T. Kidney funtion in newly diagnosed type 2 (non-insulin-dependent) diabetic patients, before and during treatment. *Diabetologia* 1989; **32**: 434–9.

10. Patrick AW, Leslie PJ, Clarke BF, Frier BM. The natural history and associations of microalbuminuria in type 2 diabetes during the first year after diagnosis. *Diabet Med* 1990; **7**: 902–8.

11. Ravid M, Savin H, Jutrin I, Bental T, Katz B, Lishner M. Long-term stabilizing effect of angiotensin converting enzyme inhibition on plasma creatinine and on proteinuria in normotensive type II diabetic patients. *Ann Intern Med* 1993; **118**: 577–81.

12. Schmitz A, Vaeth M, Mogensen CE. Systolic blood pressure relates to the rate of progression of albuminuria in NIDDM. *Diabetologia* 1994; **37**: 1251–8.

13. Cooper ME, Fraumann A, O'Brian RC et al. Progression of proteinuria in type 1 and type 2 diabetes. *Diabet Med* 1988; **5**: 361–8.

14. Christiansen JS, Gammelgaard J, Frandsen M, Parving H-H. Increased kidney size glomerular filtration rate and renal plasma flow in short-term insulin dependent diabetics. *Diabetologia* 1981; **20**: 451–6.

15. Schmitz A, Hansen HH, Christensen T. Kidney function in newly diagnosed type 2 (non-insulin-dependent) diabetic patients, before and during treatment. *Diabetologia* 1989; **32**: 434–9.

16. Hasslacher C, Borgholte G, Panradl PW Verbesserte Prognose von Typ-1- und Typ-II-Diabetikern mit Nephropathy. *Med Klin* 1990; **85**: 643–6.

17. Nowack, R, Raum E, Blum W, Ritz E. Renal hemodynamics in recent-onset type II diabetes. *Am Kidney Dis* 1992; **20**: 342–7.

18. Vora JP, Dolpen J, Dean JD et al. Renal hemodynamics in newly presenting non-insulin dependent diabetes mellitus. *Kidney Int* 1992; **41**: 829–55.

19. Hasslacher C, Ritz E, Wahl P, Michael C. Similar risks of nephropathy in patients with type I or type II diabetes mellitus. *Nephrol Dialysis Transpl* 1989; **4**: 859–63.

20. Biesenbach G, Janko O, Zazgornik J. Similar rate of progression in the predialysis phase in type I and type II diabetes mellitus. *Nephrol Dialysis Transpl* 1994; **9**: 1097–102.

21. Gall MA, Nielsen FS, Smitz, UM, Parving HH. The course of kidney function in type 2 (non-insulin-dependent) diabetic patients with diabetic nephropathy. *Diabetologia* 1993; **36**: 1071–8.

22. Hasslacher, C, Bostedt-Kiesel A, Kempe HP, Wahl P. Effect of metabolic factors and blood pressure on kidney function in proteinuric type 2 (non-insulin-dependent) diabetic patients. *Diabetologia* 1993; **36**: 1051–6.

23. EURODIAB IDDM Complications Study Group. Microvascular and acute complications in IDDM patients. The EURODIAB IDDM Complications Study. *Diabetologia* 1994; **37**: 278–85.

24. Klein R, Klein BEK, Linton KLP, Moss SE. Microalbuminuria in a population based study of diabetes. *Arch Intern Med* 1992; **152**: 153–8.

25. Joner G, Brinchman-Hansen O, Torres CG, Hanssen KF. A nationwide cross-sectional study of retinopathy and microalbuminuria in young Norwegian type 1 (insulin dependent) Diabetic patients. *Diabetologia* 1992; **35**: 1049–5.

26. Marshall SM, Alberti KGMM. Comparison of the prevalence and associated features of abnormal albumin excretion in insulin dependent and non-insulin dependent diabetes. *Q J Med* 1989; **70**: 61–71.

27. Microalbuminuria Collaborative Study Group UK. Risk factors for development of microalbuminuria in insulin dependent diabetic patients: a cohort study. *Br Med J* 1993; **306**: 1235–9.

28. Mathiesen ER, Ronn B, Storm B, Foght H, Deckert T. The natural course of microalbuminuran in insulin-dependent diabetes: a 10-year prospective study. *Diabet Med* 1995; **12**: 482–7.

29. The Diabetes Control and Complications Trial (DCCT) Research Group. Effect of intensive therapy on the development and progression of diabetic nephropathy in the Diabetes Control and Complications Trial. *Kidney Int* 1995; **47**: 1703–20.

30. Andersen AR, Sandahl Christiansen JK, Anderson JK, Kreiner S, Deckert T. Diabetic nephropathy in type 1 (insulin dependent) diabetes: an epidemiological study. *Diabetologia* 1983; **25**: 496–501.

31. Krolewski AS, Warram JH, Christlieb AR, Busick EJ, Kahn CR. The changing natural history of nephropathy in type 1 diabetes. *Am J Med* 1985; **78**: 785–94.

32. Yokoyama H, Okudaira M, Otani T et al. Higher incidence of diabetic nephropathy in type 2 than in type 1 diabetes in early-onset diabetes in Japan. *Kidney Int* 2000; **58**: 302–11.

33. Yokoyama H, Okudaira M, Otani T. High incidence of diabetic nephropathy in early-onset Japanese NIDDM patients. *Diabet Care* 1998; **21**: 1080.

34. Nordwall M, Bojestig M, Arnqvist H, Ludvigsson J. Persistent decrease in nephropathy in type 1 diabetes. *Diabetologia* 2000; **43** (1): abstr 971.

35. Harvey J, Rizvi K, Craney L, Messenger J, Shah R, Meadows P. A population-based survey of the prevalence of diabetic nephropathy. *Diabetologia* 2000; **43** (1): abstr 972.

36. Humphrey LL, Ballard DJ, Frohnert PP et al. Chronic renal failure in non-insulin-dependent diabetes mellitus; a population-based study in Rochester, Minnesota. *Ann Intern Med* 1989; **111**: 788–96.

37. Krolewski M, Eggers PW, Warram JH. Magnitude of end-stage renal disease in IDDM: a 35 year follow-up study. *J Kidney Int* 1996; **50**: 2041–6.

38. Rossing P, Rossing K, Jakosen P, Parving HH. Unchanged incidence of diabetic nephropathy in IDDM patients. *Diabetes* 1995; **44**: 739–43.

39. Klein R, Klein BEK, Moss SE, Cruickshanks KJ, Brazy PC. The 10-year incidence of renal insufficiency in people with type 1 diabetes. *Diabet Care* 1999; **22**: 743–50.

40. Sequist ER, Goetz FC, Rich S, Barbosa J. Familial clustering of diabetic kidney disease: evidence for genetic susceptibility to diabetic nephropathy. *N Engl J Med* 1989; **320**: 1161–5.

41. Borch-Johnsen K, Norgaard HE, Mathiesen ER et al. Is diabetic nephropathy an inherited complication? *Kidney Int* 1992; **41**: 719–22.

42. Pettitt DJ, Saad MF, Bennett PH, Nelson RG, Knowler WC. Familial predisposition to renal disease in two generation of Pima Indians with type 2 (non-insulin-dependent) diabetes mellitus. *Diabetologia* 1990; **33**: 438–43.

43. Krolewski AS, Canessa M, Warram JH et al. Predisposition to hypertension and susceptibility to renal disease in insulin-dependent diabetes mellitus. *N Engl J Med* 1988; **318**: 140–45.

44. Earle K, Walker J, Hill C, Viberti GC. Familial clustering of cardiovascular disease in patients with insulin-dependent diabetes and nephropathy. *N Engl J Med* 1992; **326**: 673–7.

45. Hasslacher C, Stech W, Wahl P, Ritz E. Blood pressure and metabolic control as risk factors for nephropathy in type 1 (insulin-dependent) diabetes. *Diabetologia* 1985; **28**: 6–11.
46. Hasslacher, C. Wolfrum M, Stech G, Wahl P, Ritz E. Diabetische Nephropathie bei Typ-II-Diabetes. Einfluss von Stoffwechselkontrolle und Blutdruck auf Entwicklung und Verlauf. *Dsch Med Wochr* 1987; **112**: 1445–9.
47. Forsblom CM, Groop PH, Ekstrand A et al. Predictors of progression from normoalbuminuria to microalbuminuria in NIDDM. *Diabet Care* 1998; **21**: 1932.
48. Tanaka Y, Atsumi Y, Matsuoka K et al. Role of glycemic control and blood pressure in the development and progression of nephropathy in elderly japanese NIDDM patients. *Diabet Care* 1998; **21**: 116–20.
49. Nosadini R, Velussi M, Brocco E et al. Course of renal function in type 2 diabetic patients with abnormalities of albumin excretion rate. *Diabetes* 2000; **49**: 76.
50. The Diabetes Control and Complications Trial Research Group. The absence of a glycemic threshold for the development of long-term complications: the perspective of the diabetes control and complications trial. *Diabetes* 1996; **45**: 1289.
51. Deedwania PC. Hypertension and diabetes; new therapeutic options. *Arch Intern Med* 2000; **160**: 1585.
52. Schmitz A, Vaeth M, Mogensen CE. Systolic blood pressure relates to the rate of progression of albuminuria in NIDDM. *Diabetologia* 1994; **37**: 1251–8.
53. Wang SL, Head J, Stevens L, Fuller J. Excess mortality and its relation to hypertension and proteinuria in diabetic patients. *Diabet Care* 1996; **19**: 305–12.
54. Toeller M, Buyken A, HeitkampG et al and the EURODIAB IDDM Complications Study Group. Protein intake and urinary albumin excretion rates in the EURODIAB IDDM Complications Study. *Diabetologia* 1997; **40**: 1219–26.
55. Telmer S, Christiansen JS, Andersen AR, Nerup J, Deckert T. Smoking habits and prevalence of clinical microangiopathy in insulin-dependent diabetics. *Acta Med* 1984; **215**: 63–8.
56. Norden G, Nyberg G. Smoking and diabetic nephropathy. *Acta Med Scand* 1984; **215**: 257–61.
57. Mühlhauser I. Smoking and diabetes. *Diabet Med* 1990; **7**: 10–15.
58. Olivarius ND, Andreasen AH, Keiding N, Mogensen CE. Epidemiology of renal involvement in newly-diagnosed middle-aged and elderly diabetic patients. Cross-sectional data from the population-based study, Diabetes Care in General Practice, Denmark. *Diabetologia* 1993; **36**: 1007–16.
59. Chase HP, Garg SK, Marshall G et al. Cigarette smoking increases the risk of albuminuria among subjects with type 1 diabetes. *J Ann Med Assoc* 1991; **265**: 614–61.
60. Sawicki PT, Didjurgeit U, Mühlhauser I et al. Smoking is associated with progression of diabetic nephropathy. *Diabet Care* 1994; **17**: 126–31.
61. Klein R, Klein BEK, Moss SE. Incidence of gross proteinuria in older-onset diabetes. A population-based perspective. *Diabetes* 1993; **42**: 381–9.
62. Moy CS, LaPorte RE, Dorman JS et al. Insulin-dependent diabetes mellitus mortality. The risk of cigarette smoking. *Circulation* 1990; **82**: 37–43.
63. Morrish NJ, Stevens LK, Head J et al. A prospective study of mortality among middle-aged diabetic patients (the London cohort of the WHO multinational study of vascular disease in diabetics) II: associated risk factors. *Diabetologia* 1990; **33**: 542–8.

64. Borch-Johnsen K, Nissen H, Henriksen E et al. The natural history of insulin-dependent diabetes mellitus in Denmark. 1. Long-term survival with and without late diabetic complications. *Diabet Med* 1987; **4**: 201–10.
65. Stegmayr BG. A study of patients with diabetes mellitus (type 1) and end-stage renal failure: tobacco usage may increase risk of nephropathy and death. *J Interm Med* 1990; **228**: 121–4.
66. Remuzzi G, Bertani T. Is glomerulosclerosis a consequence of altered glomerular permeability to macromolecules. *Kidney Int* 1990; **38**: 384–94.
67. Rossing P, Hommel E, Smidt UM, Parving HH. Impact of arterial blood pressure and albuminuria on the progression of diabetic nephropathy in IDDM patients. *Diabetes* 1993; **42**: 715.
68. Jakobsen P, Rossing K, Tarnow L et al. Progression of diabetic nephropathy in normotensive type 1 diabetic patients. *Kidney Int* 1999; **56**: 101–5.
70. Rossing P, Hommel E, Smidt UM, Parving HH. Reduction of albuminuria predicts a beneficial effect on diminishing the progression of human diabetic nephropathy during antihypertensive treatment. *Diabetologia* 1994; **37**: 511–16.

3

Pathogenesis of Diabetic Nephropathy: Biochemical and Functional Alterations of Glomerular Basement Membrane and Mesangium

BENITO A. YARD, NICOLE F. VAN DET AND
FOKKO J. VAN DER WOUDE
Klinikum Mannheim, University of Heidelberg, Mannheim, Germany

INTRODUCTION

Changes in the composition of the mesangium and the glomerular basement membrane (GBM) in diabetic nephropathy are thought to be responsible, at least in part, for the functional changes observed. Although these functional changes are discussed more extensively in Chapters 2 and 6, the current clinical classification of nephropathy (1) will be briefly recapitulated first in order to be able to put the biochemical and morphological alterations in context.

The classification of nephropathy into several distinct phases can be used in IDDM and NIDDM. Initial changes include glomerular hyperfiltration and hyperperfusion. A silent phase follows hyperfiltration. It has been documented that, at least in IDDM patients, there are already subtle morphological changes present during this phase, such as thickening of the glomerular basement membrane, glomerular hypertrophy, mesangial expansion and

Diabetic Nephropathy. Edited by C. Hasslacher.
© 2001 John Wiley & Sons, Ltd.

modest expansion of the tubulointerstitium (1,2). This phase is followed by a phase known as microalbuminuria, or incipient diabetic nephropathy, defined as a urinary albumin excretion rate of 20–200 μg/min (3). Micro-albuminuria is predictive of the development of overt proteinuria, particularly in IDDM. Although in these patients the stage of microalbuminuria is clinically well defined, the glomerular lesions leading to microalbuminuria are not well defined. Basement membrane thickness, as well as the volume fraction of mesangium/glomerulus, are increased as compared to IDDM patients with normoalbuminuria (4,5). For microalbuminuric patients with NIDDM, the morphological pattern is more heterogeneous, suggesting a more complex pathogenesis than in IDDM (6). After the phase of micro-albuminuria, urinary protein excretion increases with declining glomerular filtration rate. This phase is known as overt nephropathy or macroprotei-nuria. It is clear that a decreased surface of the peripheral capillary wall is causally related to declining glomerular filtration. It has been claimed that an increased mesangial volume fraction, caused by mesangial expansion, correlates best with overt nephropathy (7). However, the morphological substrate for declining renal function is probably more complex: the loss of function is seen only when all glomerular structures are markedly abnormal, including an increase of mesangial volume fraction [summarized in (2)].

Although most studies have focused on the glomerular mesangial expansion and GBM thickening, abnormalities in the glomerular cells must play a role in extracellular matrix pathology. Glomerular visceral epithelial cells (podocytes) produce the external part of the GBM and the filtration slits between podocyte foot processes are thought to be important as a barrier for albumin excretion, but there is a relative paucity of data about the role of podocytes in diabetes. It has been reported that the width of the filtration slits decreases with increasing albumin excretion (8). Moreover, concomitant podocyte loss and progression of nephropathy has been described in Pima Indians with NIDDM (9). In addition, a decreased staining for α3 β1 integrin staining at the basal plasma membrane of podocytes has recently been described in short-and long-term diabetic rats (10). Since data on podocytes are still scarce at this time, this chapter will focus on the bio-chemical abnormalities of the extracellular matrix (ECM) in GBM and mesangial matrix that have been described thus far.

As mentioned above, the major pathological changes in diabetic nephrop-athy are thickening of the GBM and mesangial matrix expansion. The glomerular capillary wall is formed by the glomerular visceral epithelial cells (GVEC) facing the urinary space, which cover the capillary loops with long finger-like extensions. The GBM is situated between the endothelial cells and the GVEC. The GBM represents the size and charge-selective barrier of the glomerulus. It is composed of a backbone of type IV collagen (α3, α4) which makes up the lamina densa, flanked on either side by layers with different composition, the lamina rara interna and externa. The lamina rara externa contains heparan sulphate proteoglycan (HSPG) and attachment proteins such as laminin, entactin and other glycoproteins. The structure and composition of the GBM is of importance for its function as a filtration barrier in the glomerulus. Mesangial cells (MC) are embedded in an ECM between the capillaries and play a critical role in the modulation of glomerular blood flow and filtration by contraction and relaxation. The mesangial matrix, although developmentally and morphologically distinct from the GBM, is composed of essentially the same components, i.e. collagen type IV (α1, α2), laminin and HSPG. Furthermore, MC have been found to produce fibronectin, entactin, collagen V and VI. Since in diabetic nephropathy most data have been reported on abnormalities in glomerular collagen type IV, laminin, fibronectin and HSPG content, these compounds will now be discussed.

COLLAGEN TYPE IV

Collagen was one of the first known constituents of the extracellular matrix; collagen type IV provides a scaffold for other ECM components, due to its network-like structure. Klein et al (11) reported that diabetic glomeruli had greater hydroxyproline content than non-diabetic glomeruli when content was expressed per glomerulus (21.9 $\pm$ 3.3 ng vs. 7.1 $\pm$ 0.5 ng) and when expressed per μg dry weight of glomeruli (44.0 $\pm$ 2.4 μg vs. 31.6 $\pm$ 1.9 μg). Glomeruli from diabetics of longest duration show the greatest increases in mass and hydroxyproline values. A pathologist's semiquantitative estimation of diffuse glomerulosclerosis revealed a high correlation between hydroxyproline values and histologic determination of the extent of the renal lesion. After the identification of the different types of collagen type IV chains, it became clear that there is a distinct distribution of the various chains in normal and diabetic GBM and mesangial matrix. The first study addressing this issue was reported by Kim et al (12). They showed that during the course of the disease, the distribution of α3(IV) segregated from that of α1(IV). In diabetic kidneys, antibodies to α3(IV) reacted intensely with the thickened GBM but not with the mesangium. In contrast, the reactivity of antibodies to various components of α1(IV) was prominent within the expanded mesangial matrix, with significant decrease in reactivity in the peripheral capillary wall. These findings have been confirmed in IDDM (13) as well as NIDDM (14) and suggest that there might be different sites of synthesis [α1 (IV) collagen from endothelial/mesangial cells and alpha 3(IV) chains from GVEC], independent control mechanisms and/or differences in degradation. An increase of type IV collagen has also been described in glomeruli of streptozotocin-treated C57BL/SJL mice, which develop histological lesions closely resembling human diabetic glomerulo-sclerosis (15). There were no glomerular lesions in diabetic mice transgenic for a growth hormone analogue that competes with native GH and results in dwarfism. Enhanced synthesis of collagen in non-renal tissues from IDDM patients with nephropathy has also been suggested (16,17). Trevisan et al (16) studied overall collagen metabolism and total protein synthesis in either normal (5 mM) or high (25 mM) glucose concentrations from 14 insulin-dependent diabetic (IDDM) patients with nephropathy, 14 IDDM patients without nephropathy and 14 healthy subjects. In high glucose concentrations (25 mM), overall collagen synthesis (measured as [3H]proline incorporation into extracellular and intracellular collagenase-sensitive material) was significantly greater in the patients with nephropathy than in the patients without nephropathy or in healthy control subjects. These findings were confirmed in an *in vivo* study (17) in which skin basement membrane from IDDM patients with and without nephropathy was studied immunohistologically. Increased staining was found for collagen type I and advanced glycosylation end products in patients with diabetic nephropathy. The skeletal muscle capillary basement membranes of IDDM patients with diabetic nephropathy were also shown to have an increased collagen type IV content (18).

Since the increased collagen content of various tissues in diabetic nephropathy in diabetic nephropathy is so well established, many investigators have sought to find a clue to pathogenesis by studying collagen synthesis and turnover. A Danish group looked at the genetic variation of a collagen IV α1-chain polymorphism in IDDM patients and found no association to nephropathy (19). Attempts to study the interaction between high glucose concentrations and collagen synthesis have been more successful: mesangial cells growing in high glucose concentrations produce more collagen types I and IV, and also more transforming growth factor-beta (TGF-β). It is now believed that TGF-β, a known prosclerotic cytokine, mediates the stimulation of ECM production in mesangial cells by high glucose in an autocrine fashion. Addition of neutralizing anti-TGF-β antibody, but not normal rabbit IgG, significantly reduced the high glucose-stimulated incorporation of 3[H]proline in mesangial cells (20). Denaturing SDS–PAGE revealed that mainly collagen types I and IV were stimulated by high (450 mg/dl) D-glucose. This high glucose-mediated increase in collagen synthesis, as well as increased levels of mRNA encoding α2(I) and α1(IV), could be reduced with anti-TGF-β antibody. Decreased mesangial cell growth and increased collagen gene expression can be induced not only by high glucose concentrations but also by increased concentrations of glycated proteins. Amadori glucose adducts in glycated albumin inhibited mesangial cell [3H]-thymidine incorporation; this effect could be inhibited with a monoclonal antibody against Amadori adducts (21, 22). Glycated serum stimulated type IV collagen gene expression and increased type IV collagen secretion, an effect also prevented by monoclonal antibodies directed against Amadori adducts. Similar results have been obtained with cultured rat glomerular endothelial cells (23). Very interesting experiments have been done in mice to study the effects of advanced glycation end-products (AGEs) *in vivo* (24). Normal mice received AGE-modified mouse serum albumin i.p. for 4 weeks, and glomerular extracellular matrix, growth factor mRNA levels and morphology were examined. AGE was found to induce an increase in $\alpha1(IV)$ collagen, laminin B1 and TGF-β mRNA levels, as well as glomerular hypertrophy. Co-administration of an AGE inhibitor, aminoguanidine, reduced all these changes. Another factor that could play a role in the increased glomerular collagen type IV content in diabetic nephropathy is insulin-like growth factor-1 (IGF-1), IGF-1 increases in the kidney early in diabetes. IGF-1 stimulates the production of laminin, fibronectin and type IV collagen in rat mesangial cells (25). This is compatible with the observation that in mice with dwarfism diabetes mellitus does not result in upregulation of glomerular type IV collagen (15). The increased glomerular type IV collagen content in diabetic nephropathy may not only be caused by increased production, but also by less degradation. It has been shown that nonenzymatic glycation of type IV collagen decreases its susceptibility to be degraded by the matrix metalloproteinases stromelysin 1 (MMP3) and gelatinase B (MMP-9) (26). Moreover, it has been shown that, in the glomeruli of patients with diabetic nephropathy, the expression of MMP-3 mRNA and tissue inhibitor of metalloproteinase (TIMP)-1 inversely correlates with mesangial expansion (27). The details of collagen degradation in diabetic nephropathy have not been extensively studied but already, on the basis of these exciting first results, it is likely that this largely unexplored field might be of great relevance to the observed thickening of GBM and mesangial matrix expansion in diabetic nephropathy.

The morphological and functional manifestations of diabetic nephropathy in the rat can be treated with glycosaminoglycan formulations (28). This can only be explained by an altered balance between collagen type IV synthesis and degradation. It was shown that, using human and murine mesangial cells, heparin could reverse a shift in the balance between $\alpha 1(IV)$, MMP-2 and TIMP-2 induced by high glucose concentrations. This reversal was mostly due to the downregulation of type IV collagen expression, rather than further increase of potential proteolysis (29). In diabetic rats it could convincingly be shown that heparin treatment reduced glomerular cell $\alpha 1 (IV)$ collagen transcript levels, mainly in mesangial cells (30).

LAMININ AND FIBRONECTIN

A medline search shows that there are 63 papers on laminin and 74 papers on fibronectin in diabetic nephropathy. The main message of most papers is that laminin and fibronectin staining in the mesangial matrix and the GBM is increased in diabetic nephropathy (e.g. 31,32). Serum laminin, fibronectin and collagen type IV, and urinary excretion of these components, have been measured to see if these parameters could be used as early markers in diabetic nephropathy (33,34). These results provide evidence that: (a) laminin concentration is increased in chronic hyperglycaemia; (b) laminin may be a marker of microangiopathic lesions; and (c) elevated laminin levels may reflect an increased synthesis and/or defective incorporation into the capillary basement membrane. The increased presence of fibronectin is thought to result from autocrine stimulation by TGF-β of mesangial cells (35) and podocytes (36). In the mesangial cells, glycated albumin stimulates TGF-β release, while in the podocytes, glucose is effective in this regard.

HEPARAN SULPHATE PROTEOGLYCANS (HSPG)

Since HSPGs are likely to play a special role in the pathogenesis of diabetic nephropathy, some hallmarks of their structure and function will be discussed here briefly. Since a complete overview is beyond the scope of this chapter, the reader is referred to (37) to learn more about classification, nomenclature, structure and function. HSPG consist of a central core protein to which heparan sulphate (HS) and glycosaminoglycan (GAG) side chains are linked by a trisaccharide. The HS–GAG side chains are constituted of repeating disaccharides. The disaccharides are the most complex of the GAGs [i.e. chondroitin sulphate (CS), dermatan sulphate (DS) or hyaluronic acid (HA)] and consist of two types of uronic acid, L-iduronic acid and D-glucuronic acid and glucosamine (Figure 3.1). Segments of one of several disaccharides, containing one type of uronic acid, are interrupted by segments containing the other. Sulphate groups are covalently bound within the HS molecule. Heparan sulphate and heparin may vary with respect to chain size, sulphation (HS contains fewer N-and O-sulphate groups and more acetyl groups than heparin) and their location. The heterogeneity in terms of dissacharide composition and sulphation in the GAGs plays an important role in the specific biological functions that these compounds play.

Reports regarding decreased expression of GAGs in diabetes appeared in the literature in the early 1980s. The possible abnormalities in GAG synthesis have been investigated for the following reasons:

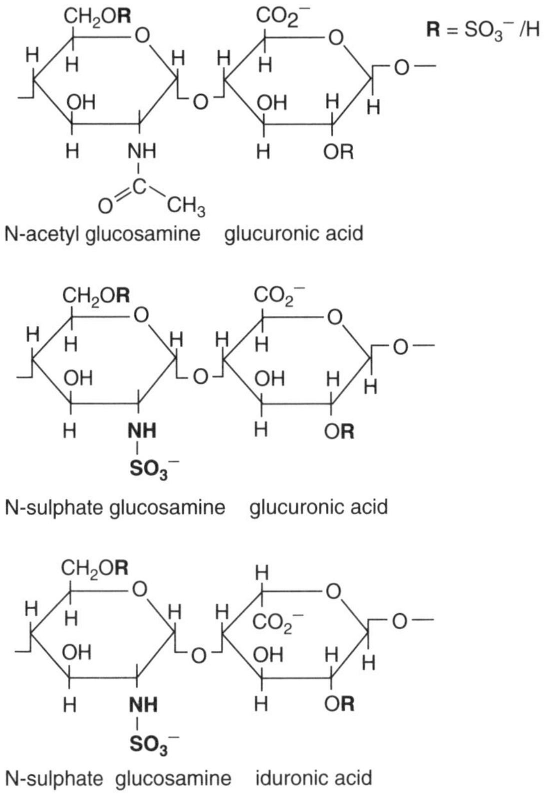

Figure 3.1 The different disaccharides in heparan sulphate

1. Albuminuria appears in DN.
2. This phenomenon implies abnormal GBM permeability.
3. GAGs, particularly HS, have an important role in determining GBM permeability.

A decreased ^{35}S-sulphate incorporation into glomerular basement membranes was found by several groups (38,39). Kanwar et al (40) reported decreased *de novo* synthesis of glomerular proteoglycans in diabetic rats, and Rohrbach et al (41,42) found changes in, and reduced synthesis of, basement membrane HSPG in diabetic mice. Parathasarathy and Spiro (43) obtained kidneys of patients with diabetes at autopsies. Histological hallmarks of glomerulopathy were present in these specimens. They observed, using biochemical techniques, that the GBM of patients with DN contained fewer GAGs than kidneys of non-diabetic controls. A few years later, their early report was confirmed (44). Deckert and co-workers put forward an hypothesis in which altered HSPG metabolism due to hyperglycaemia plays a pivotal role in the pathogenesis of diabetic nephropathy (45). A genetic heterogeneity for a key-enzyme in HS modification, i.e. N-deacetylase/N-sulphotransferase (DAST), would result in an increased vulnerability to high glucose levels in a subset of patients. This would lead to an undersulphation of HS. Resultant loss or reduced synthesis of HSPG in the GBM could provide a molecular basis for albuminuria, an early sign of diabetic nephropathy (45–47). To date, two cDNAs encoded by an 8 kb and 4 kb transcript, designated as DAST-1 and -2, respectively, have been identified (48,49). These two enzymes exhibit alternate specificities that lead to varying extents of N-sulphation. Whereas DAST-1 generates approximately 40% N-sulphation of HS, DAST-2 produces approximately 80% N-sulphation of HS (50). Glomerular N-deacetylase activity is inhibited in diabetic rats, as has been described by Koefoed-Enevoldsen (51), and thus may play an important pathogenic role in DN. It does not, however, explain why only approximately 30% of diabetic patients develop DN. Thus far, no polymorphism in the DAST gene loci has been reported. Decreased mesangial HSPG, with the resulting lack of inhibition of extracellular matrix production and of cellular proliferation, could contribute to mesangial expansion, a hallmark of nephropathy with prognostic value (52). Furthermore, regarding albuminuria as a marker for generalized vascular damage, changes of HS could be involved in altered lipoprotein lipase (LPL)-mediated lipid metabolism. Therefore, changes in HSPG metabolism induced by hyperglycaemia could be of pathogenic relevance in the development of both glomerulosclerosis and arteriosclerosis, a frequently observed combination in patients with DN. In fact, generalized loss of HSPG may also lead to an increase in vascular smooth muscle cell proliferation in the vessel and may result in arteriosclerosis. Recent studies have further explored HSPG expression in human diabetic glomerulopathy. HS and HSPG were found to be decreased (13,53,54) in patients with overt diabetic nephropathy, using newly developed monoclonal antibodies with reactivity to HS and HSPG core proteins (53). A decreased expression of GBM–HS without changes in HSPG core protein staining was found, suggesting a vulnerability in the metabolism of the negatively charged side chain of HSPG in DN. Now that it has become evident that agrin, but not perlecan, is the major HSPG present in the GBM (55), these studies have to be re-evaluated to exclude an altered expression of agrin in DN. The expression of agrin in DN has not been studied so far. Vernier et al (56) described a correlation between GBM HSPG expression and mesangial expansion, using electron microscopy morphometry and histological staining techniques. Thus, recent studies confirmed and visualized the results from the Parathasarathy and Spiro Study (43). Furthermore, they suggest that especially a decrease or alteration of HSPG GAG side chains may be of relevance in the pathogenesis of DN. Similar changes in HSPG content in the intima of the aortas of patients with diabetes mellitus have been observed (57), suggesting that the abnormalities in HSPG metabolism are not entirely restricted to the kidney.

Renal cell cultures have been used to further analyse the effect of the diabetic milieu on HS. Proteoglycan production can be studied *in vitro* using mesangial cells (58–60) and visceral epithelial cell cultures (61,62). Using an enzyme immunoassay with a specific anti-serum recognizing the core of HSPG, Olgemoller et al (63) described a decreased production of HSPG in porcine mesangial cells exposed to glucose concentrations of up to 40 mmol/l. It should be noted that such high glucose concentrations are only rarely encountered in diabetic patients. Silbiger et al (64) observed a reduction in proteoglycan charge when rat mesangial cells were grown on a non-enzymatically glycated mesangial matrix or when the cells were continuously exposed to high glucose levels for 8 weeks without passage. Moran et al (65) reported that glucose and-IGF-1 resulted in a decreased mesangial HS production. We recently combined chemical studies using ^{35}S and [^{3}H]glucosamine incorporation and column fractionation with immunochemical studies using newly developed monoclonal antibodies (66). HS proteoglycan and dermatan sulphate proteoglycan were detected in both the culture medium and the cell layer of mesangial cells. Glomerular visceral epithelial cell culture medium contained HSPG and a second proteoglycan with properties of a hybrid molecule, which contained HS and chondroitin sulphate. The cell layer contained HSPG and chondroitin sulphate proteoglycan. Detailed analysis of the hybrid molecule revealed that it has an apparent molecular mass of 400 kDa. Sodium dodecyl sulphate–polyacrylamide gel electrophoresis of the hybrid molecules, after treatment with heparitinase and chondroitinase ABC, yielded a core protein of 80 kDa. Using 1.8% polyacrylamide–0.6% agarose gel electrophoresis, we deduced that HS and chondroitin sulphate were independently attached to one core protein. We also studied the produced proteoglycans with the same monoclonal antibodies that had been used to perform immunofluorescence on diabetic kidneys (67). Anti-rat GBM HSPG monoclonal antibody (JM403) and polyclonal antihuman GBM HSPG (both antibodies were known to react with the large basement membrane HSPG, Perlecan) reacted strongly with HSPG obtained from both the mesangial cells and the glomerular visceral epithelial cells. However, the hybrid molecule did not react with these antibodies, a feature which suggest that both the HS side chains and the core protein were different from GBM HSPG. We then went on to investigate the effects of high-glucose conditions on the synthesis of HSPG by glomerular visceral epithelial cells *in vitro* (67). Human adult mesangial and glomerular visceral epithelial cells were cultured under normal (5 mM) and high-glucose (25 mM) conditions. Immunofluorescence performed on cells cultured in 25 mM glucose gave similar results, as compared with diabetic kidneys: an unaltered staining for HSPG core protein and a decreased staining for HS–GAG. Using metabolic labelling, we observed an altered proteoglycan production under high-glucose conditions, with predominantly a decrease in HS as compared with dermatan or chondoitin sulphate proteoglycan, N-sulphation analysis of HSPG produced under high-glucose conditions revealed fewer di- and tetrasaccharides as compared with larger oligosaccharides, indicating an altered sulphation pattern. Furthermore, with quantification of HSPG by enzyme-linked immunosorbent assay, a significant decrease was observed when mesangial and visceral epithelial cells were cultured under high-glucose conditions.

Mesangial expansion is the main morphological parameter related to renal function deterioration and proteinuria in diabetic nephropathy (68). Since angiotensin-converting enzyme inhibitors are known to slow the progression of diabetic nephropathy (69), and since HSPGs are thought to play a pivotal role in diabetic nephropathy, we approached the question of whether angiotensin II (ANG II) is an important mediator for mesangial HSPG production. Since ANG II was also known to stimulate extracellular matrix production through TGF-β production in rat mesangial cells (70), we also studied the role of TGF-β in this regard (71).

Metabolic labelling studies revealed that ANG II induced a decrease of HSPG synthesis, with decreases in N-sulphation of the GAG side chains. Enzyme-linked immunosorbent assay measurements with the HS-specific monoclonal antibody JM403 confirmed that ANG II decreased HS production. ANG II increased TGF-β production in a dose-dependent fashion. Specific mRNA for perlecan HSPG decreased, while mRNA for TGF-β increased after incubation with ANG II. Blockade of the subtype 1 ANG II receptor (ATRI) reversed both the effects of ANG II on HSPG and TGF-β production. Coincubation of the mesangial cells with neutralizing antibodies against TGF-β significantly reduced the production of HS as compared with controls and ANG II. These results indicate that the decrease in HS synthesis induced by ANG II is not mediated by an increase in TGF-β but, on the contrary, the increase in TGF-β partially counteracts the inhibition of HS production by ANG II. We could not demonstrate the presence of ATR1 or ATR2 in cultured visceral epithelial cells.

The Modulating Effects of HSPG on Intraglomerular Growth Factors

Overproduction and accumulation of extracellular matrix proteins, and induced proliferation within the glomerular mesangium, the glomerular basement membranes or the renal interstitium, are prominent features of almost all progressive renal diseases. Especially in diabetic nephropathy, the excessive accumulation of both basement membrane and mesangial matrix, as well as an increase in cell number, are very prominent features. Here we focus on the role of the three growth factors in glomerular matrix accumulation: ANG II, TGF-β and bFGF.

Angiotensin II

Heparin can lower the systemic blood pressure in spontaneously hypertensive and Goldblatt-hypertensive rats, and it is believed that the antihypertensive effects of heparin may be mediated by two interconnected mechanisms: (a) endothelial cell-mediated vasodilatation, and (b) blunted vascular smooth muscle cell contractility (72). Heparin suppresses ANG II-stimulated intracellular calcium mobilization in vascular smooth muscle cells (73) and thereby probably leads to vascular relaxation. It is conceivable that locally produced HSPG may have a similar effect on mesangial cells, thereby modulating the contractile response of mesangial cells after ANG II stimulation in an autocrine fashion. Although aldosterone and catecholamine levels are suppressed during the blood pressure rise observed in diabetic renal disease (74), an increase in glomerular expression of angiotensin-converting enzyme has been described in diabetic rats (75). Also, one could speculate that the decrease in glomerular and vascular HSPG observed in diabetic nephropathy makes an individual more susceptible to the haemodynamic effects of ANG II. In line with our *in vitro* findings that ANG II inhibits HSPG synthesis by mesangial cells are *in vivo* data showing that enalapril improves albuminuria by preventing glomerular loss of HS in diabetic rats (76).

Transforming Growth Factor beta (TGF-β)

Although not always consistent, *in vitro* studies have shown that TGF-β plays a role in the regulation and accumulation of some matrix components (77–80). In fact, several investigators have shown that effects of other stimuli, such as high glucose or ANG II, are mediated through an induction of TGF-β (81–84). In order to study the functional aspects of TGF-β in the kidney, Isaka et al (84) transfected normal rat glomeruli *in vivo* with cDNA for TGF-β. As compared with the contralateral, non-transfected kidney, the transfected glomeruli developed hypercellularity and expansion of the ECM. We found that ANG II inhibits HSPG production but at the same time stimulates TGF-β synthesis. TGF-β stimulates HSPG synthesis by mesangial cells. Ceol et al (85) recently found that heparin can inhibit the increase in TGF-β production induced by high glucose concentrations in rat mesangial cell cultures. Again, it is possible that HSPG present in the glomerular extracellular matrix regulates the local production of TGF-β: as far as we know, this possibility has not yet been studied.

Basic Fibroblast Growth Factor (bFGF)

bFGF was found to be a potent mitogen for both mesangial cells (86) and glomerular visceral epithelial cells (87). *In vivo* experiments have suggested that bFGF might also play a role in induction of matrix expansion, but these data are limited. For example, increase expression of bFGF was found in the thy-1.1 model of immune system-mediated mesangial proliferative nephritis, where mesangial expansion is preceded by a phase of active mesangial cell proliferation. In addition, in experimentally induced diabetic nephropathy, changes of mesangial expansion were preceded by increased expression of bFGF (88). We studied *in vitro* the effect of the interaction between glomerular heparan sulphate and bFGF on human mesangial cell proliferation and matrix production. By both reverse-transcriptase polymerase chain reaction and fluorescence-activated cell sorter analysis, expression of the bFGF receptor 1 on mesangial cells was found. Using [^{3}H]thymidine incorporation as a readout, we found that bFGF induced a two- to four-fold increase in mesangial cell proliferation. Biosynthetic labelling followed by immunoprecipitation showed that bFGF enhanced matrix synthesis of fibronectin, laminin B1 and collagen type IV. Heparin, HSPG isolated from human glomeruli, and Perecan isolated from glomerular visceral epithelial cell culture medium inhibited the mitogenic effect of bFGF on mesangial cells. So, HSPG molecules, locally present in the extracellular matrix, modulate the stimulatory effect of bFGF. bFGF can only deliver its signal after interaction with cell surface HSPG (89,90). Therefore, Perlecan normally may compete with cell surface-bound HSPG. This may be of pathogenic importance in renal diseases in which reduced levels of HSPG coincide with mesangial expansion.

Which Roles Do HSPGs Play in Diabetic Nephropathy?

Hyperglycaemia has a direct effect on HSPG metabolism; the production is inhibited, as is the sulphation of the GAG side chains (see Figure 3.2). The mechanisms underlying this phenomenon have not yet been characterized; convincing data showing that the susceptibility to develop diabetic nephropathy is associated with an altered HSPG synthesis (e.g. caused by genetic variants of DAST) have not yet been reported. In podocytes hyperglycaemia leads to decreased HSPG production, which may at least partially explain the albuminuria in diabetic nephropathy. The decrease in HSPG may also

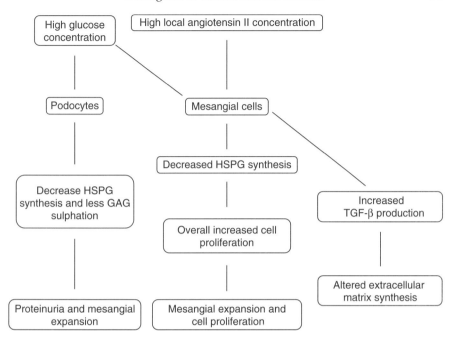

Figure 3.2 Synopsis of the possible pivotal role of HSPG in the pathogenesis of the glomerular alteration in diabetic nephropathy. There are insufficient data on glomerular endothelial cells in this respect and these cells are therefore not depicted in this diagram

contribute substantially to the TGF-β production induced by high glucose concentrations. Hyperglycaemia and an increased local ANG II production may both contribute to mesangial expansion and sclerosis. The fact that bFGF also stimulates mesangial cell proliferation is not an argument against this hypothesis, since the absolute number of mesangial cells in diabetic nephropathy has been shown to be increased (91). This mesangial expansion leads directly to loss of renal function in diabetic nephropathy.

CONCLUSIONS AND FUTURE DEVELOPMENTS

The evidence that HSPG is of relevance in diabetic nephropathy has been accumulating over the last 10 years. It is not unlikely that the decreased HSPG content in the glomeruli and in the vessel walls of

Continues

Continued

patients with diabetic nephropathy plays a pivotal role in both diabetic nephropathy and macroangiopathy (mesangial cells and vascular smooth muscle cells can be regarded as phenotypically related), leading to mesangial and smooth muscle cell perturbations, an altered permeability of glomerular and vessel walls and a disturbance of the physiological modulatory influence of HSPGs on growth factors such as ANG II, TGF-β and bFGF.

The logical consequence of this line of thought is to treat experimental animals and humans with diabetic nephropathy with heparinoids. Both experimental animal studies (92) and preliminary clinical trials (93,94) have been published, showing favourable effects of HSPG or heparin preparations. Further studies with newer, better-defined compounds are necessary to enable us to attain a better understanding of the mode of action to document and reduce possible side-effects.

REFERENCES

1. Cooper ME. Pathogenesis, prevention, and treatment of diabetic nephropathy. *Lancet* 1998; **352**: 213–19.
2. Parving HH, Österby R, Anderson PW, Hsueh WA. Diabetic nephropathy. In *The Kidney*, 5th edn, Brenner BM (ed.). Saunders: Philadelphia, PA, 1996; 1864–92.
3. Mogensen CE, Keane WF, Bennet PH et al. Prevention of diabetic renal disease with special reference to microalbuminuria. *Lancet* 1995; **346**: 1080–84.
4. Walker JD, Close CF, Jones SL et al. Glomerular structure in type 1 (insulin-dependent) diabetic patients with normo- and microalbuminuria. *Kidney Int* 1992; **41**: 741–8.
5. Bangstad HJ, Osterby R, Dahl-Jorgensen K et al. Early glomerulopathy is present in young, type 1 (insulin-dependent) diabetic patients with microalbuminuria. *Diabetologia* 1993; **36**: 523–9.
6. Fioretto P, Mauer M, Brocco E et al. Patterns of renal injury in NIDDM patients with macroalbuminuria. *Diabetologia* 1996; **39**: 1569–76.
7. Mauer SM, Steffes MW, Ellis EN. Structural–functional relationships in diabetic nephropathy. *J Clin Invest* 1984; **74**: 1143–55.
8. Osterby R, Bangstad HJ, Hanssen KF. Interrelation of glomerular structure and abnormal albuminuria in IDDM. *J Diabet Complicat* 1992; **6**: 5–7.
9. Pagtalunan ME, Miller PL, Jumping-Eagle S et al. Podocyte loss and progressive glomerular injury in type II diabetes. *J Clin Invest* 1997; **99**: 342–8.
10. Regoli M, Bendayan M. Alterations in the expression of the α3 β1 integrin in certain membrane domains of the glomerular epithelial cells (podocytes) in diabetes mellitus. *Diabetologia* 1997; **40**: 15–22.
11. Klein L, Butcher DL, Sudilovsky O, Kikkawa R, Miller M. Quantification of collagen in renal glomeruli isolated from human nondiabetic and diabetic kidneys. *Diabetes* 1975; **24**: 1057–65.

12. Kim Y, Kleppel MM, Butkowski R et al. Differential expression of basement membrane collagen chains in diabetic nephropathy. *Am J Pathol* 1991; **138**: 413–20.

13. Tamsma JT, van den Born J, Bruijn JA et al. Expression of glomerular extracellular matrix components in human diabetic nephropathy: decrease of heparan sulphate in the glomerular basement membrane. *Diabetologia* 1994; **37**: 313–20.

14. Yagame M, Kim Y, Zhu D et al. Differential distribution of type IV collagen chains in patients with diabetic nephropathy in non-insulin-dependent diabetes mellitus. *Nephron* 1995; **70**: 42–8.

15. Striker GE, Eastman RD, Striker LJ. Diabetic nephropathy: molecular analysis of extracellular matrix and clinical studies update. *Nephrol Dial Transpl* 1996; **11** (5): 58–61.

16. Trevisan R, Yip J, Sarika L, Li LK, Viberti G. Enhanced collagen synthesis in cultured skin fibroblasts from insulin-dependent diabetic patients with nephropathy. *J Am Soc Nephrol* 1997; **8**: 1133–9.

17. Van der Pijl JW, Daha MR, van den Born J et al. Extracellular matrix in human diabetic nephropathy: reduced expression of heparan sulphate in skin basement membrane. *Diabetologia* 1998; **41**: 791–8.

18. Yokoyama H, Hoyer PE, Hansen PM et al. Immunohistochemical quantification of heparan sulphate proteoglycan and collagen type IV in skeletal muscle capillary basement membranes of patients with diabetic nephropathy. *Diabetes* 1997; **46**: 1875–80.

19. Chen JW, Hansen PM, Tarnow L, Hellgren A, Deckert T, Pociot F. Genetic variation of a collagen IV α1-chain gene polymorphism in Danish insulin-dependent diabetes mellitus (IDDM) patients: lack of association to nephropathy and proliferative retinopathy. *Diabet Med* 1997; **14**: 143–7.

20. Ziyadeh FN, Sharma K, Ericksen M, Wolf G. Stimulation of collagen gene expression and protein synthesis in murine mesangial cells by high glucose is mediated by autocrine activation of transforming growth factor-beta. *J Clin Invest* 1994; **93**: 536–42.

21. Cohen MP, Zidyadeh FN. Amadori glucose adducts modulate mesangial cell growth and collagen gene expression. *Kidney Int* 1994; **45**: 475–84.

22. Cohen MP, Hud E, Wu VY, Ziyadeh FN. Albumin modified by Amadori glucose adducts activates mesangial cell type IV collagen gene transcription. *Mol Cell Biochem* 1995; **151**: 61–7.

23. Cohen MP, Wu VY, Cohen JA. Glycated albumin stimulates fibronectin and collagen IV production by glomerular endothelial cells under normoglycemic conditions. *Biochem Biophys Res Commun* 1997; **239**: 91–4.

24. Yang CW, Vlassara H, Peten EP et al. Advanced glycation end products upregulate gene expression found in diabetic glomerular disease. *Proc Natl Acad Sci USA* 1994; **91**: 9436–40.

25. Schreiber BD, Hughes ML, Groggel GC. Insulin-like growth factor-1 stimulates production of mesangial cell matrix components. *Clin Nephrol* 1995; **43**: 368–74.

26. Mott JD, Khalifah RG, Nagase H et al. Non-enzymatic glycation of type IV collagen and matrix metalloproteinase susceptibility. *Kidney Int* 1997; **52**: 1302–12.

27. Suzuki D, Miyazaki M, Jinde K et al. *In situ* hybridization studies of matrix metalloproteinase-3, tissue inhibitor of metalloproteinase-1 and type IV collagen in diabetic nephropathy. *Kidney Int* 1997; **52**: 111–19.

28. Gambaro G, Venturini AP, Noonan DM et al. Treatment with a glycosaminoglycan formulation ameliorates experimental diabetic nephropathy. *Kidney Int* 1994; **46**: 797–806.
29. Caenazzo C, Garbista S, Onisto M et al. Effect of glucose and heparin on mesangial alpha 1(IV) COLL and MMP-2/TIMP-2 mRNA expression. *Nephrol Dial Transplant* 1997; **12**: 443–8.
30. Ceol M, Nerlich A, Baggio B et al. Increased glomerular alpha 1(IV) collagen expression and deposition in long-term diabetic rats is prevented by chronic glycosaminoglycan treatment. *Lab Invest* 1996; **74**: 484–95.
31. Dixon AJ, Burns J, Dunnil MS, McGee JO. Distribution of fibronectin in normal and diseased human kidneys. *J Clin Pathol* 1980; **33**: 1021–8.
32. Nerlich A, Schleicher E. Immunohistochemical localisation of extracellular matrix components in human diabetic glomerular lesions. *Am J Pathol* 1991; **139**: 889–99.
33. Jackle-Meyer I, Szukics B, Neubauer K et al. Extracellular matrix proteins as early markers in diabetic nephropathy. *Eur J Clin Chem Biochem* 1995; **33**: 211–19.
34. Werle E, Diehl E, Hasslacher C. Levels and molecular size distribution of serum laminin in adult type I diabetic patients with and without microangiopathy. *Metabolism* 1998; **47**: 63–9.
35. Ziyadeh FN, Han DC, Cohen JA, Guo J, Cohen MP. Glycated albumin stimulates fibronectin gene expression in glomerular mesangial cells: involvement of the transforming growth factor-beta system. *Kidney Int* 1998; **53**: 631–8.
36. Van Det NF, Verhagen NA, Tamsma JT et al. Regulation of glomerular epithelial cell production of fibronectin and transforming growth factor-beta by high glucose, not by angiotensin II. *Diabetes* 1997; **46**: 834–40.
37. Kjellen L, Lindahl U. Proteoglycans: structures and Interactions. *Ann Rev Biochem* 1991; **60**: 443–75.
38. Cohen MP, Surma ML. 35 S-sulfate incorporation into glomerular basement membrane glycosaminoglycans is decreased in experimental diabetes. *J Lab Clin Med* 1981; **98**: 715–22.
39. Brown DM, Klein DJ, Michael AF, Oegema TR. 35S-glycosaminoglycan and 35S-glycopeptide metabolism by diabetic glomeruli and aorta. *Diabetes* 1995; **31**: 418–25.
40. Kanwar YS, Jabukowski ML, Rosenzweig LJ. Distribution of sulfated glycosaminoglycans in the glomerular basement membrane and mesangial matrix. *Eur J Cell Biol* 1983; **31**: 290–96.
41. Rohrbach DH, Hassel JR, Kleinman HK, Martin GR. Alteration in the basement membrane (heparan sulfate) proteoglycan in diabetic mice. *Diabetes* 1982; **31**: 185–8.
42. Rohrbach DH, Wagner CW, Star VL et al. Reduced synthesis of basement membrane heparan sulfate proteoglycans in streptozotocin-induced diabetic mice. *J Biol Chem* 1983; **258**: 11672–7.
43. Parathasarathy N, Spiro R. Effect of diabetes on the glycosaminoglycan component of the human glomerular basement membrane. *Diabetes* 1982; **8**: 3279–82.
44. Shimomura H, Spiro R. Studies on macromolecular components of human glomerular basement membrane and alterations in diabetes: decreased levels of heparan sulfate proteoglycan and laminin. *Diabetes* 1987; **36**: 374–81.
45. Olson JL. Diabetes Mellitus. In *Pathology of the Kidney*, Heptinstall RH (ed.). Boston: Little, Brown, 1995; 1715–63.

46. Tisher CC, Hostetter TH. Diabetic Nepropathy. In *Renal Pathology*, Tisher CC, Brenner BM (eds). Lippincott: Philadelphia, PA, 1991; 1387–412.

47. Hostetter TH. Diabetic Nephropathy. In *The Kidney*, Brenner BM, Rector FC (eds). WB Saunders: Philadelphia, PA, 1991; 1695–727.

48. Dixon J, Loftus SK, Galdwin AJ et al. Cloning of the human heparan sulfate-N-deacetylase/N-sulfotransferase gene from the Treacher Collins syndrome candidate region at 5q32–q33.1. *Genomics* 1995; **26**: 239–4.

49. Kusche-Gullberg M, Eriksson I, Pikas DS, Kjellen L. Identification and expression of two heparan sulfate glucosamyl N-deacetylase/n-sulfotransferase genes. *J Biol Chem* 1998; **273**: 11902–7.

50. Rosenberg RD. Heparan sulfate proteoglycans of the cardiovascular system. *J Clin Invest* 1997; **99**: 2062–70.

51. Kofoed-Enevoldsen A. Inhibition of glomerular glucosamyl N-deacetylase in diabetic rats. *Kidney Int* 1992; **41**: 1021–8.

52. Mauer SM. Structural–functional correlations of diabetic nephropathy. *Kidney Int* 1994; **45**: 612–22.

53. Van den Born J, van den Heuvel LPWJ, Bakker MAH et al. Monoclonal antibodies against the protein core and glycosaminoglycan side chain of glomerular basement membrane heparan sulfate proteoglycan: characterization and immunohistological application in human tissues. *J Histochem Cytochem* 1994; **42**: 89–102.

54. Van den Born J, van den Heuvel LPWJ, Bakker MAH et al. Distribution of GBM heparan sulfate proteoglycan core protein and side cahins in human glomerular diseases. *Kidney Int* 1993; **43**: 454–63.

55. Groffen AJ, Ruegg MA, Dijkman H et al. Agrin is a major heparn sulfate proteoglycan in the human glomerular basement membrane. *J Histochan Cytochem* 1998; **46**: 1–9.

56. Vernier RL, Steffes MW, Sisson-Ross S, Mauer M. Heparan sulfate proteoglycan in the glomerular basement membrane in type I diabetes mellitus. *Kidney Int* 1992; **41**: 1070–80.

57. Wasty F, Alavi MZ, Moore S. Distribution of glycosaminoglycans in the intima of human aortas: changes in artherosclerosis and diabetes mellitus. *Diabetologia* 1993; **36**: 316–22.

58. Yaoita E, Oguri K, Okayama E. Isolation and characterization of proteoglycans synthesized by cultured mesangial cells. *J Biol Chem* 1990; **265**: 522–31.

59. Groggel GC, Hovingh P, Linker A. Proteoglycan and glycosaminoglycansynthesis by cultured rat mesangial cells. *J Cell Physiol* 1991; **147**: 455–9.

60. Thomas GJ, Mason RM, Davies M. Characterization of proteoglycans synthesized by human adult mesangial cells in cultures. *Biochem J* 1991; **277**: 81–8.

61. Klein DJ, Oegema TR, Fredeen TS et al. Partial characterization of proteoglycans synthesized by human glomerular epithelial cells in culture. *Biochem Biophys* 1990; **277**: 389–401.

62. Stow JL, Soroka CJ, Mackay K, Striker L, Farquhar MG. Basement membrane heparan sulfate proteoglycan is the main proteoglycan synthesized by glomerular epithelial cells in culture. *Am J Pathol* 1989; **135**: 637–46.

63. Olgemoller B, Schwaabe S, Gerbitz KD, Schleicher ED. Elevated glucoses decrease the content of a basement membrane associated heparan sulfate proteoglycan in proliferating porcine mesangial cells. *Diabetologia* 1992; **35**: 183–6.

64. Silbiger S, Schlondorff D, Crowley S et al. The effect of glucose on proteoglycans produced by cultured mesangial cells. *Diabetes* 1993; **42**: 185–2.

65. Moran A, Brown DM, Kim Y, Klein DJ. Effects of IgF-1 and glucose on protein and proteoglycan synthesis by human fetal mesangial cells in culture. *Diabetes* 1992; **40**: 1346–54.
66. van Det NF, van den Born J, Tamsma JT et al. Proteoglycan production by human glomerular visceral epithelial cells and mesangial cells *in vitro. Biochem J* 1995; **307**: 759–68.
67. van Det NF, van den Born J, Tamsma JT et al. Effects of high glucose on the production of heparan sulfate proteoglycan by human mesangial and glomerular visceral epithelial cells *in vitro. Kidney Int* 1996; **49**: 1079–89.
68. Mauer SM, Steffes MW, Ellis EN et al. Structural–functional relationships in diabetic nephropathy. *J Clin Invest* 1984; **74**: 1143–55.
69. Lewis EJ, Hunsicker LG, Bain RP, Rohde RD. The effect of angiotensin-converting enzyme inhibition on diabetic nephropathy. *N Eng J Med* 1993; **329**: 1456–62.
70. Kagami S, Border WA, Miller DE, Noble NA. Angiotensin II stimulates extracellular matrix protein synthesis through induction of transforming growth factor-β expression in rat glomerular mesangial cells. *J Clin Invest* 1994; **93**: 2431–7.
71. van Det NF, Tamsma JT, van den Born J et al. Differential effects of angiotensin II and transforming growth factor-β on the production of heparan sulfate proteoglycans by mesangial cells *in vitro. J Am Soc Nephrol* 1996; **7**: 1015–23.
72. Mandal AK, Lyden TW, Sakalayen MG. Heparin lowers blood pressure: biological and clinical perspectives. *Kidney Int* 1995; **47**: 1017–30.
73. Zaragoza R, Battle-Tracy KM, Owen NE. Heparin inhibits Na^+H^+ exchange in vascular smooth muscle cells. *Am J Physiol* 1990; **258**: C46–53.
74. Feldt-Rasmussen B, Mathiesen ER, Deckert T et al. Central role of sodium in the pathogenesis of blood pressure changes independent of angiotensin, aldosterone and catecholamines in type I (insulin-dependent) diabetes mellitus. *Diabetologia* 1987; **30**: 610–17.
75. Anderson S, Jung FF, Ingelfinger JR. Renal renin–angiotensin system in diabetes: functional, immunochemical and biological correlations. *Am J Physiol* 1993; **265**: F477–86.
76. Reddi A, Ramamurthi R, Miller M, Dhuper S, Lasker N. Enalapril improves albuminuria by preventing glomerular loss of heparan sulfate in diabetic rats. *Biochem Med Metab Biol* 1991; **45**: 119–31.
77. Nakamura T, Miller D, Ruoslathi E, Border WA. Production of extracellular matrix by glomerular epithelial cells is regulated by transforming growth factor-β1. *Kidney Int* 1992; **41**: 1213–21.
78. Humes HD, Nakamura T, Cieslinski DA, Emmons RV, Border WA. Role of proteoglycans and cytoskeleton in the effects of TGF-β on renal proximal tubule cells. *Kidney Int* 1993; **41**: 575–84.
79. Border WA, Okuda S, Languino LR, Ruoslathi E. Transforming growth factor-β regulates production of proteoglycans by mesangial cells. *Kidney Int* 1990; **37**: 689–95.
80. Kagami S, Border WA, Miller DE, Noble NA. Angiotensin II stimulates extracellular matrix protein synthesis through the production of transforming growth factor-β expression in rat glomerular mesangial cells. *J Clin Invest* 1994; **93**: 2431–7.
81. Ziyadeh FN, Sharma K, Ericksen M, Wolf G. Stimulation of collagen gene expression and protein synthesis in murine mesangial cells by high glucose is

mediated by autocrine activation of transforming growth factor-β. *J Clin Invest* 1994; **93**: 536–42.

82. Bollineni JS, Reddi AS. Transforming growth factor-β1 enhances glomerular collagen synthesis in diabetic rats. *Diabetes* 1993; **42**: 1673–7.

83. Kashgarian M, Oshima S, Takeuchi A, Throckmorton D, Rasmussen H. The contribution of mesangial cell collagen synthesis to the pathogenesis of diabetic nephropathy. *Contrib Nephrol Basel Krage* 1994; **107**: 132–9.

84. Isaka M, Akai Y, Fujii Y, Doki Y. Glomerulosclerosis induced by *in vivo* transfection of transforming growth factor beta or platelet-derived growth factor gene into the rat kidney. *J Clin Invest* 1993; **92**: 2597–601.

85. Ceol M, Gambaro G, Sauer U et al. TGFβ1 renal overexpression in long-term diabetic rats and in high glucose mesangial cell cultures: inhibition by heparinoid (abstr). Congress of the European Diabetic Nephropathy Study Group Upsala, Sweden, 1996; 70.

86. Jaffer F, Saunders C, Schultz P et al. Regulation of mesangial cell growth by polypeptide mitogens: inhibitory role of transforming growth factor β. *Am J Pathol* 1989; **135**: 261–9.

87. Takeuchi A, Yoshizywa N, Yamamoto M et al. Basic fibroblast growth factor promotes proliferation of rat glomerular visceral epithelial cells *in vitro*. *Am J Pathol* 1992; **141**: 107–16.

88. Young BA, Johnson RJJ, Alpers CE et al. Cellular events in the evolution of experimental diabetic nephropathy. *Kidney Int* 1995; **47**: 935–44.

89. Maccarana M, Casu B, Lindahl U. Minimal sequence in heparin/heparan sulfate required for binding of basic fibroblast growth factor. *J Biol Chem* 1993; **268**: 23898–905.

90. Turnbull JE, Fernig DG, Ke Y, Wilkinson MC, Gallagher JT. Identification of the basic fibroblast growth factor sequence in fibroblast heparan sulfate. *J Biol Chem* 1992; **267**: 10337–41.

91. Steffes M, Pluth R, Schmidt D, McCrey R. Glomerular and mesangial cell number in insulin dependent diabetes (abstract). Congress of the European Diabetic Study Group Upsala, Sweden, 1996; 27.

92. Gambaro G, Cavazzana AO, Luzi P et al. Glycosaminoglycans prevent morphological renal alterations and albuminuria in diabetic rats. *Kidney Int* 1992; **42**: 285–91.

93. Myrup B, Hansen PM, Jensen T et al. Effect of low dose heparin on urinary albumin excretion in insulin-dependent diabetes mellitus. *Lancet* 1995; **345**: 421–2.

94. Tamsma JT, van der Woude FJ, Lemkes HHPJ. Effects of sulphated glycosaminoglycans on albuminuria in patients with overt type II nephropathy. *Nephrol Dial Transpl* 1996; **11**: 182–5.

4

Pathogenesis of Diabetic Nephropathy: Haemodynamic Alterations

HENK J.G. BILO[1], PIET M. TER WEE[2] AND RIJK O.B. GANS[3]

[1]Department of Internal Medicine, Isala Clinics, Zwolle,[2] University Hospital, Groningen, and [3]Department of Nephrology, Free University Hospital, Amsterdam, The Netherlands

The pathophysiological mechanisms that contribute to the development of diabetic nephropathy have not yet been fully explained. Studies in recent decades based on animal and human populations demonstrate clearly that, aside from biochemical factors, haemodynamic factors play an important role.

ANIMAL STUDIES

Micropuncture studies in rats have disclosed that four factors regulate glomerular ultrafiltration (9). The first determinant of glomerular ultrafiltration is the glomerular blood flow, Q_A. The second determinant is the transcapillary hydrostatic pressure difference (ΔP), which is the difference between the hydrostatic pressure in the glomerular capillary and the hydrostatic pressure in Bowman's space. A third factor is the oncotic pressure (π) in the glomerular capillary, which is opposed by ΔP. The final factor is the ultrafiltration coefficient (K_f) of the glomerular basement membrane. The ongoing ultrafiltration along the glomerular capillary causes π to rise, which

Diabetic Nephropathy. Edited by C. Hasslacher.
© 2001 John Wiley & Sons, Ltd.

opposes Δ P, resulting in a gradual decrease in ultrafiltration (shaded area in Figure 4.1). In rats, π counterbalances Δ P completely before the end of the glomerular capillary loop and so-called "filtration equilibrium" is reached. Whether such a filtration equilibrium is present in man is still a matter of debate. Tucker and Blantz (51) have shown that Q_A is the most important determinant of glomerular ultrafiltration in both filtration equilibrium and filtration disequilibrium states, since increments in Q_A will shift the equilibrium point (dotted line in Figure 4.1).

In rats, a loss of renal mass, as provoked by (subtotal) nephrectomy, induces glomerular hyperfiltration in order to compensate for the decrease in the number of functioning nephrons (3, 30). Such a rise in single nephron glomerular filtration rate (GFR) results from increments in Q_A and Δ P. However, those rats with a loss in renal mass will subsequently develop hypertension, proteinuria and, ultimately, endstage renal failure (11, 25, 27). Additional studies have resolved that the progressive decline in renal function, subsequent to a reduction in renal mass, is primarily induced by the compensatory rise in Δ P (1, 37). Rats with a reduced renal mass treated with an angiotensin I converting enzyme inhibitor manifested a persistently elevated Q_A but a Δ P indistinguishable from control rats. In those rats, the development of proteinuria and the deterioration of renal function was markedly reduced. Likewise, treatment with a low-protein diet prevented the deterioration of renal function of rats with a reduced renal mass

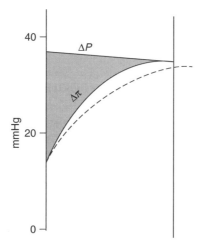

Figure 4.1 Depiction of haemodynamic forces along the length of the glomerular capillary loop. ΔP, hydrostatic pressure difference between the capillary lumen and Bowman's capsule. $\Delta\pi$, change of the oncotic pressure. Note that with ongoing ultrafiltration π increases and counterbalances ΔP

(10, 26, 28). Thus, it was concluded that an elevated Δ P, or in other words glomerular hypertension, is harmful to the glomerulus and should be prevented.

Rats with untreated diabetes mellitus also show glomerular hyperfiltration. Micropuncture studies revealed that this glomerular hyperfiltration was also the resultant of an elevated Q_A and Δ P (24). This was induced by a fall in renal vascular resistance as the result of a decrease in tone of the afferent arteriole (24). These observations suggest a loss of renal autoregulation. Indeed, it has been demonstrated that autoregulation of renal blood flow is impaired (21) and/or even reset to a lower blood pressure range in diabetic rats (17). Utilizing a videomicroscopic technique, it has been demonstrated in isolated perfused hydronephrotic kidneys that afferent arterioles of 4–6 week-old diabetic rat kidneys did not constrict in response to stepwise elevations in renal arterial pressure from 80 to 180 mmHg (Figure 4.2) (22). In 1 week-old diabetic rats, afferent arteriolar responsiveness to increments in renal arterial pressure was markedly attenuated but not completely blunted (Figure 4.2) (46). Altogether, these observations imply that diameters of renal resistance vessels will be larger at a lower blood pressure, resulting in a rise in glomerular blood flow and an unbuf-

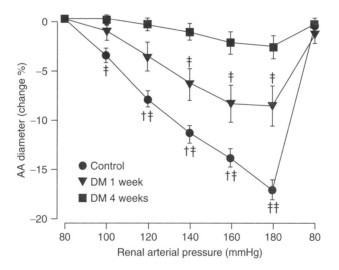

Figure 4.2 Data comparing afferent arteriolar responses to an elevation in renal arterial pressure in kidneys isolated from control rats, 1-week diabetic rats (DM 1 week) and 4–6 week-old diabetic rats (DM 4 weeks). Pressure-induced vasoconstriction was abolished in 4–6 week-old diabetic rats and attenuated in 1 week-old diabetic kidneys. Results are mean ± SE. [†] $3p < 0.05$ control vs. DM 1 week; [‡] $3p < 0.05$ vs. DM 4 weeks

fered transmission of systemic blood pressure to the glomerulus, thus causing glomerular hyperfiltration.

In isolated perfused kidneys of control and diabetic rats, glucose infusion induces a rise in effective renal plasma flow (ERPF) and GFR (29). This effect of glucose may result from a disturbed tubuloglomerular feedback mechanism (6), downregulation of receptors of vasoconstrictors such as angiotensin II (57), enhanced production of vasodilating substances such as prostaglandins (29), impaired contractility of mesangial cells (19) and, finally, enhanced metabolism of glucose via the polyol pathway (57). In the hydronephrotic kidney it has been demonstrated that galactose feeding completely abolishes afferent arteriolar responsiveness to increasing renal arterial pressure, indicating an impaired myogenic responsiveness. This could be prevented by pretreatment with an aldose reductase inhibitor (47). The effects of insulin *per se* on glomerular dynamics have not been elucidated. Tucker et al (52,53) demonstrated in awake 1 and 6 week-old diabetic rats that insulin infusion acutely lowered ERPF and GFR. In contrast, other investigators found vasodilation after the administration of insulin (16). Thus, additional studies are warranted to clarify the exact role of insulin on renal haemodynamics.

A possible explication for the altered renal haemodynamics of the diabetic state could be a modified balance between vasoconstricting and vasodilating agents. On one hand, a reduced synthesis of vasoconstrictors or a decreased susceptibility of diabetic vessels to vasoconstrictors might exist, whereas on the other hand, the synthesis of vasodilating agents could be enhanced. It has been demonstrated that afferent arteriolar responsiveness to angiotensin II had already been diminished after 1 week of diabetes mellitus (46). It is of interest that after 1 day of diabetes the angiotensin II receptor density was found to be already decreased, which was still the case after 4–6 weeks of diabetes (2). Insulin treatment prevented this decline in angiotensin II receptor density. Likewise, downregulation of vasopressin receptors has been documented (57). Craven et al (14) demonstrated glomerular hyperfiltration in 2-week diabetic rats. In these rats the production of vasodilating prostaglandins was enhanced but also that of thromboxane A_2. After 4 weeks of diabetes mellitus glomerular hyperfiltration persisted, which could not be affected by non-steroidal antiinflammatory drugs (15). In these rats the production of vasodilating prostaglandins was reduced to normal levels, whereas the production of thromboxane A_2 was still elevated. These observations indicate that in the early stage of untreated diabetes mellitus glomerular hyperfiltration might (at least partially) originate from an increased production of vasodilating prostaglandins but not at later stages. Furthermore, the persistent hyperfiltration despite an enhanced production of thromboxane A_2 might point to a decreased susceptibility to this agent. Finally, other study results indicate that an increased production of nitric oxide may contribute to (renal) vasodilation early in the course of experimental diabetes mellitus (49).

In summary, in untreated diabetic rats glomerular hyperfiltration originates from glomerular hyperperfusion and glomerular hypertension as the result of predominant afferent vasodilation. The underlying mechanisms have not been fully elucidated, but the diabetic state seems to be associated with a modified balance between vasoconstrictor and vasodilator effects, resulting in net vasodilation.

HUMAN STUDIES

In the initial phase of type 1 DM renal haemodynamic derangements include increases in both GFR and ERPF (32, 42), although quite often GFR shows a larger increase than ERPF, thus leading to an increased filtration fraction (FF). A rise in FF suggests that predominantly afferent vasodilation also plays a role in humans. Both the increase in GFR and the rise in FF are seen as associated with intraglomerular hypertension.

Increased GFR and ERPF levels are most expressly seen in patients with poor metabolic control and improvements in metabolic control are associated with decreases, but not often normalization, of GFR and ERPF. In a subset of patients, however, such glomerular hyperfiltration persists despite optimizing glycaemic control (32, 42). This glomerular hyperfiltration has been proven to be an independent marker for the development of diabetic nephropathy (38). Other studies also demonstrate that a large number of patients with type 2 DM manifest elevated values of GFR and ERPF at the time of diagnosis (55). Like in patients with type 1 DM, a subset of those patients also disclosed persistently elevated values for GFR and ERPF despite an improvement in glycaemic control (56). This observation suggests that glomerular hyperfiltration could be a marker for future development of diabetic nephropathy in patients with type 2 DM too. The degree of hyperfiltration and the course of the GFR in type 2 DM was prospectively evaluated in detail in Pima Indians (34). The results were remarkable (Table 4.1).

It should be emphasized that the rate of fall in the group with overt proteinuria was 0.93 ml/month, a rate comparable to that seen in type 1 DM. Still, despite such evident results in Pima Indians, it is somewhat confusing that hyperfiltration in African-Americans with type 2 DM apparently does not identify patients at risk for deterioration in renal function, even with a follow-up of up to 15 years (13).

Whether the glomerular hyperfiltration in man is or is not the result of glomerular hypertension can only be investigated indirectly, utilizing the determination of albuminuria/proteinuria and by clearance techniques to determine GFR and ERPF. Subsequently, the filtration fraction (FF =

Table 4.1   Baseline GFR and changes after 4 years follow-up in Pima Indians (34)

At baseline:	(n)	Mean GFR (ml/min)	Δ at follow-up (%)
Normal GTT*	31	123	–
Impaired GTT	29	135	+ 14
Newly diagnosed type 2 DM	30	143	+ 18
Overt type 2 DM, over 5 years	70		
Normo- and microalbuminuria		153	Stable
Overt proteinuria		124	– 35

*Glucose tolerance test.

GFR/ERPF) is calculated and frequently used as a surrogate marker for changes in Δ P. The latter may be hazardous, since Carmines et al (12), utilizing a mathematical model, have pointed out that proportional similar decrements in afferent and efferent arteriolar resistance are associated with an increase in renal blood flow and a fall in FF without affecting Δ P. Because the changes in renal haemodynamics of patients with diabetes mellitus include a proportionally similar change in ERPF and GFR, and therefore an unchanged FF, this implies that changes in Δ P (based on predominant afferent vasodilation) and/or changes in the ultrafiltration coefficient of the glomerular membrane must have occurred. An increase in glomerular surface area, possibly enlarging K_f, has been demonstrated in hyperfiltering diabetic subjects (31). The latter cannot completely account for the rise in GFR, however, as optimizing glycaemic control lowered the GFR, whereas the glomerular surface area was not affected. The observation that improvement of glycaemic control results not only in a reduction of glomerular hyperfiltration but also in a decrease in albuminuria might indicate that the renal derangements of hyperfiltering diabetic subjects are at least partially based on a rise in Δ P.

Further indirect support for the assumption that the elevated GFR of hyperfiltering diabetic patients is partially based on a rise in Δ P is provided by studies on so-called renal reserve filtration capacity (7). It has been shown that GFR and ERPF can be acutely affected by the separate or combined administration of low-dose dopamine and amino acids (or a meat meal) (44, 48). Dopamine infusion induces a disproportional rise in ERPF compared to GFR. Consequently, FF falls. This may be explained by dopamine-induced proportional decrements in afferent and efferent arteriolar vasodilation or even a predominantly efferent vasodilation. On the other hand, protein loading by either amino acid infusion or a meat meal induces parallel changes in GFR and ERPF, resulting in an unchanged or slightly elevated FF. These observations are explained by predominantly afferent vasodilation. In normofiltering diabetic subjects, the effect of protein loading on renal haemodynamics did not differ from that of control subjects (5). In contrast, as can be seen in Figure 4.3, hyperfiltering subjects with type 1 DM did not respond to amino acid infusion with a further rise in GFR (45). In normofiltering and hyperfiltering patients with type 1 DM the dopamine-induced rises in GFR and ERPF were similar to those of control subjects (44, 45). Thus, these observations are in accord with the assumption that glomerular hyperfiltration of diabetic subjects is at least partially based on a rise in Δ P, probably resulting from a predominant afferent vasodilation.

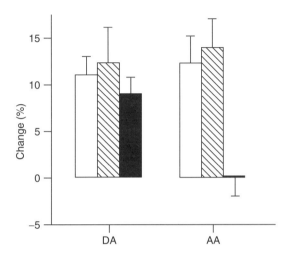

Figure 4.3   Percentage dopamine (DA)-induced and amino acid (AA)-induced changes in GFR of control subjects (open bars), normofiltering IDDM patients (hatched bars) and hyperfiltering IDDM patients (solid bars). Note the lack of AA-induced changes in hyperfiltering IDDM patients

PROPOSED MECHANISMS FOR HYPERFILTRATION IN HUMANS WITH DM

Hormones may play a role in the development (and prevention) of hyperfiltration. Insulin-like growth factor-1 (IGF-1) can give renal vasodilation and a rise in GFR when infused in non-diabetic subjects (23), whereas the administration of octreotide to subjects with type 1 DM partially reverses the early hyperfiltration and increase in renal size (43). However, administration of growth hormone leads to an increase in GFR (41). Glucagon has been implicated as well, and appears to be able to increase GFR (35). The exact mechanisms behind these observations are not clear, despite some interesting hypotheses by the various authors.

A role for prostaglandins is supposed, as already alluded to when discussing the animal models. GFR often decreases when NSAIDs are used by subjects with DM, again suggesting a role for prostaglandins in renal hae-modynamics in diabetes.

Hyperinsulinaemia and hyperglycaemia can stimulate sodium reabsorp-tion, thus contributing to extracellular volume expansion. Some suggest that this rise in extracellular volume may be an additional factor contributing to the rise in GFR (20,54). Whether there is a role for a high insulin level itself as a contributor for hyperfiltration is not clear. Insulin treatment, leading to improved metabolic control, does reverse hyperfiltration. In rats, however, hyperinsulinaemia in a state of euglycaemia induces hyperfiltration (52).

Intracellular accumulation of sorbitol after conversion of intracellular glucose by aldose reductase might also play a role. Chronic administration of an aldose reductase inhibitor lowers GFR to normal in hyperfiltering subjects with type 1 DM (36). Glycosylation products seem to play a role: when non-diabetic rats are infused with early glycosylation products, glom-erular hyperfiltration is the result (39). There are no studies in humans known, however.

Actual blood glucose levels do play a role in the degree of hyperfiltration in humans: when testing even moderately controlled subjects with type 1 DM under near-normoglycaemic circumstances, GFR was only slightly elevated compared to non-diabetic controls (5). Rises in actual glucose levels are associated with a concomitant rise in GFR, thus suggesting a momentary effect, resulting in especially afferent vasodilation (58).

There also is a role for ketone bodies, with a rise in GFR when ketone bodies are present (50). It is suggested that not only the glomerular hyper-filtration but also the lack of renal reserve filtration capacity (RRFC) might play a role in the ultimate damage of the kidney by hyperfiltration (8). This lack in RRFC is especially prominent with hyperglycaemia, and restoration of RRFC is possible when returning to near-normoglycaemia (5). Such information provides a further argument for strict metabolic control.

The role of catecholamines is not clear. Despite an early report of vascular hyporesponsiveness to catecholamines (33), suggesting a decreased ability of the renal vascular system to contract and dilate when necessary, others report an increased responsiveness, even to endogeneous catecholamines, especially in poorly controlled subjects (4).

CONCLUSION

Results from animal studies indicate that in untreated diabetic rats renal autoregulation is impaired, causing predominantly afferent vasodilation. Consequently, systemic pressure is transferred to the

Continues

Continued

glomerular capillary loop, resulting in glomerular hypertension and glomerular hyperfiltration. Results from studies in man are in accord with the assumption that in patients with diabetes mellitus glomerular hyperfiltration is also caused by predominant afferent vasodilation, causing a rise in ΔP and Q_A. Studies in rats with non-diabetic and diabetic renal disease have revealed that, especially, an elevated ΔP, i.e. glomerular hypertension, may contribute to or even initiate glomerular damage, leading to a progressive loss of renal function. Proposed mechanisms for the occurrence of hyperfiltration include hormonal influences, changes in prostaglandin production, actual blood glucose levels and ketone body concentrations, enhanced tubular sodium reabsorption and intracellular sorbitol accumulation.

Treatment strategies for preventing the development of progressive (diabetic) nephropathy should be aimed on eliminating glomerular hypertension. Treatment strategies will be described elsewhere.

REFERENCES

1. Anderson S, Rennke HG, Brenner BM. In arresting progressive renal disease, all anti-hypertensive drugs are not created equal. *Kidney Int* 1986; **29**: 314.
2. Ballerman BJ, Skorecki KL, Brenner BM. Reduced glomerular angiotensin II receptor density in early untreated diabetes mellitus in the rat. *Am J Physiol* 1984; **247**: F110–16.
3. Bank N, Aynedjian HS. Individual nephron function in experimental bilateral nephritis. I. Glomerular filtration rate and proximal tubule sodium, potassium and water reabsorption. *J Lab Clin Med* 1966; **68**: 713–27.
4. Bilo HJG, Gans ROB, Polee MB et al. Catecholamines and blood glucose control in Type 1 diabetes. *Diabet Med* 1991a; **8**: S108–112.
5. Bilo HJG, van Ballegooie E, Hazenberg HJA, Gans ROB, Donker AJM. Renal function and renal function reserve in insulin-dependent diabetic patients during near-normoglycaemia. *Nephron* 1991b; **58**: 295–9.
6. Blantz RC, Peterson OW, Gushwa L, Tucker BJ. Effect of modest hyperglycemia on tubuloglomerular feedback activity. *Kidney Int* 1982; **22**: S206–12.
7. Bosch JP, Saccagi AS, Lauer A et al. Renal functional reserve in humans. *Am J Med* 1983; **75**: 943–9.
8. Bosch JP, Lew S, Glabman S, Lauer A. Renal hemodynamic changes in humans. Response to protein loading in normal and diseased kidneys. *Am J Med* 1986; **81**: 809–15.
9. Brenner BM, Humes HD. Mechanisms of glomerular ultrafiltration. *N Engl J Med* 1977; **297**: 148–54.
10. Brenner BM, Meyer TM, Hostetter TH. Dietary protein intake and the progressive nature of kidney disease. *N Engl J Med* 1982; **307**: 652–9.
11. Brenner BM. Nephron adaptation to renal injury or ablation. *Am J Physiol* 1985; **249**: F324–37.

12. Carmines PK, Perry MD, Hazelrig JB, Navar LG. Effects of preglomerular and postglomerular vascular resistance alterations on filtration fraction. *Kidney Int* 1987; **31** (20): S229–32.
13. Chaiken RL, Eckert-Norton M, Bard M et al. Hyperfiltration in African-American patients with type 2 diabetes. *Diabet Care* 1998; **21**: 2129–34.
14. Craven PA, Caines MA, DeRubertis F. Sequential alterations in glomerular prostaglandin and thromboxane synthesis in diabetic rats: relationship to the hyperfiltration of early diabetes. *Metabolism* 1987; **36**: 95–103.
15. Craven PA, DeRubertis FR. Role for local prostaglandin and thromboxane production in the regulation of glomerular filtration rate in the rat with streptozotocin-induced diabetes. *J Lab Clin Med* 1989; **113**: 674–81.
16. Cohen AJ, McCarthy DM, Stoff JS. Direct hemodynamic effect of insulin in the isolated perfused kidney. *Am J Physiol* 1989; **257**: F580–85.
17. De Micheli AG, Forster H, Duncan RC, Epstein M. A quantitative assessment of renal blood flow autoregulation in experimental diabetes. *Nephron* 68: 245–251.
18. Forster HG, ter Wee PM, Takena, Epstein M. Impairment of afferent arteriolar myogenic responsiveness in the galactose-fed rats. *Proc Soc Exp Biol Med* 1994; **206**: 365–74.
19. Haneda M, Kikkawa R, Koya D et al. Alteration of masangial response to ANP and angiotensin II by glucose. *Kidney Int* 1995; **44**: 518–26.
20. Hannedouche TP, Delgado AG, Gnionsahe DA et al. Renal hemodynamics and segmental tubular reabsorption in early type 1 diabetes. *Kidney Int* 1990; **37**: 1126–33.
21. Hashimoto Y, Wedra T, Yoshimura A, Koshikawa S. Autoregulation of renal blood flow in streptozotocin-induced diabetic rats. *Diabetes* 1989; **38**: 1109–13.
22. Hayashi K, Epstein M, Loutzenhiser R, Forster H. Impaired myogenic responsiveness of the afferent arteriole in streptozotocin-induced diabetic rats: role of eicosanoid derangements. *J Am Soc Nephrol* 1992; **2**: 1578–86.
23. Hirschberg R, Brunori G, Kopple JD, Guler HP. Effects of insulin-like growth factor I on renal function in normal men. *Kidney Int* 1993; **43**: 387–97.
24. Hostetter TH, Troy JL, Brenner BM. Glomerular hemodynamics in experimental diabetes mellitus. *Kidney Int* 1981a; **19**: 410–15.
25. Hostetter TH, Olson JL, Rennke HG, Venkatachalam MA, Brenner BM. Hyperfiltration in remnant nephrons: a potentially adverse response to renal ablation. *Am J Physiol* 1981b; **241**: F85–93.
26. Hostetter TH, Rennke HG, Brenner BM. Compensatory renal hemodynamic injury: a final common pathway of residual nephron destruction. *Am J Kidney Dis* 1982; **1**: 310–14.
27. Hostetter TH. The hyperfiltering glomerulus. *Med Clin N Am* 1985; **68**: 387–98.
28. Hostetter TH, Meyer TW, Rennke HG, Brenner BM. Chronic effects of dietary protein in the rat with intact and reduced renal mass. *Kidney Int* 1986; **30**: 509–17.
29. Kasiske BL, O'Donnell MP, Keane WF. Glucose-induced increases in renal hemodynamic function. Possible modulation by renal prostaglandins. *Diabetes* 1985; **34**: 360–64.
30. Kaufman JM, Sugel NJ, Hayslett JP. Functional and hemodynamic adaptation to progressive renal ablation. *Circ Res* 1975; **36**: 286–93.
31. Kroustrup JP, Gundersen HJG, Osterby R. Glomerular size and structure in diabetes mellitus III. Early enlargement of the capillary surface. *Diabetologia* 1997; **13**: 207–10.

32. Mogensen CE, Andersen MJF. Increased kidney size and glomerular filtration rate in juvenile diabetes: normalization by insulin-treatment. *Diabetologia* 11: 221–4.

33. Nakamura T, Fukui M, Ebihara E et al. mRNA expression of growth factors in glomeruli from diabetic rats. *Diabetes* 1993; **42**: 450–56.

34. Nelson DG, Bennett PH, Beck GJ et al. Development and progression of renal disease in Pima Indians with non-insulin-dependent diabetes mellitus. *N Engl J Med* 1991; **335**: 1636–42.

35. Parving H-H, Sandahl-Christiansen J, Noar J, Tronier B, Mogensen CE. The effect of glucagon infusion on kidney function in short-term insulin-dependent juvenile diabetics. *Diabetologia* 1980; **19**: 350–54.

36. Passariello N, Sepe J, Marazzo G et al. Effect of aldose reductase inhibitor (tolrestat) on urinary albumin excretion rate and glomerular filtration rate in IDDM subjects with nephropathy. *Diabet Care* 1993; **16**: 789–95.

37. Raij L, Chiou XC, Owens R, Wrigley B. Therapeutic implications of enalapril and a combination of hydralazine, reserpine, and hydrochlorothiazide in an experimental model. *Am J Med* 1985; **79** (3C): 37–41.

38. Rudberg S, Persson B, Dahlquist G. Increased glomerular filtration rate as a predictor of diabetic nephropathy—an 8-year prospective study. *Kidney Int* 1992; **41**: 822–8.

39. Sabbatini M, Sansone G, Uccello F et al. Early glycosylation products induce glomerular hyperfiltration in normal rats. *Kidney Int* 1992; **42**: 875–81.

40. Sandahl-Christiansen J, Gammelgaard J, Frandsen M, Parving H-H. Increased kidney size, glomerular filtration rate and renal plasma flow in short-term insulin-dependent diabetics. *Diabetologia* 1981; **20**: 451–6.

41. Sandahl-Christiansen J, Gammelgaard J, Frandsen M, Orskov H, Parvin H-H. Kidney function and size in type I diabetic patients before and during growth hormone administration for one week. *Diabetologia* 1982; **22**: 333–7.

42. Sandahl-Christiansen J. On the pathogenesis of the increased glomerular filtration rate in short-term insulin-dependent diabetes. *Dan Med Bull* 1984; **31**: 349–61.

43. Serri O, Beauregard H, Brazeau P et al. Somatostatin analogue, octreotide, reduces increased glomerular filtration rate and kidney size in insulin-dependent diabetics. *J Am Med Assoc* 1991; **265**: 888–92.

44. ter Wee PM, Rosman JB, van der Geest S, Sluiter WJ, Donker AJM. Renal hemodynamics during separate and combined infusion of amino acids and dopamine. *Kidney Int* 1986; **29**: 870–74.

45. ter Wee PM, van Ballegooie E, Donker AJM. Renal reserve filtration capacity in patients with type 1 (insulin-dependent) diabetes mellitus. *Nephrol Dialysis Transpl* 1987; **2**: 504–9.

46. ter Wee PM, Forster H, Epstein M. Rapid initiation of attenuated pressure-and angiotensin II (AII)-induced vasoconstriction of rat afferent arterioles (AA) in untreated diabetes mellitus (DM). *Am J Soc Nephrol* 1992; **3**: 767(A).

47. ter Wee PM, Forster H, Epstein M. Impairment of afferent arteriolar (AA) responsiveness to pressure in galactose-fed rats is prevented by tolrestat. *J Am Soc Nephrol* 1993; **4**: 804(A).

48. ter Wee PM, Tegzess AM, Donker AJM. Pair-tested renal reserve filtration capacity in kidney recipients and their donors. *J Am Soc Nephrol* 1994; **4**: 1798–808.

49. Tilton RG, Chang K, Hasan KS et al. Prevention of diabetic vascular dysfunction by guanidines. Inhibition of nitric oxide synthase versus advanced glycation end-product formation. *Diabetes* 1993; **42**: 221–32.

50. Trevisan R, Nosadini R, Fioretto P et al. Metabolic control of kidney hemody-namics in normal and insulin-dependent diabetic patients. *Diabetes* **36**: 1073–81.
51. Tucker BJ, Blantz RC. An analysis of the determinants of nephron filtration rate. *Am J Physiol* 1977; **232**: F477–83.
52. Tucker BJ, Anderson CM, Thies RS, Collins RC, Blantz RC. Glomerular hemo-dynamic alterations during acute hyperinsulinemia in normal and diabetic rats. *Kidney Int* 1992; **42**: 1160–68.
53. Tucker BJ, Mendonca MM, Blantz RC. Contrasting effects of acute insulin infusion on renal function in awake non-diabetic and diabetic rats. *J Am Soc Nephrol* 1993; **3**: 1686–93.
54. Vallon V, Richter K, Blantz RC et al. Glomerular hyperfiltration in experimental diabetes mellitus: potential role of tubular reabsorption. *J Am Soc Nephrol* 1999; **10**: 2569–76.
55. Vora JP, Dolben J, Dean JD et al. Renal hemodynamics in newly presenting non-insulin dependent diabetes mellitus. *Kidney Int* 1992; **41**: 829–35.
56. Vora JP, Dolben J, Williams JD, Peters JR, Owens DR. Impact of initial treatment on renal function in newly-diagnosed type 2 (non-insulin-dependent) diabetes mellitus. *Diabetologia* 1993; **36**: 734–40.
57. Williams B, Tsai P, Schrier RW. Glucose-induced downregulation of angio-tensin II and arginine vasopressin receptors in cultured rat aortic vascular smooth muscle cells. Role of protein kinase C. *J Clin Invest* 1992; **90**: 1992–9.
58. Wiseman MJ, Mangili R, Alberetto M, Keen H, Viberti GC. Glomerular response mechanisms to glycaemic changes in insulin-dependent diabetics. *Kidney Int* 1981; **31**: 1012–18.

5

Renal Structural Damage in IDDM and NIDDM— Functional Relationships

RUDY BILOUS

University of Newcastle upon Tyne, UK

INTRODUCTION

Although the classical glomerular pathological lesions of nodules and diffuse mesangial expansion were recognized in patients with nephropathy in the 1930s and 1940s, structural abnormalities in the diabetic kidney had been noted 50 years earlier (1). The first of these was glycogen deposition in the tubules, reported in 1877, and this was quickly followed by descriptions of glomerular and interstitial abnormalities long before the seminal observation of nodules by Kimmelstiel and Wilson in 1936 (2). By 1960, early studies with the electron microscope had revealed marked glomerular basement membrane thickening (GBMT) in diabetic patients, and this finding is now recognized as a *sine qua non* for diabetic glomerulopathy. For the most part, the pathological changes in the diabetic kidney are similar for both IDDM (type 1) and NIDDM (type 2). Indeed, the first descriptions were in the pre-insulin era and must of necessity have been in NIDDM patients. This chapter will briefly outline the pathological changes in the diabetic kidney seen in both types of diabetes, but will point out any contrasts between IDDM and NIDDM where they occur. It will use the definitions of *nephropathy*, as a clinical diagnosis based upon the finding of proteinuria, and *glomerulopathy*, which describes the pathological changes occurring in the glomerulus.

Diabetic Nephropathy. Edited by C. Hasslacher.
© 2001 John Wiley & Sons, Ltd.

MACROSCOPIC CHANGES IN THE DIABETIC KIDNEY

Whole kidney enlargement (nephromegaly) is an early feature of both experimental and human diabetes (3,4). In animals, nephromegaly occurs within 4 days of diabetes onset and most IDDM patients have large kidneys at diagnosis. This enlargement is mostly due to a combination of tubular hypertrophy and hyperplasia and interstitial expansion, and is probably a response to increased glucose and fluid filtration and their active reabsorption.

Glomeruli only account for 1% of total kidney volume, so their contribution to whole organ enlargement is insignificant.

Renal scarring and papillary necrosis are more common in diabetic patients, especially women, and may result from an increased prevalence of urinary tract infection (5). Rates of bacteriuria of up to 20% have been reported in some hospital series.

Finally, atherosclerosis of the renal arteries severe enough to cause functional renal artery stenosis has been described in some NIDDM patients (6).

MICROSCOPIC CHANGES

Glomerulus—Light Microscopy

There are $350–1050 \times 10^6$ glomeruli in the normal kidney (7), and each comprises a convoluted knot of capillaries supported on a scaffold of mesangium, made up of cellular and matrix components (Figure 5.1a). Blood enters the glomerulus via one or more afferent arterioles and leaves via usually one efferent vessel. Each capillary comprises a basement membrane, which is continuous with the mesangium and is lined by a fenestrated endothelium (Figure 5.2). The outer surface of the basement membrane is covered by an epithelium of interdigitating foot processes (Figure 5.3). No two adjacent foot processes arise from the same epithelial cell, and they are separated by a narrow filtration slit and membrane. The glomerular tuft is surrounded by Bowman's capsule, which is continuous with the basement membrane of the proximal convoluted tubule. Haemofiltration occurs from within the capillary, through the endothelial fenestrae, across the basement membrane, through the filtration slits and across the filtration membrane, into the urinary space defined by Bowman's capsule, and thus into the tubular part of the nephron.

Like global nephromegaly, glomerular enlargement occurs within days of onset of experimental diabetes (8). It is also a feature of IDDM patients with short diabetes duration. Animal studies suggest that most of the enlargement is due to an increase in capillary length and diameter, although minor

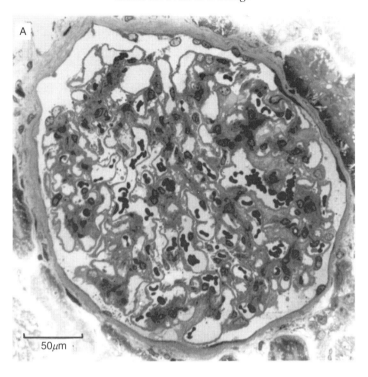

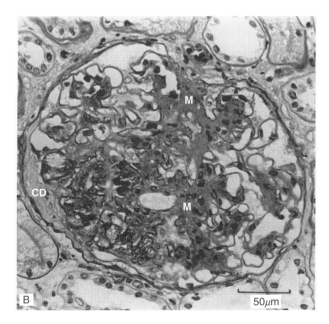

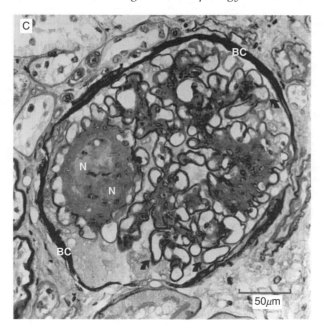

Figure 5.1 PAS-stained light micrographs of semi-thin sections. (A) Normal renal glomerulus. (B) Diffuse mesangial expansion (M). Note reduction in number of open capillary loops. Also present is a capsular drop (CD). (C) Kimmelstiel–Wilson nodule (N). Note also thickened Bowman's capsule (BC) and capillary basement membrane (arrowed)

increases in mesangial volume have also been described. GBMT is unchanged over this period, which implies a significant increase in the production of matrix material in order to accommodate the observed change in capillary dimensions (8).

Glomerular enlargement is also a feature of late diabetic nephropathy, particularly in NIDDM patients (9). Mean values of up to $4 \times 10^6 \, \mu m^3$ in IDDM and $> 6 \times 10^6 \, \mu m^3$ in NIDDM have been reported. These contrast with values of 1–$2.3 \times 10^6 \, \mu m^3$ reported in non-diabetic control subjects of the same studies (9, 10). Why NIDDM patients with nephropathy should demonstrate a greater capacity for glomerular enlargement is unclear. Indeed, the mechanisms underpinning increases in glomerular size are unknown. Early changes may be secondary to haemodynamic perturbations, whereas later enlargement may be a compensatory response to capillary loss due to mesangial expansion and global glomerulosclerosis.

Diffuse mesangial expansion, with or without nodule formation, is the hallmark of diabetic glomerulopathy (1). An accumulation of periodic acid–

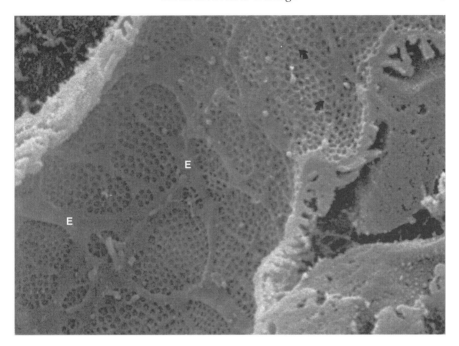

Figure 5.2 Scanning electron micrograph from a freeze-fractured rat glomerulus revealing the endothelial lining of a capillary. Note fenestrated endothelium (arrowed). E, endothelial cell

Schiff (PAS)-positive staining matrix material is seen to a greater or lesser extent in all patients with nephropathy. In its early stages, the accumulation tends to be in the centre of the glomerular tuft, and the capillary loops become marginalized to the periphery (Figure 5.1b). Eventually, the remaining capillaries are also obliterated by mesangial tissue encroaching along the endothelial surface.

The end result of advanced glomerulopathy is a hyalinized glomerulus with no obvious capillary loops. This global sclerosis is probably secondary to two processes that may occur in differing proportions in individual glomeruli and different patients; these are ischaemia secondary to arteriolar hyalinosis, and obliteration secondary to mesangial expansion (11). The former process results in a collapsed-looking glomerulus with crenated basement membranes, while the latter results in a larger, more amorphous structure. Eventually, such glomeruli are completely reabsorbed.

Nodule formation is highly specific for diabetic glomerulopathy, but is not an invariable finding and always occurs on the background of diffuse mesangial expansion. Nodules appear as acellular, eosinophilic, lamellated

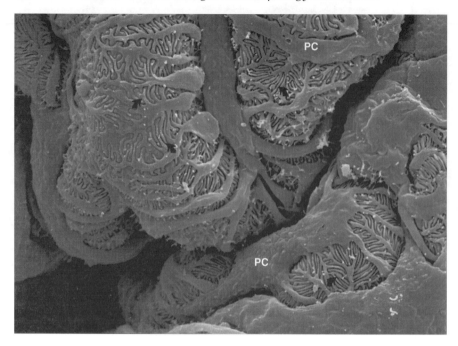

Figure 5.3 Scanning electron micrograph from a freeze-fractured rat glomerulus showing interdigitating foot processes (arrowed) on the epithelial side of a capillary. PC, podocyte

structures and are usually located at the periphery of the tuft (1, 2) (Figure 5.1c). This location is distinct from the pattern of lesion seen in other glomerulopathies, where most of the abnormalities are more central (12). The pathogenesis of nodules is unclear but they may represent obliterated capillary micro-aneurysms. An alternative hypothesis is that mesangial expansion disrupts endothelial cell attachment, resulting in them ballooning into the capillary lumen, quickly followed by mesangial matrix material (13).

Finally, it is not uncommon to see accumulations of PAS-positive material arranged in so-called "capsular drops" between the basement membrane and parietal epithelial cells of Bowman's capsule (Figure 5.1b). Their presence is non-specific, however, and their pathological significance unclear.

Glomerulus—Electron Microscopy

With the greater magnification possible with the electron microscope, much of the mesangial expansion can be seen to be due to an accumulation of amorphous matrix material (Figure 5.4). Normally, mesangial matrix com

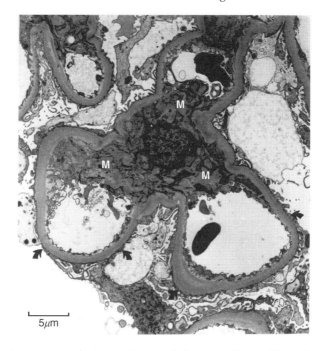

Figure 5.4 Low-power electron micrograph from a patient with nephropathy showing a glomerular lobule comprising three capillaries with thickened glomerular basement membrane (arrowed). Note the central mesangium (M) expanding into the capillaries, reducing the available filtration surface area of the peripheral basement membrane

prises predominantly type IV collagen, with smaller proportions of laminin, fibronectin and entactin, and the proteoglycans chondroitin and dermatan sulphate (1). This matrix is arranged around a dense mesh of microfibrils, which form a plexus around the mesangial cells. At the mesangial–endothelial cell interface and the attachment points of the capillary basement membrane, the microfibrils are much more tightly organized (14). This arrangement lends itself to the various functions of the mesangium, such as providing a support for the capillaries that is contractile and thus able to adjust the tension in the basement membrane, and forming a mesh that can entrap, neutralize and dispose of circulating macromolecules and pathogens. Matrix is produced by epithelial and endothelial cells on the surface of the GBM, and also by the mesangial cells themselves (15). Degradation and recycling is a function of the mesangium and also possibly macrophages.

In diabetes, the increase in matrix is secondary to a combination of excess production and decreased degradation. In addition, its composition differs from normal, with more type VI collagen and a reduction in proteoglycans, particularly heparan sulphate (16). Moreover, matrix accumulation disrupts the microfibrillar structure, altering the porous nature of the mesangium and weakening the attachments to the endothelium and the GBM. In tissue culture experiments, these changes can be induced by high ambient glucose, growth factors such as TGF-β (17), prostanoids such as thromboxane (18), and advanced glycation end products.

The other obvious feature of glomerulopathy visible using the electron microscope is capillary basement membrane thickening (Figures 5.4, 5.5). Normally, the GBM has an electron-dense middle (lamina densa) and less dense inner (lamina rara interna) and outer (lamina rara externa) layers. It comprises mainly matrix material of a similar composition to the mesangium and is continuous with it. The main proteoglycan constituent is heparan sulphate, specifically perlecan. The type IV collagen chains are arranged in a tight lattice, leaving a small number of pores with a functional size of approximately 60 Å. Much of the permselectivity to circulating macromolecules is dependent upon this structure.

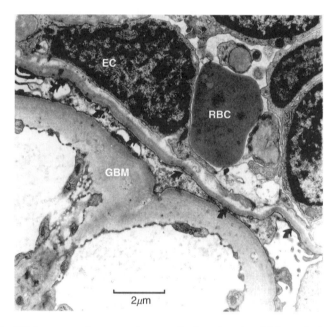

Figure 5.5 High-power electron micrograph showing the thickened glomerular basement membrane (GBM) adjacent to the thin segment (arrowed). Note the contrasting electron density appearing as two distinct layers in the thin segment. RBC, red blood cell; EC, endothelial cell

GBM thickening can be demonstrated in most patients with diabetes, irrespective of their nephropathy status, although those with heavier proteinuria tend to have thicker membranes (19). It is therefore not as specific a feature of glomerulopathy as mesangial expansion or nodule formation. Most of the increase in matrix is due to type IV collagen accumulation. There is, however, a net loss of proteoglycan, which is also more dispersed throughout the thicker membranes (20). This loss is thought to result in a loss of negative electrostatic charge and thus permit the passage of positively charged proteins such as albumin.

Mesangial matrix accumulation can be prevented and reversed in experimental animals treated with insulin or islet transplantation. GBM thickening can certainly be prevented but resolution is much slower (21). In man, mesangial expansion and GBMT have been shown to reverse after 10 years of normoglycaemia induced by pancreas transplantation (22). These observations emphasize the slowness of the rate of turnover of matrix *in vivo*—the lesions take almost as long to resolve as they do to develop. Studies of the impact of antihypertensive therapy on renal structure have failed to show any impact on the lesions, perhaps because the duration between biopsies was just 3 years (23, 24).

Very much thinner segments of GBM have been seen in some patients with established nephropathy (25). (Figure 5.5). These segments occasionally appear "lumpy" and irregular and are lined with an abnormal endothelium. Their origin is obscure but they could represent micro-aneurysms or even new capillary growth. They have been associated with asymptomatic haematuria in non-diabetic subjects (26), but their significance in diabetes is uncertain. They could provide an area of non-selective leakage of proteins.

There are no obvious changes in endothelial or epithelial cells in glomerulopathy, except that there is a widening of podocyte foot processes. This development may be a ubiquitous response to increased protein passage across the GBM, as it is seen in other proteinuric states. The total number of epithelial cells may also be reduced in patients with glomerulopathy, and this reduction does not appear to be amenable to glycaemic correction (27).

Tubulo-interstitium—Light Microscopy

The tubular portion of the nephron arises from Bowman's capsule and continues to the connecting ducts in the renal medulla. Glycogen-rich granules can be seen in the proximal tubular cells in acute diabetes and are the result of massive glucose reabsorption. They do not occur in insulin-treated animals (28) and are rarely seen in man. In experimental diabetes there is an initial tubular hyperplasia of approximately 11%, but after 2 days of hyperglycaemia hypertrophy predominates (29). These changes are mediated via growth factors such as TGF-β and IGF$_1$. Hypertrophy is partly reversible by insulin, but cell numbers remain increased. In man, it is likely that similar processes underpin nephromegaly, but glycaemic correction does not reverse long-standing, whole kidney enlargement (30). Tubular cell atrophy is a feature of advanced nephropathy and is largely secondary to glomerular loss, secondary to global glomerulosclerosis.

Arteriolar hyalinosis is a common feature and is particularly noticeable in hypertensive patients (31). Involvement of the glomerular efferent arteriole is said to be specific to diabetes, and this may play a role in increasing intra-glomerular capillary pressure, which is thought to be of critical importance in the pathophysiology of glomerulopathy.

The interstitial space is increased as a part of kidney enlargement in both human and experimental diabetes. Apart from fluid, this space also contains immunologically active cells and fibroblasts, and these cells are thought to be responsible for the fibrotic changes seen in advanced nephropathy. There is a clear link between the severity of these changes and those seen in the glomeruli but it is not certain which occur first.

Tubulo-interstitium—Electron Microscopy

Subtle changes in the macula densa cells of the juxtaglomerular apparatus (JGA) of the rat can be seen within hours of developing glycosuria (32). It is hypothesized that they may represent a signalling pathway that could control glomerular blood flow and thus GFR. Careful observation of the JGA in diabetic man has also revealed changes from normal but their significance is unclear.

Tubular basement membrane (TBM) is thought to have a similar composition and structure to GBM but is almost twice as wide. Diabetic patients develop TBM thickening about two to three times the value seen in their non-diabetic siblings (33) and it is common to see splitting under both light and electron microscopy. The significance of this is unclear, but macromolecular penetration of the interstitial space may activate fibrosis and would be facilitated by disruption of the TBM. Advanced glycation end products have been shown to increase pore size in bovine TBM, which may also result in increased protein permeation (34).

Arteriolar hyaline appears to be similar to mesangial matrix in its composition. It is present in significantly greater amounts in microalbuminuric IDDM compared to normoalbuminuric controls, and is positively correlated with GBM width.

Interstitial changes appear to be responsive to antihypertensive therapy with angiotensin-converting enzyme inhibitors (ACEI), at least in NIDDM patients. Two small studies showed an increase in interstitium in conventionally treated patients that was not observed in those given ACEI (23, 24). These results imply that an important pathological abnormality of nephropathy is able to be influenced by antihypertensive treatment—perhaps by inhibition of growth factors—and may provide clues as to the pathophysiology of nephropathy.

FUNCTIONAL RELATIONSHIPS WITH RENAL STRUCTURE

Clinical diabetic nephropathy is characterized by a steady, relentless decline in GFR, increasing albuminuria and increasing systemic blood pressure. There have been many attempts to relate the pathological changes seen in the kidney at post mortem to the clinical features of the patient in life (1). Latterly, percutaneous renal biopsy has meant that the progression of the disease can be related to the progression of the lesions, and in this way lead to a greater understanding of the pathophysiology of renal failure in diabetes. The use of the electron microscope, and more precise quantitation of the pathology by morphometric measurement (35), has increased our understanding of the structural–functional relationships in diabetic nephropathy. This section will outline the determinants of GFR and albuminuria and describe the pathological correlates.

Glomerular Filtration Rate

GFR is determined by the product of the ultrafiltration pressure (P_{uf}), capillary wall permeability (k), and the surface area of the capillary wall available for filtration (s).

$$GFR = P_{uf} \cdot k \cdot s$$

The ultrafiltration pressure is determined by the hydrostatic pressure across the capillary wall (P) and the osmotic pressure of the plasma proteins (π). Furthermore, P is determined, in turn, by the difference between the hydrostatic pressure within the glomerular capillary (P_{gc}) and the filtrate (P_{tf}); and π by the difference between the osmotic pressure in plasma (π_{gc}) and the filtrate (π_{tf}). Thus:

$$GFR = k \cdot s \cdot [(P_{gc} - P_{tf}) - (\pi_{gc} - \pi_{tf})]$$

The product $k.s$ is termed the ultrafiltration coefficient (K_f).

The most important glomerular structure determining GFR is therefore capillary surface area. It is possible to estimate this from photomicrographs of the glomerular tuft by using morphometric techniques (35). In this way a surface area per unit volume of glomerulus can be derived, and this measure is called surface density or S_v. The product of S_v and glomerular volume (also able to be derived from micrographs) is the surface area of capillary for that glomerulus. By estimating the surface areas in several glomeruli, an average filtration surface per glomerulus can be estimated. Positive correlations between this surface area and GFR (specifically creatinine clearance) have been reported, with $r^2 > 50\%$ (Figure 5.6) (36,37).

The average filtration surface per glomerulus has been shown to be determined by a combination of the mesangial and glomerular volumes, giving a combined r of 0.93 (36). As mesangial expansion increases, filtration surface declines, and this effect is ameliorated by glomerular enlargement. Careful scrutiny of Figure 5.6, however, reveals that the relationship between average filtration surface per glomerulus and GFR is not that

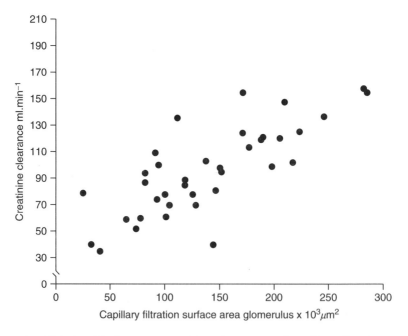

Figure 5.6   Relationship between creatinine clearance and capillary filtration surface area per glomerulus in 37 type 1 diabetic patients with differing severities of nephropathy ($r = 0.79$; $p = 0.001$). Note the wide range of filtration surface area per glomerulus for any given creatinine clearance. Reproduced from (36), by permission of the editor and publishers of *Kidney International*

precise. For example, for a given creatinine clearance of 80 ml/min, filtration surface per glomerulus can vary three-fold (< 50–150×10^3 μm^2). Part of the explanation lies in the fact that glomerular number also varies more than three-fold between individuals, and it is, of course, the total available filtration surface per patient that determines GFR (i.e. the product of average filtration surface per glomerulus and glomerular number). The final structural determinant of filtration surface in patients with nephropathy is the percentage of globally sclerosed (and non-functioning) glomeruli. Negative correlations of > 0.60 have been reported (36, 37).

Thus filtration surface area is itself affected by four main structural parameters:

1. *Mean glomerular volume*: possibly determined by haemodynamic factors, at least in short-duration diabetes.
2. *Mesangial volume*: matrix accumulation related to glycaemia and mediated via growth factors, such as TGF-β, and possibly mechanical factors, such as stretch (38).
3. *Total number of glomeruli*: probably genetically determined (see below).
4. *Percentage of sclerosed glomeruli*: related to arteriolar hyalinosis (ischaemia) and mesangial volume (internal obliteration) (11).

The factors governing total glomerular number in man are unknown. There is a great deal of debate surrounding the foetal programming hypothesis of Barker and others (39). These workers propose that foetal malnutrition leads to low birth weight and arrested development of key organs such as renal glomeruli and pancreatic islets. Thus, the individual is "programmed" from birth to be at risk of developing renal disease, hypertension and diabetes.

There are only limited published data on birth weight and glomerular number in man and these have shown no significant relationship, although none of the individuals in that study weighed < 2.5 kg at birth (40). The same workers have also found no relationship between post mortem glomerular number in persons with and without diabetes, and with and without nephropathy (41). A major difficulty in testing the foetal programming idea lies in the problem of obtaining accurate estimates of glomerular number in living man.

From the studies of structure and function, the following hypothesis has been proposed. Patients with large numbers (more at birth, less global sclerosis) or large glomeruli (greater inherent capacity for enlargement) could accommodate an expanding mesangium and therefore have a greater tendency to preserve GFR, compared to persons with smaller numbers of smaller glomeruli. Thus, variability in glomerular number, structure and adaptability could provide a structural basis for determining the clinical course of nephropathy, and possibly the risk of developing it in the first place.

Most of these deductions have been made from cross-sectional studies in IDDM patients. The few longitudinal repeat biopsy reports suggest that the rate of GBM thickening slows in advanced nephropathy, but that mesangial expansion continues, with a resulting loss in filtration surface (42). Longer natural history studies of renal structure and function are ongoing and their results eagerly awaited.

Two other factors that influence GFR have to be considered. Firstly, there is a renal reserve of functional capacity, probably determined by limiting blood flow to a population of glomeruli, and only recruiting them for active filtration at times of need, e.g. diuresis, protein loading (43). Obviously, pathological examination cannot take this into account and is reliant on the estimate of GFR to be as close as possible to the maximum.

Secondly, the role of the tubulo-interstitium in determining GFR is only just being explored (44). A positive correlation between serum creatinine and interstitial volume was demonstrated years ago (45) and has been confirmed since. However, the pathophysiology of tubulo-interstitial nephritis and fibrosis is probably multifactorial and, until it is better understood, it is hard to draw firm conclusions about the nature of the relationship with progressive renal impairment in diabetes.

Albuminuria

GFR is an important determinant of protein filtration but there are many other factors that affect the amount of protein that appears in urine. Circulating macromolecules have to pass through the endothelial fenestrae, the GBM and between the epithelial foot processes before appearing in the filtrate, and each of these structures provides both a size and an electrostatic barrier. Their combined selective property is termed "the permselectivity of the glomerulus". Thereafter, proteins are subject to reabsorption by tubular cells, and this process has a high degree of individual variability between different tubules and different proteins (46). Some proteins can be secreted by tubules, and finally, any process that leads to blood loss into, or inflammation of, the urinary tract and bladder can also increase proteinuria.

Experiments with electrically neutral dextran molecules of differing sizes has shown that there is unrestricted permselectivity of the GBM for molecules < 60 000 molecular weight and which have an effective radius of < 24 Å (47). The physical characteristics of albumin (radius 36 Å) therefore make albuminuria a sensitive marker of disordered permselectivity. There is probably little effective prevention of protein filtration by the endothelial fenestrae; however, the GBM provides both a size restriction in the form of the collagen meshwork and a negatively charged electrostatic barrier of proteoglycan molecules (48). The negative charge sites are concentrated in the lamina rara interna and externa in normal man, but in the thickened, diabetic GBM the number and density of these sites are reduced, leading to an increased passage of positively-charged molecules, such as albumin. Significant negative correlations between charge site number and albuminuria have been reported in IDDM patients.

Mathematical modelling in patients with heavy proteinuria has suggested a heteroporous model of permselectivity (49). The increase in non-selective proteinuria that is seen in progressive clinical nephropathy can be explained by the development of a population of large pores < 10 nm diameter and occupying just 2% of the total filtration surface area. No such pores have been identified by the electron microscope, but this may be because they are too small and too widely scattered. Some workers have suggested that the thin segments of the GBM may act as the large pores, but there is no confirmation of this and thin GBM does not cause heavy proteinuria in non-diabetic subjects. There is a consistent but weak correlation, of the order of 34%, between overall GBM width and proteinuria in both IDDM and NIDDM (50), and it is likely that disruption of the collagen mesh by an accumulation of excess matrix material creates functional wide pores beyond the resolution of the electron microscope (51).

Epithelial cells change shape in response to proteinuria with widening of the foot processes. This effectively shortens the length of the filtration slit and thus reduces the available filtration path. Both mean foot process width and filtration slit length correlate with albuminuria (52) and filtration slit width with GFR (53). There are also charge sites on the podocyte cell surface, but no quantitative data on their density in diabetes.

Tubular reabsorption of albumin is thought to be fully saturated at physiological levels of albumin filtration (54). Thus, any excess caused by altered permselectivity is likely to be detected in the urine. However, there is no known method of estimating tubular reabsorption of proteins in living man and, at low levels of albuminuria (10–30 µg/min), it is possible that some of the observed day-to-day variability of excretion is determined by variable tubular function.

There are correlations between estimates of tubulo-interstitial disease and albuminuria. Moreover, recent ideas about the pathophysiology of progressive nephropathies have proposed increased tubular protein trafficking as a potential mechanism (54).

The relative lack of precision in the observed relationship between albuminuria and measures of structural damage (19) may therefore be due to a number of factors. First, patients with "normal" albuminuria may develop pathological changes prior to increasing albumin excretion. Second, the variability in protein reabsorption may mean that, for a given severity of glomerulopathy leading to excess albumin filtration, some patients will show "abnormal" albuminuria while others will not. Third, the structural basis for protein passage may be beyond the resolution of the electron microscope. Fourth, demonstration and quantitation of charge sites in the GBM remains technically difficult. Finally, the net result of albuminuria is due to change in many structures at different parts of the nephron and their relative importance is not known.

Despite these caveats, it is important to remember that the reason why patients enter end stage renal failure is because of loss of nephrons. Thus, a greater understanding of the pathological processes that lead to nephron loss is essential if a reduction in the numbers of diabetic patients requiring renal replacement therapy is to be achieved. To this end, carefully controlled and planned studies of renal structure and function using prospective kidney biopsy and unbiased quantitative analysis are necessary (55).

ACKNOWLEDGEMENTS

My thanks to Mrs K. White, of the Biomedical Electron Microscopy Unit of the University of Newcastle upon Tyne, for providing the photomicrogaphs

REFERENCES

1. Bilous R W. The pathology of diabetic nephropathy. In *International Textbook of Diabetes Mellitus*, 2nd edn, Alberti KGMM, Zimmet P, DeFronzo RA, Keen H (eds). Wiley: Chichester, 1997; 1349–62.
2. Kimmelstiel P, Wilson C. Intercapillary lesions in the glomeruli of the kidney. *Am J Pathol* 1936; **12**: 83–97.
3. Seyer-Hansen K, Gundersen HJG. Renal hypertrophy in experimental diabetes. A morphometric study. *Diabetologia* 1980; **18**: 501–5.
4. Mogensen CEF, Andersen MJF. Increased kidney size and glomerular filtration rate in early juvenile diabetes. *Diabetes* 1973; **22**: 706–12.
5. Eknoyan G, Qunibi WY, Grissom RT, Tuma SN, Ayus JC. Renal papillary necrosis: an update. *Medicine (Baltimore)* 1982; **61**: 55–73.
6. Ritchie CM, McIlrath E, Hadden DR et al. Renal artery stenosis in hypertensive diabetic patients. *Diabet Med* 1988; **5**: 265–7.
7. Nyengaard JR, Bendtsen TF. Number and size of glomeruli, kidney weight and body surface area in normal human beings. *Anat Rec* 1992; **232**: 194–201.
8. Osterby R, Gundersen HJG. Fast accumulation of basement membrane material and the rate of morphological changes in acute experimental diabetic glomerular hypertrophy. *Diabetologia* 1980; **18**: 493–500.
9. Schmitz A, Nyengaard JR, Bendtsen TF. Glomerular volume in type 2 (non-insulin dependent) diabetes estimated by a direct and unbiased stereologic method. *Lab Invest* 1990; **62**: 108–13.

10. Bilous RW, Mauer SM, Sutherland DER, Steffes MW. Mean glomerular volume and the rate of development od diabetic nephropathy. *Diabetes* 1989; **38**: 1142–7.
11. Harris RD, Steffes MW, Bilous RW, Sutherland DER, Mauer SM. Global glomerular sclerosis and glomerular arteriolar hyalinosis in insulin dependent diabetes. *Kidney Int* 1991; **40**: 107–14.
12. Sandison A, Newbold KM, Howie AJ. Evidence for unique distribution of Kimmelstiel–Wilson nodules in glomeruli. *Diabetes* 1992; **41**: 952–5.
13. Stout LC, Kumar S, Whorton EB. Focal mesangiolysis and the pathogenesis of the Kimmelstiel–Wilson nodule. *Hum Pathol* 1993; **24**: 77–89.
14. Rosenblum ND. The mesangial matrix in the normal and sclerotic glomerulus. *Kidney Int* 1994; **45**: S73–7.
15. Beavan LA, Davies M, Couchman JR, Williams MA, Mason RM. *In vivo* turnover of the basement membrane and other heparan sulphate proteoglycans of rat glomerulus. *Arch Biochem Biophys* 1989; **269**: 576–85.
16. Ziyadeh FN. The extracellular matrix in diabetic nephropathy. *Am J Kidney Dis* 1993; **22**: 736–44.
17. Sharma K, Ziyadeh FN. Hyperglycaemia and diabetic kidney disease. The case for transforming growth factor β as a key mediator. *Diabetes* 1995; **44**: 1139–46.
18. DeRubertis FR, Craven PA. Eicosanoids in the pathogenesis of the functional and structural alterations of the kidney in diabetes. *Am J Kidney Dis* 1993; **22**: 727–35.
19. Fioretto P, Steffes MW, Mauer SM. Glomerular structure in non-proteinuric IDDM patients with various levels of albuminuria. *Diabetes* 1994; **43**: 1358–64.
20. Tamsma JT, van den Born J, Bruijn JA et al. Expression of glomerular extracellular matrix components in human diabetic nephropathy: decrease of heparan sulphate in the glomerular basement membrane. *Diabetologia* 1994; **37**: 313–20.
21. Mauer SM, Steffes MW, Sutherland DER et al. Studies of the rate of regression of the glomerular lesions in diabetic rats treated with pancreatic islet transplantation. *Diabetes* 1975; **24**: 280–85.
22. Fioretto P, Steffes MW, Sutherland DER, Goetz FC, Mauer SM. Reversal of lesions of diabetic nephropathy after pancreas transplantation. *N Engl J Med* 1998; **339**: 69–75.
23. Cordonnier DJ, Pinel N, Barro C et al. Expansion of cortical interstitium is limited by converting enzyme inhibition in type 2 diabetic patients with glomerulosclerosis. *J Am Soc Nephrol* 1999; **10**: 1253–63.
24. Nankervis A, Nicholls K, Kilmartin G et al. Effects of perindopril on renal histomorphometry in diabetic subjects with microalbuminuria: a 3-year placebo controlled biopsy study. *Metabolism* 1998; **47** (1): 12–15.
25. Osterby R, Gundersen HJG, Nyberg G, Aurell M. Advanced diabetic glomerulopathy. Quantitative structural characterization of non-occluded glomeruli. *Diabetes* 1987; **36**: 612–19.
26. Cosio FG, Falkenhain ME, Sedmak DD. Association of thin glomerular basement membrane with other glomerulopathies. *Kidney Int* 1994; **46**: 471–4.
27. Pagtalunan ME, Miller PL, Jumping Eagle S et al. Podocyte loss and progressive glomerular injury in type II diabetes. *J Clin Invest* 1997; **99**: 342–8.
28. Rasch R, Gotzsche O. Regression of glycogen nephrosis in experimental diabetes after pancreatic islet transplantation. *APMIS* 1988; **96**: 749–54.
29. Nyengaard JR, Flyvbjerg A, Rasch R. The impact of renal growth, regression and regrowth in experimental diabetes mellitus on number and size of proximal and distal tubular cells in the rat kidney. *Diabetologia* 1993; **36**: 1126–31.

30. Wiseman MJ, Saunders AJ, Keen H, Viberti GC. Effect of blood glucose control on increased glomerular filtration rate and kidney size in insulin dependent diabetes. *N Engl J Med* 1985; **312**: 617–21.
31. Osterby R, Bangstad H-J, Nyberg G, Walker JD, and Viberti GC. A quantitative ultrastructural study of the juxtaglomerular arterioles in IDDM patients with micro- and normoalbuminuria. *Diabetologia* 1995; **38**: 1320–27.
32. Rasch R, Holck P. Ultrastructure of the macula densa in streptozotocin diabetic rats. *Lab Invest* 1988; **59**: 666–72.
33. Steffes MW, Sutherland DER, Goetz FC, Rich SS, Mauer SM. Studies of kidney and muscle biopsy specimens from identical twins discordant for type 1 diabetes mellitus. *N Engl J Med* 1985; **312**: 1282–7.
34. Anderson SS, Tsilibary EC, Charonis AS. Non-enzymatic glycosylation-induced modifications of intact bovine tubular basement membrane. *J Clin Invest* 1993; **92**: 3045–52.
35. Gundersen HJG, Bendtsen TF, Korbo L et al. Some new simple and efficient stereological methods and their use in pathological research and diagnosis. *APMIS* 1988; **96**: 379–94.
36. Ellis EN, Steffes MW, Goetz FC, Sutherland DER, Mauer SM. Glomerular filtration surface in type 1 diabetes mellitus. *Kidney Int* 1986; **29**: 889–94.
37. Osterby R, Parving H-H, Nyberg G et al. A strong correlation between glomerular filtration rate and filtration surface in diabetic nephropathy. *Diabetologia* 1988; **31**: 265–70.
38. Cortes P, Riser BL, Yee J, Narins RG. Mechanical strain of glomerular mesangial cells in the pathogenesis of glomerulosclerosis: clinical implications. *Nephrol Dial Transpl* 1999; **14**: 1351–4.
39. Barker DJ, Hales CN, Fall CH et al. Type II (non-insulin dependent) diabetes mellitus, hypertension and hyperlipidaemia (syndrome X): relation to reduced fetal growth. *Diabetologia* 1993; **36**: 62–7.
40. Nyengaard JR, Bendtsen TF, Mogensen CE. Low birth weight—is it associated with few and smal glomeruli in normal persons and NIDDM (non-insulin dependent diabetes mellitus) patients? *Diabetologia* 1996; **39**: 1634–7.
41. Bendtsen TF, Nyengaard JR. The number of glomeruli in type 1 (insulin dependent) and type 2 (non-insulin dependent) diabetic patients. *Diabetologia* 1992; **35**: 844–50.
42. Fioretto P, Steffes MW, Sutherland DER, Mauer SM. Sequential renal biopsies in insulin dependent diabetic patients: structural factors associated with clinical progression. *Kidney Int* 1995; **48**: 1929–35.
43. Trevisan R, Nosadini R, Fioretto P et al. Ketone bodies increase glomerular filtration rate in normal man and in patients with type 1 (insulin dependent) diabetes mellitus. *Diabetologia* 1987; **30**: 214–21.
44. Ziyadeh FN, Goldfarb S. The renal tubulo-interstitium in diabetes mellitus. *Kidney Int* 1991; **39**: 464–75.
45. Bader R, Bader H, Grund KE et al. Structure and function of the kidney in diabetic glomerulosclerosis. Correlations between morphological and functional parameters. *Pathol Res Pract* 1980; **167**: 204–16.
46. Scandling JD, Myers BD. Glomerular size-selectivity and microalbuminuria in early diabetic glomerular disease. *Kidney Int* 1992; **41**: 840–46.
47. Myers BD, Winetz JA, Chui F, Michaels AS. Mechanisms of proteinuria in diabetic nephropathy: a study of glomerular barrier function. *Kidney Int* 1982; **21**: 633–41.

48. Goode NP, Shires M, Crellin DM, Aparicio SR, Davison AM. Alterations of glomerular basement membrane charge and structure in diabetic nephropathy. *Diabetologia* 1995; **38**: 1455–65.
49. Deen WM, Bridges CR, Brenner BM, Myers BD. A heteroporous model of size selectivity: application to normal and nephrotic humans. *Am J Physiol (Renal Fluid Electrol Physiol)* 1985; **249**: F374–89.
50. Steffes MW, Bilous RW, Sutherland DER, Mauer SM. Cell and matrix components of the glomerular mesangium in type 1 diabetes. *Diabetes* 1992; **41**: 679–84.
51. Makino H, Yamasaki Y, Haramoto T et al. Ultrastructural changes of extracellular matrices in diabetic nephropathy revealed high resolution scanning and immunoelectron microscopy. *Lab Invest* 1993; **68**: 45–55.
52. Ellis EN, Steffes MW, Chavers B, Mauer SM. Observations of glomerular epithelial cell structure in patients with type 1 diabetes mellitus. *Kidney Int* 1987; **32**: 736–41.
53. Bjorn SF, Bangstad H-J, Hanssen KP et al. Glomerular epithelial foot processes and filtration slits in IDDM patients. *Diabetologia* 1995; **38**: 1197–1204.
54. Remuzzi G, Bertani T. Pathophysiology of progressive nephropathies. *N Engl J Med* 1998; **339**: 1448–56.
55. Mauer SM, Chavers BM, Steffes MW. Should there be an expanded role for kidney biopsy in the management of patients with type 1 diabetes? *Am J Kidney Dis* 1990; **16**: 96–100.

6

Diabetic Nephropathy in Children and Adolescents

THOMAS DANNE[1], ELISABETH ENGELMANN[2] and OLGA KORDONOURI[2]

[1]Kinderkrankenhaus auf der Bult, Hannover, Germany, [2]Humboldt-Universität, Berlin, Germany

Diabetic angiopathy in children and adolescents is caused predominantly by microangiopathy, representing structural changes in the microvascular system, leading mainly to detectable abnormalities in the eye and the kidney (1). The patho-anatomical correlate of advanced diabetic nephropathy, i.e. glomerulosclerosis, is rarely found in the paediatric population. However, characteristic histological changes associated with microalbuminuria, such as basement membrane thickening and mesangial expansion reflecting early glomerulopathy, can be seen when biopsies are taken. Two studies in young people with a mean age around 18 years demonstrated such findings after a mean diabetes duration of 7 and 16 years, respectively (2, 3).

While overt proteinuria is found in less than 1% of paediatric patients (4, 5) microalbuminuria may be detected in 5–20% of young adults with diabetes, sometimes beginning during early puberty (1, 6–8) (Table 6.1). The discrepancies in the prevalence of microalbuminuria in paediatric populations may partly be explained by characteristics of the study population, such as age range, diabetes duration and glycaemic control, as well as differing microalbuminuria definitions and sampling procedures. However, there is agreement that microalbuminuria is rarely found before puberty and hormonal and metabolic changes during this period may be important for its development. In particular, IGF-1 and growth hormone

Diabetic Nephropathy. Edited by C. Hasslacher.
© 2001 John Wiley & Sons, Ltd.

Table 6.1   Prevalence of microalbuminuria in children, adolescents and young adults with type 1 diabetes in different studies

Reference	Population (n)	Prevalence of microalbuminuria (%)	Age group (years)	Mean diabetes duration (years)	Screening procedure
(51)	Clinic (97)	20	7–18	10	AER, overnight
(7)	Clinic (129)	20	7–23	10	AER, overnight
(24)	Clinic (113)	15	1–18	9	AER, 24 h-urine
(4)	Nationwide (957)	4	2–19	6	AER, overnight
(5)	Community (371)	12	8–30	10.5	AER, overnight
(1)	Clinic/ follow-up (249)	Transient: 2 Intermittent: 3 Permanent: 5	7–18	Onset: 4 Follow-up: 9	AER, overnight
(8)	Clinic/ follow-up (233)	Intermittent: 9 Permanent: 14	13–18	Onset: 4 Follow-up: 7	ACR, morning spot urine

may contribute significantly to the pathogenesis of early diabetic nephropathy (9) and may explain why puberty is an independent risk factor for the progression of microalbuminuria (10).

DIAGNOSIS OF INCIPIENT NEPHROPATHY IN CHILDREN AND ADOLESCENTS

At least two out of three consecutive samples should have tested positive for an elevated albumin excretion before the diagnosis of microalbuminuria is considered (11). The high intra-individual variation of albumin excretion with a variation coefficient of close to 50% limits the prognostic value of an elevated albumin excretion in single urine samples. The preferred urine collection method depends on local circumstances, but several methodological problems should be considered (12). In many centres a screening is performed using a timed overnight urine collection (1, 6, 7), which is easy for children and their parents to understand. Urine collection at resting conditions also excludes influences of physical exercise, as observed following daytime urine collections (13). While the upper limit of normal in timed overnight urine samples in adults in 20 µg/min (11), studies in healthy children have indicated an upper limit of normal 5–10 µg/min lower than that, irrespective of age, if corrected for the standard body surface area of

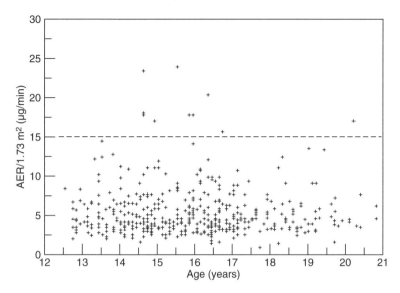

Figure 6.1 Individual timed overnight albumin excretion rates of 449 healthy children and adolescents, demonstrating no influence of age when corrected for standard body surface area. Data taken from (14)

$1.73\,m^2$ (14) (Figure 6.1). Nevertheless, the reference value of $20\,\mu g/min$ adjusted for body surface area appears to be useful in predicting the development of permanent microalbuminuria, while the prognostic relevance of albumin excretion rates slightly above the 95th centile of healthy controls but below $20\,\mu g/min$ is controversial.

Some centres use the albumin:creatinine ratio (ACR) in morning spot urine samples for screening. The ACR differs significantly between boys and girls beyond puberty, due to muscle mass-related differences in creatinine excretion. Therefore, sex-specific normal ranges have to be considered (Figure 6.2). However, a high day-to-day variability of both albumin and creatinine excretion makes this parameter less reliable than the albumin analysis in overnight urine samples.

Apart from albumin, a pathological urinary excretion of other proteins of glomerular (transferrin, IgG) and tubular origin (α1-microglobulin, β-2-microglobulin, Tamm–Horsfall protein, N-acetyl-β-D-glucosaminidase, etc.) can also be detected without, sometimes before, microalbuminuria. Although recent evidence points to persistently elevated NAG excretion predicting the later development of microalbuminuria (15), the prognostic and diagnostic relevance of tubular markers remains to be elucidated (16).

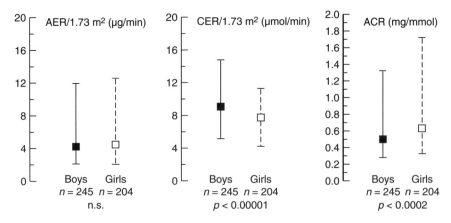

Figure 6.2 Albumin excretion rates (AER), creatinine excretion rates (CER) and albumin: creatinine ratios (ACR) of boys and girls (medians and ranges from 3rd to 97th centiles). AER is similar in boys and girls, while the ACR differs significantly due to significant differences in creatinine excretion. Data taken from (14)

There is increasing evidence that 20–30% of patients with microalbuminuria may never progress to nephropathy without pharmacological intervention (17). Some patients develop microalbuminuria after a relatively short diabetes duration (18). Others show elevated albumin excretion only intermittently (19). In the Berlin Retinopathy Study, for example, out of 249 patients with a mean age of 13 at the initial urinary albumin determination, 12 developed persistent, seven intermittent and five only a transient elevation of urinary albumin excretion during a follow-up of 3–9 years (1) (Table 6.1). Therefore, other clinical parameters need to be taken into account in order to distinguish those patients with transient functional disturbances from those with likely permanent abnormalities when renoprotective pharmacological therapy is considered. In agreement with another study in adolescents (20), the Berlin patients with permanent microalbuminuria had a significantly poorer metabolic control, higher blood pressure, longer diabetes duration and more frequent background retinopathy than those with transient elevations of the albumin excretion rate (21). Clinical data of patients with intermittent microalbuminuria were non-homogeneous, possibly indicating that some of these patients may proceed to permanent microalbuminuria. Such differences in the definition of microalbuminuria, the sampling procedures and the methods of albumin determination hamper the evaluation of different intervention studies.

POTENTIAL INTERVENTIONS IN ADOLESCENTS WITH INCIPIENT NEPHROPATHY

Despite evidence for the importance of genetic factors in the development of nephropathy (22), the long-term follow-up of children with diabetes in a Swedish community (where the genetic background is not likely to have changed during the study period) gives reason for believing that a lot can be achieved by the patient and the therapeutic team. Comparing the outcome of all 213 children aged below 15 years at diabetes onset during 1961–1980, the improvement of diabetes care was associated with a decline in the incidence of diabetes-related nephropathy from 30% to less than 10% during this time period (23). Four different therapeutic strategies are currently clinically relevant for adolescents with incipient nephropathy:

- Improvement of glycaemic control.
- Decrease in protein intake.
- Smoking cessation.
- "Renoprotective" therapy with antihypertensive agents.

Glycaemic Control

Several studies have provided conclusive evidence that the development of microalbuminuria is associated with long-term poor metabolic control (24), with final evidence coming from the DCCT study, in both the total cohort and the adolescent subgroup [$n = 195$, age 15 (13–17 years) at the onset of the study] (25). In a study with renal biopsies of young adults ($n = 15$, mean age 18 years, diabetes duration 6–16 years) evaluating the impact of long-term metabolic control, blood pressure and initial GFR on the degree of glomerular structural changes in the transitional stage from normoalbuminuria to microalbuminuria (i.e. 15–30 μg/min), it was found that the 5 year mean HbA_{1c}, diabetes duration and the initial GFR were independent predictors of basement membrane thickness, while blood pressure did not emerge as an independent predictor (26). Even in the stage before the occurrence of permanent microalbuminuria in adolescents, a correlation between the extent of early histological abnormalities and the degree of the previous long-term metabolic compensation has been described (27). Controversy exists about whether achieving a cutpoint of control may constitute some threshold changing the rate of microvascular complications (28). In the case of a non-linear relationship, there may be a limited therapeutic window between therapy-related disturbances of the psychosocial development of children, on the one hand, and the long-term risk to develop secondary complications, on the other. An "optimal" benefit of improved control would be achieved if the long-term values of glycated haemoglobin remained below that threshold, even if not reaching an optimum. Krolewski et al (29) suggested a non-linear model for the relationship between glycaemic control and microalbuminuria, showing a steep increase beyond a HbA_{1c} value of 8.1%. Similar observations were reported from a 10-year prospective study in 211 patients from the Steno Memorial Hospital (30). The issue of a glycaemic threshold remains controversial and even the most recent additional analyses from the DCCT group argued against its presence (31).

In a study following young patients with renal biopsies, improving glycaemic control slowed down the further advancement of histologic changes (32). Moreover, in a 10-year follow-up of 109 young adult patients (mean age at baseline, 17 years), 15 of 27 patients initially showing microalbuminuria were normoalbuminuric upon follow-up (17). These patients were able to improve their glycaemic control from baseline to follow-up (mean HbA_{1c}, 7.5–6.6%, $p = 0.01$). Despite the efforts of paediatric diabetologists all over the world, however, one can extrapolate from the multinational, multicentre Hvidore Childhood Diabetes Study that the desired level of control (i.e. HbA_{1c} below 8%) is currently not reached by more than half of children living in countries with advanced medical care (33).

Smoking Cessation

Cigarette smoking has been demonstrated as an important independent variable for the development of microalbuminuria for 20 years. In a group of young adults (mean age, 20 years; diabetes duration, 11 years) with pathological albuminuria and high normal AER ($> 7.6\,\mu g/min$), smokers had a 2.2-fold risk for progression of albuminuria, which remained significant after correction for other confounding factors, such as HbA_1 (34). Although there is evidence that addictive behaviour may be less frequent in adolescents with diabetes than in their peers, tobacco consumption is prevalent in a substantial number of young adults with diabetes (35) and should be addressed and discouraged as early as possible. Nevertheless, the limited success of such interventions has been discouraging.

Reduction the Dietary Protein Content

Dietary protein intake influences the glomerular filtration rate through prostaglandin effects. In addition, high protein diets are associated with elevated renin levels, which have also been described to be related to nephropathy in adolescents with diabetes (36). In a recent meta-analysis of five studies of protein restriction in a total of 108 patients with type I diabetes and nephropathy, a positive effect comparable to that in non-diabetic renal diseases was shown (37). It appeared to be independent of glycaemic control and blood pressure. However, only one study included normotensive patients, with microalbuminuria exhibiting a 10% reduction from the baseline AER during 24 months of a diet with a protein intake of 0.68 g/kg body weight/day. Two major problems are associated with a prescription of such a diet to adolescents, namely protein/calorie malnutrition and compliance. Even in adults, the achieved protein content was 0.23 g/kg/day higher than that prescribed (38). The problem of protein malnutrition may be pertinent, especially for growing children. A protein intake of 1 g/kg/day is also sufficient in growing children, while in most children in industrialized countries the protein content is approximately 20% of the daily caloric intake, i.e. 1.5–2.0 g/kg. No data is available on whether a reduction of protein to 12% of the total caloric intake would be feasible and beneficial in adolescents at risk for nephropathy, but these aspects may be considered during the individual consultation. Such a meal composition can only be reached in a more or less vegetarian diet. In any case, there is a heterogeneity in the response of GFR following the introduction of a low protein diet (39); thus, the potential therapeutic effect should be monitored and "non-responders" could continue with their normal diet.

Antihypertensive and "Renoprotective" Pharmacological Treatment

There is abundant evidence for the importance of haemodynamic changes in the pathogenesis of nephropathy. Associational studies in young people have indicated that the presence of high-normal diastolic blood pressure results in a higher incidence of microalbuminuria (40). Moreover, higher blood pressure during adolescence predisposes to the later development of advanced nephropathy. Early echocardiographic signs of diabetes-related cardiomyopathy in young adults with a mean age of 18 years were found to be associated with increased blood pressure and microalbuminuria (41). It remains controversial, however, whether elevated blood pressure is a concomitant or secondary phenomenon (18) or whether it contributes independently to the development of microalbuminuria. Recently, a matched-pairs study indicated significantly higher blood pressure values in adolescents 3 years prior to the detection of microalbuminuria compared to age- and diabetes-matched controls, who remained normoalbuminuric (42). Therefore, blood pressure, "tracking", i.e. follow-up of periodic random measurements at every clinic visit appears to be important for the early detection of consistent blood pressure increases within the normal percentiles predisposing to overt hypertension and diabetes-related nephropathy (43).

A practical problem has been so-called "white-coat hypertension", referring to elevated blood pressure measurements caused by the medical consultation (44). Ambulatory 24 hour blood pressure measurement (ABPM) allows such patients to be distinguished from those with true hypertension. Therefore, ABPM should be performed in every patient with blood pressure values above the respective age-(height-)related 90th centile of systolic or diastolic blood pressure before hypertension is suspected and treated. Normal values of ABPM for the paediatric age group have now been established (45). A comparison of daytime means of both systolic and diastolic blood pressure of ABPM with random office values indicated that systolic office values in particular are frequently overrated (1). In addition, ABPM allows the physiological nocturnal blood pressure dip to be evaluated; this may be severely blunted in patients with diabetes-related autonomic dysfunction (46). This blunted nocturnal decline has also been described in the transitional phase from normoalbuminuria to micro-albuminuria (47). Preliminary data showed an association between 24 h blood pressure levels, basement membrane thickness and mesangial volume in normoalbuminuric adolescents, where nocturnal "non-dippers" had the worst glomerular changes (48). However, it is controversial whether this blood pressure abnormality is related to microalbuminuria in young patients (44).

There remains some debate whether ACE-inhibitors are superior to other antihypertensive medications for the treatment of arterial hypertension in adults with diabetes concerning the progression of diabetic nephropathy. Recently a group of experts in diabetic nephropathy have recommended ACE-inhibitor treatment also for normotensive patients, suggesting that this may have some renoprotective effect (11). This treatment has also been recommended for the paediatric age group (6).

In a placebo-controlled study, a 3-monthly treatment with ACE-inhibitors was able to reduce microalbuminuria in 10 of 12 normotensive adolescents with diabetes (49). There remains no doubt that ACE-inhibitors are able to reduce the albumin excretion rate also in young patients with diabetes. However, the change in the GFR is a more suitable surrogate endpoint for the follow-up of pharmacological intervention than the albumin excretion rate. However, none of the studies to date have shown convincingly that this treatment ameliorates the change of GFR. It has to be kept in mind that the longest follow-up trial in young normotensive patients with microalbuminuria has been 8 years (50), showing significant differences in the rate of development of macroproteinuria (9/23 in the control vs. 2/21 in the captopril group) but no differences in the GFR between both groups. Although there is widespread experience in the paediatric age group and ACE-inhibitor therapy has been associated with few side effects, long-term data evaluating the impact of potential side effects of treatment and the influence on end stage renal disease and mortality are lacking. In particular the absence of a clear-cut effect on GFR in the long-term studies is troubling.

Therefore, the decision to start a pharmacological treatment of microalbuminuria in adolescents should always be made individually (21). Non-pharmacological aspects, such as improved glycaemic control, reduced protein intake and discouragement from smoking, should require primary consideration. In the case of elevated blood pressure values, a thorough evaluation of potential non-diabetes-related causes for arterial hypertension is mandatory. The results of at least three determinations of the albumin excretion rate (preferably timed collections under standardized conditions), routine check-up for the presence of other diabetes-related complications (especially retinal changes) and risk factors for microangiopathy (1) and the ambulatory 24 h blood pressure profile should be the basis for a decision.

Although it is likely that better glycaemic control during childhood would have prevented the onset of incipient nephropathy, one has to keep in mind that normoglycaemia frequently can not be reached in the paediatric age group (33). Therefore, additional therapeutic options have to be initiated, as has been outlined above. In view of the multiplicity of medical, but also pedagogical and psychological aspects of paediatric diabetology, it appears likely that the current therapeutic optimum may only be reached by a competent multidisciplinary team in centres with expertise for the care of children and adolescents supporting local practitioners. It is one of the tasks for the future to join all efforts in order to provide access to such treatment facilities for all children with diabetes, and to reduce the impact of diabetic nephropathy on the prognosis of childhood-onset type 1 diabetes.

REFERENCES

1. Danne T, Kordonouri O, Hövener G, Weber B. Diabetic angiopathy in children. *Diabet Med* 1997; **14**: 1012–25.
2. Silverstein JH, Fenell R, Donelly W et al. Correlates of biopsy-studied nephropathy in young patients with insulin dependent diabetes mellitus. *J Pediatr* 1985; **106**: 196–201.
3. Bangstad HJ, Osterby R, Dahl-Jorgensen K et al. Early glomerulopathy is present in young, type 1 (insulin-dependent) diabetic patients with microalbuminuria. *Diabetologia* 1993; **36**: 523–9.
4. Mortensen HB, Hougaard P, Ibsen KK et al. A nationwide cross-sectional study of urinary albumin excretion rate, arterial blood pressure and blood glucose control in Danish children with type 1 diabetes. *Diabet Med* 1990; **7**: 887–97.
5. Joner G, Brinchmann-Hansen O, Torres CG, Hanssen KF. A nationwide cross-sectional study of retinopathy and microalbuminuria in young Norwegian type 1 (insulin-dependent) diabetic patients. *Diabetologia* 1992; **35**: 1049–54.

6. Mortensen HB. Microalbuminuria in young patients with type 1 diabetes. *In The Kidney and Hypertension in Diabetes Mellitus*, 3rd edn, Mogensen CE ed. Kluwer Academic: Boston, 1996; 331–340.
7. Dahlquist G, Rudberg S. The prevalence of microalbuminuria in diabetic children and adolescents and its relation to puberty. *Acta Pediatr Scand* 1987; **76**: 795–800.
8. Jones CA, Leese GP, Kerr S et al. Development and progression of microalbuminuria in a clinic sample of patients with insulin dependent diabetes mellitus. *Arch Dis Child* 1998; **78**: 518–23.
9. Cummings EA, Sochett EB, Dekker MG, Lawson ML, Daneman D. Contribution of growth hormone and IGF-1 to early diabetic nephropathy in type 1 diabetes. *Diabetes* 1998; **47**: 1341–6.
10. Barkai L, Vamosi I, Lukacs K. Enhanced progression of urinary albumin excretion in IDDM during puberty. *Diabet Care* 1998; **21**: 1019–23.
11. Mogensen CE, Keane WF, Bennett PH et al. Prevention of diabetic renal disease with special reference to microalbuminuria. *Lancet* 1995; **346**: 1080–84.
12. Mogensen CE, Vestbo E, Logstrup Poulsen P et al. Microalbuminuria and potential confounders. A review and some observations on variability of urinary albumin excretion. *Diabet Care* 1995; **18**: 572–81.
13. Houser MT, Jahn MF, Kobayashi A, Walburn J. Assessment of urinary protein excretion in the adolescent: effect of body position and exercise. *J Pediatr* 1986; **109**: 556–61.
14. Klipping, E, Danne T, Weber B. Nächtliche Albuminausscheidung unterhalb der Albustix-Grenze bei gesunden Kindern und Jugendlichen (abstr). *Akt Endokr Stoffw* 1989; **10**: 103.
15. Kordonouri O, Hartmann R, Müller C, Danne T, Weber B. Predictive value of tubular markers for the development of microalbuminuria in adolescents with diabetes. *Horm Res* 1998; **50**: 23–7.
16. Kordonouri O, Hopfenmüller W, Danne T, Müller C, Weber B. Proteinuria of glomerular and tubular origin: risk factors for the development of diabetic nephropathy? In *Structural and Functional Abnormalities in Subclinical Diabetic Angiopathy*, Weber B, Burger W, Danne T (eds). Karger: Basel, *Pediatr Adolesc Endocr* 1992; **22**: 117–23.
17. Bojestig M, Arnquist HJ, Karlberg BE, Ludvigsson J. Glycemic control and prognosis in type I diabetic patients with microalbuminuria. *Diabet Care* 1996; **19**: 313–17.
18. Rudberg S, Ullman E, Dahlqiust G. Relationship between early metabolic control and the development of microalbuminuria—a longitudinal study in children with type 1 (insulin-dependent) diabetes. *Diabetologia* 1993; **36**: 1309–14.
19. Mullis P, Köchli HP, Zuppinger K, Schwarz HP. Intermittent microalbuminuria in children with type 1 diabetes mellitus without clinical evidence of nephropathy. *Eur J Pediatr* 1988; **147**: 385–8.
20. Rudberg S, Dahlquist G. Determinants of progression to microalbuminuria in adolescents with IDDM. *Diabet Care* 1996; **19**: 369–71.
21. Danne T, Kordonouri O. Controversis in the pathogenesis of diabetic angiopathy: which treatment for normotensive adolescents with microalbuminuria and type 1 diabetes. *J Pediatr Endocrinol Metab* 1998; **11** (2): 347–63.
22. The Diabetes Control and Complications Study Group. Clustering of long-term complications in families with diabetes in the diabetes control and complications trial. *Diabetes* 1997; **46**: 1829–39.

23. Bojestig M, Arnqvist HJ, Hermansson G, Karlberg BE, Ludvigsson J. Declining incidence of nephropathy in insulin-dependent diabetes mellitus. *N Engl J Med* 1994; **330**: 15–18.
24. Norgaard K, Storm B, Grae M, Feldt-Rasmussen B. Elevated albumin excretion and retinal changes in children with type I diabetes are related to long-term poor blood glucose control. *Diabet Med* 1989; **6**: 325–8.
25. DCCT Research Group. Effect of intensive diabetes treatment on the development and progression of long-term complications in adolescents with insulin-dependent diabetes mellitus: Diabetes Control and Complications Trial. *J Pediatr* 1994; **125**: 177–88.
26. Rudberg S, Osterby R, Dahlquist G, Nyberg G, Persson B. Predictors of renal morphological changes in the early stage of microalbuminuria in adolescents with IDDM. *Diabet Care* 1997; **20**: 265–71.
27. Berg UB, Torbjörnsdotter TB, Jaremko G, Thalme B. Kidney and morphological changes in relation to long-term renal function and metabolic control in adolescents with IDDM. *Diabetologia* 1998; **41**: 1047–56.
28. Danne Th, Weber B, Dinesen B, Mortensen HB. Threshold of HbA1c for the effect of hyperglycemia on the risk of diabetic microangiopathy (letter). *Diabet Care* 1996; **19**: 183.
29. Krolewski AS, Laffel LMB, Krolewski M, Quinn M, Warram JH. Glycosylated haemoglobin and the risk of microalbuminuria in patients with insulin-dependent diabetes mellitus. *N Engl J Med* 1995; **332**: 1251–5.
30. Mathiesen ER, Ronn B, Strom B, Foght V, Deckert T. The natural course of microalbuminuria in insulin-dependent diabetes: a ten year prospective study. *Diabet Med* 1995; **12**: 482–7.
31. DCCT Research Group. The absence of a glycemic threshold for the development of long-term complications: the perspective of the Diabetes Control and Complications Trial. *Diabetes* 1996; **45**: 1289–98.
32. Bangstad HJ, Osterby R, Dahl-Jorgensen K et al. Improvement of blood glucose control in IDDM patients retards the progression of morphological changes in early diabetic nephropathy. *Diabetologia* 1994; **37**: 483–90.
33. Mortensen HB, Hougaard P, for the Hvidore Study Group on Childhood Diabetes. Comparison of metabolic control in a cross-sectional study of 2873 children and adolescents with insulin-dependent diabetes from 18 nations. *Diabet Care* 1997; **20**: 714–20.
34. Chase HP, Garg SK, Marshall G et al. Cigarette smoking increases the risk of albuminuria among subjects with type 1 diabetes. *J Am—Hed Assoc* 1991; **265**: 614–17.
35. Masson EA, MacFarlane IA, Priestley CJ, Wallymahmed ME, Flavell HJ. Failure to prevent nicotine addiction in young people with diabetes. *Arch Dis Child* 1992; **67**: 100–102.
36. Daneman D, Crompton CH, Balfe JW et al. Plasma prorenin as an early marker of nephropathy in diabetic (IDDM) adolescents. *Kidney Int* 1994; **46**: 1154–9.
37. Pedrini MT, Levey AS, Lau J, Chalmers TC, Wang PH. The effect of dietary protein restriction on the progression of diabetic and non-diabetic renal diseases. *Ann Int Med* 1996; **124**: 627–32.
38. Locatelli F, Alberti D, Graziani G et al. Prospective randomized multicentre trial of effect of protein restriction on progression of chronic renal insufficiency. *Lancet* 1991; **337**: 1299–304.
39. Walker JD, Bendig JJ, Dodds RA et al. Restriction of dietary protein and progression of renal failure in diabetic nephropathy. *Lancet* 1989; **ii**: 1411–14.

40. Mortensen HB, Hougaard P, Ibsen KK et al. Relationship between blood pressure and urinary excretion rate in young Danish type 1 diabetic patients: comparison to non-diabetic children. *Diabetic Med* 1994; **11**: 155–61.
41. Kimball TR, Daniels SR, Khoury PR et al. Cardiovascular status in young patients with insulin-dependent diabetes mellitus. *Circulation* 1994; **90**: 357–61.
42. Kordonouri O, Danne T, Hopfenmüller W et al. Lipid profiles and blood pressure: are they risk factors for the developemt of early background retinopathy and incipient nephropathy in children with insulin-dependent diabetes mellitus? *Acta Paediatr* 1996; **85**: 43–8.
43. Virdis R, Vanelli M, Street M et al. Blood pressure tracking in adolescents with insulin-dependent diabetes mellitus. *J Hum Hypertens* 1994; **8**: 313–17.
44. Holl RW, Pavlovic M, Heinze E, Thon A. Circadian blood pressure during the early course of type 1 diabetes. Analysis of 1011 ambulatory blood pressure recordings in 354 adolescents and young adults. *Diabet Care* 1999; **22**: 1151–7.
45. Soergel M, Kirschstein M, Busch C et al. Oscillometric twenty-four hour ambulatory blood pressure values in healthy children and adolescents: a multicenter trial including 1141 subjects. *J Pediatr* 1997; **130**: 178–84.
46. Madacsy L, Yasar A, Tulassay T et al. Relative nocturnal hypertension in children with insulin-dependent diabetes mellitus. *Acta Paediatr* 1994; **83**: 414–17.
47. Poulsen PI, Hansen KW, Mogensen CE. Ambulatory blood pressure in the transition from normo-to microalbuminuria, a longitudinal study in IDDM patients. *Diabetes* 1995; **43**: 1248–53.
48. Rudberg S, Osterby R. Diabetic glomerulopathy in young IDDM patients. Preventive and diagnostic aspects. Horm Res 1998; **50** (1): 17–22.
49. Cook J, Daneman D, Spino M Angiotensin converting enzyme inhibitor therapy to decrease microalbuminuria in normotensive children with diabetes mellitus. *J Pediatr* 1990; **117**: 39–45.
50. Mathiesen ER, Hommel E, Smith U, Parving HH. Efficacy of captopril in normotensive diabetic patients with microalbuminuria—8 years follow-up (abstr). *Diabetologia* 1995; **38**: 1746.
51. Mathiesen ER, Saurbrey N, Hommel E, Parving HH. Prevalence of microalbuminuria in children with type 1 (insulin-dependent) diabetes mellitus. *Diabetologia* 1986; **29**: 640–643.

7

Genetic Predictors and Markers of Diabetic Nephropathy

RUGGERO MANGILI

Istituto Scientifico San Raffaele, Milano, Italy

The idea that genetic factors may play a role in the pathogenesis of diabetic nephropathy was first outlined almost two decades ago by studies in prospective cohorts of patients with insulin-dependent diabetes mellitus (IDDM). Should the onset of long-term complications of diabetes be a simple function of exposure to hyperglycaemia, a linear relationship of their cumulative incidence with time would be expected. In fact, the cumulative incidence of diabetic retinopathy is a linear function of the duration of diabetes, with a potential for the recruitment of all patients after about 50 years of metabolic abnormalities (1). In contrast, the cumulative incidence of persistent proteinuria rises until about 30 years of duration of diabetes but levels off thereafter, leaving over 50% of the patients free from the destiny of endstage renal failure despite poor glycaemic control. In other words, one or more among the metabolic abnormalities of diabetes can trigger kidney disease by an unknown pathogenic mechanism that operates in susceptible individuals and is defective among the majority, who are protected from this complication.

The contribution of genetic factors to this phenomenon has been emphasized by the observation of a strong family clustering of nephropathy, both in IDDM and in non-insulin-dependent diabetes mellitus (NIDDM), e.g. (2, 3). Interestingly, raised urinary albumin excretion *per se* can be heritable

Diabetic Nephropathy. Edited by C. Hasslacher.
© 2001 John Wiley & Sons, Ltd.

among the non-diabetic first-degree relatives of patients with NIDDM (4). Furthermore, an association of diabetic nephropathy with family history of conditions that are known to be compounded by heritable components, such as essential hypertension, cardiovascular disease and type 2 diabetes, has been recently confirmed (5–7). Understanding the nature of this genetic component is not a mere academic point. As extensively discussed elsewhere in this book, both the onset and the progression of renal disease can be favourably modulated by therapeutic interventions, but cannot be halted at any stage of diabetic nephropathy. Thus, there is hope that studies of the genetic background may lead to understanding the pathogenesis of diabetic nephropathy, to develop markers of susceptibility and to tailor more effective preventive strategies in the subset of patients with a poor renal prognosis.

There are two general strategies to analyse the genetic component in diabetic nephropathy. A conservative approach stems from the phenotype to detect the genotype, and is defined as "functional cloning". This examines the phenotypic level and the intermediate phenotypes of diabetic nephropathy in the hope of clarifying the pathogenesis of this complication, identifying the molecular abnormalities that are involved, and to identify the corresponding genes to explain genetic susceptibility on a pathophysiologic basis.

Although this approach remains very important, the progressive increase in knowledge and availability of molecular biology techniques has more recently given the possibility of investigating and scanning the human genome to characterize alleles at known loci and their genotype frequency and distribution, and to examine their association with the phenotype. By this approach, much is termed "positional cloning", one can identify the chromosomal regions that are likely to contain the genes responsible for diabetic renal disease and also look for the corresponding biological defects. As a straightforward outcome, qualitative markers of susceptibility may be identified and may become relevant to clinical practice even before the molecular and biochemical abnormalities of pathogenic relevance are understood.

These strategies are not mutually exclusive and they will eventually merge. This review will discuss the intermediate phenotypes of diabetic nephropathy and will summarize the candidate genes examined in diabetic nephropathy, to set current knowledge in perspective and briefly mention methodological issues.

INTERMEDIATE PHENOTYPES OF DIABETIC NEPHROPATHY

Given that diabetic nephropathy can be partly due to an inherited component, the characterization of an intermediate phenotype of nephropathy should, in principle, follow evidence of a family distribution of the corresponding abnormality, so that heritable components can be suggested to predominate on the environmental determinants of the molecular abnormality.

So far, the only variable that fulfils the above definition is the activity rate of erythrocyte sodium–lithium countertransport (SLC), which has been shown to be elevated in both IDDM and NIDDM patients with nephropathy (8). Elevated SLC activity is a quantitative genetic trait and is the most consistent cation transport abnormality that associates with an increased risk of essential hypertension (9). Smaller studies have also shown a similar parental component in IDDM (10, 11). Furthermore, there is evidence that potential environmental confounders of this abnormality, such as poor glycaemic control and serum triglycerides, do not account for the elevated activity rates found in diabetic nephropathy (12, 13). Finally, two prospective studies have recently reported that progression to microalbuminuria can be predicted by elevated SLC activity rates, suggesting that this abnormality can precede nephropathy, independent of poor glycaemic control (14, 15). However, a considerable overlap in the distribution of SLC rates between cases and controls is usually present (12), and heterogeneity in the relatively complex measurement techniques made this a controversial issue (8). Such factors pose limitations to the use of this abnormality as a marker of susceptibility. Furthermore, the molecular mediator of this transport is not known. Functional cation transport studies have recently suggested the molecular independence of SLC from the amiloride-sensitive isoform 1 of the sodium–hydrogen exchanger (NHE-1) (16). This can in fact mediate sodium–lithium exchange but, unlike SLC, NHE-1 is phloretin-insensitive. Similar studies have recently described a novel phloretin-sensitive (and amiloride-insensitive) NHE activity in human erythrocytes (17), as well as a novel sodium–lithium exchange of human skin fibroblasts that may be functionally similar to SLC, based on a majority of kinetic properties and on its sensitivity to inhibitors (18). It is to be hoped that the genes that codify for these exchangers can soon be cloned, offering the possibility of learning more about their pathophysiology and relevance to SLC, and the genetic background of diabetic nephropathy.

Some of the abnormalities that have been associated to diabetic nephropathy can be observed in case-control studies of cultured cells, e.g. skin fibroblasts or immortalized lymphoblasts, after several passages *in vitro*. Under the assumption that growth *in vitro*, using standardized media for a few weeks, can be enough to remove the influence of previous (*in vivo*) environment, a predominantly genetic component of these abnormalities can be postulated. This is the case for the elevated activity of NHE-1 and excess proliferation rate. Several studies have shown that these abnormalities appear to characterize diabetic nephropathy (19–21), as well as essential hypertension in non-diabetic individuals (22). In particular, elevated activity of the amiloride-sensitive NHE-1 has been found also in fresh cells, such as erythrocytes and circulating lymphomonocyte preparations, and has been suggested to predict the progression from normoalbuminuria to microalbuminuria by a prospective study in IDDM (23), thus paralleling the above-mentioned findings for SLC.

However, both the pathophysiology of cell growth and the molecular nature and regulation of the amiloride-sensitive NHE-1 are better known, and are functionally linked by the increase in NHE activity that parallels cell growth and replication in response to growth factors or mitogenic stimuli (24).

Whether this may be relevant to one or more among the growth factor receptors or to the complex intracellular mitogen-activated protein-kinase signalling pathways (25), dependent either on tyrosine kinase or on G-proteins, must be established. For example, excess NHE-1 activity seems to be due to overphosphorylation of the exchanger in essential hypertension (26) but not in diabetic nephropathy (20). More recently, overactivity of NHE-1 has been associated with enhanced signal transduction due to pertussis toxin-sensitive G proteins in cells from patients with essential hypertension (27), possibly in association with a polymorphism in exon 10, which encodes the β3 subunit of the molecule (28). Cells from patients with diabetic nephropathy also exhibit enhanced signal transduction through this pathway (29), but the corresponding polymorphism seems to show no linkage with this phenotype (30). Thus, despite similarity in the intermediate phenotype, two clinical conditions may recognize diverse molecular determinants and genetic factors. In the process of understanding the molecular mechanisms of complex genetic diseases, this is the point where future studies will have to weigh the contribution of candidate genes, not only to the phenotype but also to the derangement of cellular and biochemical functions, i.e. the intermediate phenotypes, which are suspected to play a pathogenetic role. The recent development of the differential display technique (31) gives the possibility of addressing the differential expression of genes in cells from probands, as compared to the cells of control patients. Hopefully, this will provide a considerable expansion in our knowledge of the intermediate phenotypes of diabetic nephropathy.

LINKAGE ANALYSIS WITH CANDIDATE GENES

Before undertaking the genetic analysis of a disease, one should ideally have a heritability estimate of the phenotype, in order to establish whether the phenotype is determined by a major gene effect or by a polygenic effect (with several genes that add to determine the phenotype). Unfortunately, diabetic nephropathy cannot be thoroughly analysed in this respect, because access to several pedigrees in which all of the family members express diabetes is necessary to dissect the heritability of nephropathy. Such pedigrees are exceedingly rare in the Caucasoid population, and only among the secluded population of the Pima Indians is the prevalence of diabetes sufficiently high to allow the observation of such families (32). However, the high degree of concordance (about 70%) in renal destiny among sib-pairs with IDDM (2) seems to allow speculation that a major gene may be involved in conferring susceptibility to nephropathy, with the contribution of some minor gene effects (33). In general, the larger the effect of a major gene on the phenotype, the smaller the sample size required for detection. Under this assumption, several groups have addressed the identification of a major gene effect by the candidate gene approach.

The simplest method for a candidate gene study accounts for a cross-sectional, case-control design, where the allelic and genotypic distribution of the candidate gene among cases (usually about 200) are compared with those of a similar number of control patients at low risk of developing nephropathy because of the persistence of normoalbuminuria and normal renal function after a long duration of diabetes. This design has the advantage of feasibility, as it requires at most a few outpatient clinics in order to select a sufficiently large population of patients. The choice of an appropriate gene is an obviously essential part of this task, but our poor knowledge of the pathogenesis of nephropathy currently allows us to base the choice most often on syllogisms. In fact, the rationale to nominate a gene for association with diabetic nephropathy may not strictly follow the derangements that are found in cellular pathophysiology. For example, diabetic nephropathy occurs only in diabetic patients, and both IDDM and NIDDM are known to have strong genetic components. Thus, it could be postulated that the genes predisposing to nephropathy can be partially in linkage disequilibrium with those that predispose to diabetes. This idea has been particularly supported in favour of genes predisposing to insulin resistance, in view of the recent finding of a higher prevalence of non-insulin-dependent diabetes among the parents of probands with insulin-dependent diabetes and nephropathy than among the parents of normoalbuminuric patients with insulin-dependent diabetes of long duration (7).

Similar syllogisms apply to identifying several other genes. Many are those that are progressively found to associate with essential hypertension and cardiovascular disease, but also those which could theoretically lead to abnormal glucose metabolism (e.g. genes in the aldose reductase region, or those that may affect the catabolism of advanced glycation end-products), and those that may regulate the metabolism of the structural components of the mesangial matrix and glomerular endothelial basement membranes, such as proteoglycans. The rationale for setting each one of these items in perspective has been detailed a few years ago (1) and can be found in other chapters of this book.

Examples of the polymorphisms that have been addressed over the past few years are provided in Table 7.1, and this list may increase considerably in the near future. Unfortunately, most studies have provided controversial or negative results. The insertion/deletion (I/D) polymorphism of intron 16 of the angiotensin-converting enzyme gene was the first candidate gene examined, with a small but significant association of the II genotype with normoalbuminuria (34). It is also for this reason that this is the most extensively investigated gene, both in IDDM and in NIDDM. Although several studies failed to reconfirm the association of nephropathy with carriers of the D allele, a recent meta-analysis has concluded that the corresponding chromosomal region may be involved in the genetic background of nephropathy (35). Also, there is evidence that, among patients with overt nephropathy, the serum levels of ACE are higher (36) and response to ACE inhibitors lower (37), among patients who are homozygous for the D allele, which appeared then to express a worse prognosis according to these initial data.

However, in a recent prospective study, the onset of microalbuminuria was more frequent among those who were homozygous for the I allele (38). Interestingly, when patients are studied with their family and parental genotypes can be accounted for, using the transmission disequilibrium test (TDT), results may be consistent with the latter finding (39). The TDT consists in the collection of DNA from the proband and both parents, but

Table 7.1 Recent association studies of genetic polymorphism with diabetic nephropathy

Gene	Chromosome	Association
Angiotensin-converting enzyme (35, 38, 39)	17q	Controversial
Angiotensinogen (45)	1q	Controversial
Angiotensin II receptor 1 (45, 47, 48)	3q	Controversial
Aldose reductase (49–51)	7q	Controversial
Methylenetetrahydrofolate reductase (52, 53)	1p	Undetected
TGF-β1 (54)	19q	Undetected
Interleukin, receptor antagonist (55–57)	2q	Controversial
β3-adrenoceptor (58, 59)	8p	Controversial
G-protein β3 subunit (30)	12p	Undetected
ANP (60, 61)	1p	Controversial
Apolipoprotein E (62, 63)	19q	Requires confirmation
Collagen IV -α (64)	13q	Undetected
Kallikrein (65)	19q	Requires confirmation
Perlecan (66)	1p	Requires confirmation
Glucose transporter 1 (67)	1p	Requires confirmation
Preliminary genomic screening data (46)	3q, 7q, 9q, 20q	Requires confirmation

only families in which both parents are heterozygous for a diallelic polymorphism of a candidate gene (as in the D/I polymorphism of the ACE
gene region) are eventually considered for analysis (40). Under these conditions, the expected allele frequency occurs among the probands of 50% for
each allele if there is no association with nephropathy. In the above study,
the II genotype was found to associate with nephropathy, particularly
among patients who developed nephropathy early in the course of IDDM
(39). A possible interpretation of these findings is that the I allele may
contribute to an early onset of nephropathy and/or to an early mortality
after the onset of nephropathy, so that the D allele may be relatively more
frequent among the survivors (35). While more studies are required to
clarify the issue, this is an outstanding example of how case-control association studies may suffer selection bias, suggesting that alternative strategies
are required. The TDT can be usefully applied to examine the association of
candidate genes, but it requires usually that the locus of the gene is specific.
Then, the methods to investigate the genetic component of complex traits
may require a different approach (41, 42).

GENOMIC SCREENING TECHNIQUES

The availability of so-called microsatellite probes and genetic markers has
made it possible to scan the human genome to identify the chromosomal
region that is likely to include the gene that links to a particular genetic trait
in a given population. This technique is valuable in the study of complex
traits (43). In brief, a microsatellite probe is a relatively short DNA sequence
that can be entirely anonymous (i.e. it does not correspond to any known
complete intronic or exonic gene), but is characterized by a unique locus
(position) in the human genome. Several microsatellite probes have been
developed that are evenly scattered along the human genome, each one thus
mapping a chromosomal region. Microsatellite probes that have polymorphism in the population are suitable for identifying the chromosomal
region that, because of linkage disequilibrium, may contain the gene that
associates with the phenotype. This can be pursued by the analysis of a
sufficient number of sib pairs that can be either concordant (41) or discordant (44) in the expression of the phenotype. The affected sib-pair analysis
tests the null hypothesis that the likelihood of sharing an allele is 50% when
the corresponding locus is not associated with nephropathy, and it is greater
than 50% when an association with nephropathy is present (41). The
discordant sib-pair analysis has been recently found to be an efficient alternative when the recurrence of the phenotype among sibs is high, as it is in
IDDM or in Pima Indians with nephropathy (44). Using these techniques,
a region in chromosome 3q, close to the gene for the angiotensin IAT1

receptor, has been suggested to include a susceptibility gene for nephr-opathy in IDDM (45). A similar result has been obtained in Pima Indians, where the chromosomal region 3q has been found of potential relevance to nephropathy, along with regions 7q, 9q and 20q (46). These exciting results should be cautiously interpreted, however, because only the conventional levels of statistical significance were obtained. In view of the very high number of chromosomal regions that are addressed in each study, allow-ance for multiple comparisons demands very high levels of significance in order to confirm linkage.

CONCLUSIONS

There is now initial evidence of the association of some genes and chromosomic region 3q with diabetic nephropathy. The selection of concordant and discordant sib-pairs in large numbers and having access to their parents seems crucial to identifying the chromosomal regions and the gene(s) predisposing to nephropathy. Accessing families for TDT in which more genes will be candidated is also essential. In this respect, the families of patients with NIDDM are less accessible. This is mainly because by the age these patients develop nephropathy, their parents have usually died. Conversely, IDDM is far less prevalent in the population, and the recruitment of useful sib-pairs and their families in sufficient numbers may require a multinational approach to obtain a sample size that will not suffer statistical power restrictions. The results of linkage studies will then require confirmation in large series of patients, and will eventually have to be consolidated in the setting of prospective studies, such as the DCCT and UKPDS, in order to calculate the relative risk expressed by the genetic markers of susceptibility and their viability in clinical practice to predict microalbuminuria and overt nephropathy.

REFERENCES

1. Doria A, Warram JH, Krolewski AS. Genetic susceptibility to nephropathy in insulin-dependent diabetes: from epidemiology to molecular genetics. *Diabet Metabol Rev* 1995; **11**: 287–314.
2. Quinn M, Angelico MC, Warram JH, Krolewski AS. Familial factors determine the development of diabetic nephropathy in patients with IDDM. *Diabetologia* 1996; **39**: 940–45.
3. Canani LH, Gerchman F, Gross JL. Familial clustering of diabetic nephropathy in Brazilian type 2 diabetic patients. *Diabetes* 1999; **48**: 909–13.

4. Gruden G, Cavallo-Perin P, Olivetti C et al. Albumin excretion rate levels in non-diabetic offspring of NIDDM patients with and without nephropathy. *Diabetologia* 1995; **38**: 1218–22.

5. Fagerudd JA, Tarnow L, Jacobsen P et al. Predisposition to essential hypertension and development of diabetic nephropathy in IDDM patients. *Diabetes* 1998; **47**: 439–44.

6. Lindsay RS, Little J, Jaap AJ et al. Diabetic nephropathy is associated with an increased familial risk of stroke. *Diabet Care* 1999; **22**: 422–5.

7. Fagerudd JA, Pettersson-Fernholm KJ, Gronhagen-Riska C, Groop PH. The impact of a family history of type II (non-insulin-dependent) diabetes mellitus on the risk of diabetic nephropathy in patients with type I (insulin-dependent) diabetes mellitus. *Diabetologia* 1999; **42**: 519–26.

8. Mangili R. Cation transport, hypertension and diabetic nephropathy. In *The Kidney and Hypertension in Diabetes Mellitus* 3rd edn, Mogensen CE (ed.). Boston: Kluwer Academic, 1997: 321–30.

9. Cirillo M, Laurenzi M, Trevisan M et al. Sodium–lithium countertransport independently predicts 6-year incidence of hypertension in the Gubbio Population Study. *J Am Soc Nephrol* 1994; **5**: 538–50.

10. Walker J, Tariq T, Viberti G. Sodium–lithium countertransport activity in red cells of patients with insulin dependent diabetes and nephropathy and their parents. *Br Med J* 1990; **301**: 635–8.

11. Chiarelli F, Verrotti A, Kalter-Leibovici O, Laron Z, Morgese G. Genetic predisposition to hypertension (as detected by Na/Li countertransport) and risk of nephropathy in childhood diabetes. *J Paediatr Child Health* 1994; **30**: 547–9.

12. Krolewski AS, Canessa M, Warram JH et al. Predisposition to hypertension and susceptibility to renal disease in insulin-dependent diabetes mellitus. *N Engl J Med* 1988; **318**: 140–45.

13. Mangili R, Zerbini G, Barlassina C, Cusi D, Pozza G. Sodium–lithium countertransport and triglycerides in diabetic nephropathy. *Kidney Int* 1993; **44**: 127–33.

14. Monciotti CG, Semplicini A, Morocutti A et al. Elevated sodium–lithium countertransport activity in erythrocytes is predictive of the development of microalbuminuria in IDDM. *Diabetologia* 1997; **40**: 654–61.

15. Chiarelli F, Catino M, Tumini S et al. Increased Na/Li countertransport activity may help to identify type 1 diabetic adolescents and young adults at risk for developing persistent microalbuminuria. *Diabet Care* 1999; **22**: 1158–64.

16. Zerbini G, Mangili R, Pozza G. Independence of dimethylamiloride-sensitive Li^+ efflux pathways and Na^+–Li^+ countertransport in human erythrocytes. *Biochim Biophys Acta* 1998; **1371**: 129–33.

17. Zerbini G, Maestroni A, Mangili R, Pozza G. Amiloride-insensitive Na^+–H^+ exchange: a candidate mediator of erythrocyte Na^+–Li^+ countertransport. *J Am Soc Nephrol* 1998; **9**: 2203–11.

18. Zerbini G, Mangili R, Gabellini D, Pozza G. Modes of operation of an electroneutral Na^+/Li^+ countertransport in human skin fibroblasts. *Am J Physiol* 1997; **272** (*Cell Physiol* **41**): C1373–9.

19. Davies J, Ng L, Kofoed-Enevoldsen A et al. Intracellular pH and Na^+/H^+ antiport activity of cultured skin fibroblasts from diabetics. *Kidney Int* 1992; **42**: 1184–90.

20. Sweeney F, Siczkowski M, Davies J et al. Phosphorylation and activity of Na/H exchanger isoform 1 of immortalized lymphoblasts in diabetic nephropathy. *Diabetes* 1995; **44**: 1180–85.

21. Lurbe A, Fioretto P, Mauer M, LaPointe MS, Battle D. Growth phenotype of cultured skin fibroblasts from patients with insulin-dependent diabetes mellitus with and without nephropathy and its association to overactivity of the Na^+/H^+ antiporter. *Kidney Int* 1996; **50**: 1684–93.
22. Rosskopf D, Frömter E, Siffert W. Hypertensive sodium-proton exchanger phenotype persists in immortalized lymphoblasts from essential hypertensive patients. *J Clin Invest* 1993; **92**: 2553–9.
23. Koren W, Koldanov R, Pronin VS et al. Enhanced erythrocyte Na^+/H^+ exchange predicts diabetic nephropathy in patients with IDDM. *Diabetologia* 1998; **41**: 201–5.
24. Noël J, Pouysségur J. Hormonal regulation, pharmacology, and membrane sorting of vertebrate Na/H exchanger isoforms. *Am J Physiol* 1995; **268**: C283–96.
25. Tomlinson DR. Mitogen-activated protein kinases as glucose transducers for diabetic complications. *Diabetologia* 1999; **42**: 1271–81.
26. Ng LL, Sweeney FP, Siczkowski M et al. Na^+-H^+ antiporter phenotype, abundance and phosphorylation of immortalized lymphoblasts from humans with hypertension. *Hypertension* 1995; **25**: 971–7.
27. Siffert W. G proteins and hypertension: an alternative candidate gene approach. *Kidney Int* 1998; **53**: 1466–70.
28. Siffert W, Rosskopf D, Siffert G et al. Association of a G protein β3 subunit variant with hypertension. *Nature Genet* 1998; **18**: 45–8.
29. Pietruck F, Spleiter S, Daul A et al. Enhanced G protein activation in diabetic nephropathy. *Diabetologia* 1998; **41**: 94–100.
30. Fogarty DG, Zychma MJ, Scott L, Warram JH, Krolewski AS. Polymorphism in the human G-protein β3 subunit gene and diabetic nephropathy in IDDM. *Diabetologia* 1998; **41**: 1304–8.
31. Page R, Morris C, Williams J, von Ruhland C, Malik AN. Isolation of diabetes-associated kidney genes using differnetial display. *Biochem Biophys Res Commun* 1997; **232**: 49–53.
32. Pettitt DJ, Saad MF, Bennett PH, Nelson RG, Knowler WC. Family predisposition to renal disease in two generations of Pima Indians with type 2 (non-insulin-dependent) diabetes mellitus. *Diabetologia* 1990; **33**: 438–43.
33. Krolewski AS. Genetics of diabetic nephropathy: evidence for major and minor gene effects. *Kidney Int* 1999; **55**: 1582–96.
34. Marre M, Bernadet P, Gallois Y et al. Relationships between angiotensin I converting enzyme gene polymorphism, plasma levels and diabetic retinal and renal complications. *Diabetes* 1994; **43**: 384–8.
35. Fujisawa T, Ikegami H, Kawaguchi I et al. Meta-analysis of association of insertion/deletion polymorphism of angiotensin I-converting enzyme gene with diabetic nephropathy and retinopathy. *Diabetologia* 1998; **41**: 47–53.
36. Villard E, Tiret L, Visvikis S et al. Identification of new polymorphisms of the angiotensin I converting enzyme (ACE) gene, and study of their relationship to plasma ACE levels by two-QTL segregation-linkage analysis. *Am J Hum Genet* 1996; **58**: 1268–78.
37. Parving HH, Jacobsen P, Tarnow L et al. Effect of deletion polymorphism of angiotensin converting enzyme gene on progression of diabetic nephropathy during inhibition of angiotensin converting enzyme: observational follow-up study. *Br Med J* 1996; **313**: 591–4.
38. Penno G, Chaturvedi N, Talmudd PJ et al. Effect of angiotensin-converting enzyme (ACE) gene polymorphism on progression of renal disease and the influence of ACE inhibition in IDDM patients. *Diabetes* 1998; **47**: 1507–11.

39. Rogus JJ, Moczulski DK, Freire MB et al. Diabetic nephropathy is associated with AGT polymorphism T235: results of a family-based study. *Hypertension* 1998; **31**: 627–31.
40. Spielman RS, Mcginnis RE, Exens WJ. Transmission test for linkage disequilibrium: the insulin gene region and insulin-dependent diabetes mellitus (IDDM). *Am J Hum Genet* 1993; **52**: 506–16.
41. Lander E, Schork N. Genetic dissection of complex traits. *Science* 1994; **265**: 2037–48.
42. Clerget-Darpoux F. Overview of strategies for complex genetic diseases. *Kidney Int* 1998; **53**: 1441–5.
43. Risch N, Merikangas K. The future of genetic studies of complex human diseases. *Science* 1996; **273**: 1516–17.
44. Rogus JJ, Krolewski AS. Using discordant sib pairs to map loci for qualitative traits with high sibling recurrence risk. *Am J Hum Genet* 1996; **59**: 1376–81.
45. Moczulski DK, Rogus JJ, Antonellis A, Warram JH, Krolewski AS. Major susceptibility locus for nephropathy in type 1 diabetes on chromosome 3q. *Diabetes* 1998; **47**: 1164–9.
46. Imperatore G, Hanson RL, Pettitt DJ et al. Sib-pair linkage analysis for susceptibility genes for microvascular complications among Pima Indians with type 2 diabetes. *Diabetes* 1998; **47**: 821–30.
47. Doria A, Onuma T, Warram JH, Krolewski AS. Synergistic effect of angiotensin II type 1 receptor genotype and poor glycaemic control on risk of nephropathy in IDDM. *Diabetologia* 1997; **40**: 1293–9.
48. Chowdhury TA, Dyer PH, Kumar S et al. Lack of association of angiotensin II type 1 receptor gene polymorphism with diabetic nephropathy in insulin-dependent diabetes mellitus. *Diabet Med* 1997; **14**: 837–40.
49. Maeda S, Haneda M, Yasuda H et al. Diabetic nephropathy is not associated with the dinucleotide repeat polymorphism upstream of the aldose reductase (ALR2) gene but with erythrocyte aldose reductase content in Japanese subjects with type 2 diabetes. *Diabetes* 1999; **48**: 420–22.
50. Moczulski DK, Burak W, Doria A et al. The role of aldose reductase gene in the susceptibility to diabetic nephropathy in type II (non-insulin-dependent) diabetes mellitus. *Diabetologia* 1999; **42**: 94–7.
51. Heesom AE, Hibberd ML, Millward A, Demaine AG. Polymorphism of the 5′-end of the aldose reductase gene is strongly associated with the development of diabetic nephropathy in type 1 diabetes. *Diabetes* 1997; **46**: 287–91.
52. Bluthner M, Bruntgens A, Schmidt S et al. Association of methylenetetrahydrofolate reductase gene polymorphism and diabetic nephropathy in type 2 diabetes? *Nephrol Dialysis Transpl* 1999; **14**: 56–7.
53. Odawara M, Yamashita K. A common mutation of the methylenetetrahydrofolate reductase gene as a risk factor for diabetic nephropathy. *Diabetologia* 1999; **42**: 631.
54. Pociot F, Hansen PM, Karlsen AE et al. TGF-beta1 gene mutations in insulin-dependent diabetes mellitus and diabetic nephropathy. *J Am Soc Nephrol* 1998; **9**: 2302–7.
55. Blakemore AIF, Cox A, Gonzalez AM et al. Interleukin-1 receptor antagonist allele (IL-1RN*2) associated with nephropathy in diabetes mellitus. *Hum Genet* 1996; **97**: 369–74.
56. Loughrey BV, Maxwell AP, Fogarty DG et al. An interleukin 1B allele, which correlates with a high secretor phenotype, is associated with diabetic nephropathy. *Cytokine* 1998; **10**: 984–8.

57. Tarnow L, Pociot F, Hansen PM et al. Polymorphisms in the interleukin-1 gene cluster do not contribute to the genetic susceptibility of diabetic nephropathy in Caucasian patients with IDDM. *Diabetes* 1997; **46**: 1075–6.
58. Sakane N, Yoshida T, Yoshioka K et al. Trp64Arg mutation of β3 adrenoceptor gene is associated with diabetic nephropathy in type II diabetes mellitus. *Diabetologia* 1998; **41**: 1533–4.
59. Grzeszczak W, Saucha W, Zychma MJ et al. Is Trp64Arg polymorphism of β3-adrenergic receptor a clinically useful marker for the predisposition to diabetic nephropathy in type II diabetic patients? *Diabetologia* 1999; **42**: 632.
60. Nannipieri M, Penno G, Pucci L et al. Pronatriodilatin gene polymorphisms, microvascular permeability and diabetic nephropathy in type 1 diabetes mellitus. *J Am Soc Nephrol* 1999; **10**: 1530–41.
61. Schmidt S, Bluthner M, Giessel R et al. A polymorphism in the gene for the atrial natriuretic peptide and diabetic nephropathy. *Nephrol Dialysis Transpl* 1998; **13**: 1807–10.
62. Werle E, Fiehn W, Hasslacher C. Apolipoprotein E polymorphism and renal function in German type 1 and type 2 diabetic patients. *Diabet Care* 1998; **21**: 994–8.
63. Kimura H, Suzuki Y, Gejyo F et al. Apolipoprotein E4 reduces risk of nephropathy in patients with NIDDM. *Am J Kidney Dis* 1998; **31**: 666–73.
64. Chen JW, Hansen PM, Tarnow L et al. Genetic variation of a collagen IV alpha-1 chain gene polymorphism in Danish insulin-dependent diabetes mellitus (IDDM) patients: lack of association to nephropathy and proliferative retinopathy. *Diabet Med* 1997; **14**: 143–7.
65. Yu H, Bowden DW, Spray BJ, Rich SS, Freedman BI. Identification of human plasma kallikrein gene polymorphisms and evaluation of their role in end-stage renal disease. *Hypertension* 1998; **31**: 906–11.
66. Hansen PM, Chowdhury TA, Deckert T et al. Genetic variation of the heparan sulfate proteoglycan gene (Perlecan gene): association with urinary albumin excretion in IDDM patients. *Diabetes* 1997; **46**: 1658–9.
67. Liu ZH, Guan TJ, Li LS. Glucose transporter (GLUT1) allele (XbaI) associated with nephropathy in non-insulin-dependent diabetes mellitus. *Kidney Int* 1999; **55**: 1843–8.

Part II

Clinical Problems And Concomitant Diseases

8

Screening for and Diagnosis of Incipient Diabetic Nephropathy (IDN) in Diabetes

MANFRED GANZ[1], RAINER PROETZSCH[1] AND
CHRISTOPH HASSLACHER[2]

[1]Roche Diagnostics GmbH, Mannheim, Germany, [2]St Josefskrankenhaus,
Heidelberg, Germany

INTRODUCTION

Occurrence of persistent microalbuminuria (MAU) is an early feature of excessive capillary leakage (1) and can be regarded today as the first marker of impaired kidney function in patients with type 1 diabetes (= incipient diabetic nephropathy) (2). Unless relevant therapeutic interventions take place, the disease process will progress, albumin excretion will increase (''macroalbuminuria'') and endstage renal disease will finally ensue.

In patients with type 2 diabetes who predominantly are hypertensive, diagnosis of IDN is difficult, since in these patients MAU can be a marker of generalized macrovascular disease. Therefore, in type 2 diabetics, MAU identifies a patient cohort with an increased risk not only of renal but also of cardiovascular disease (3). The occurrence of macroalbuminuria in these patients points to already advanced glomerular damage. Since the rising numbers of patients receiving dialysis are primarily patients with type 2 diabetes, early detection and state-of-the-art therapy in this group of patients is becoming more important than ever.

Diabetic Nephropathy. Edited by C. Hasslacher.
© 2001 John Wiley & Sons, Ltd.

Clinical Problems and Concomitant Diseases

URINARY ALBUMIN EXCRETION

Under physiological conditions, albumin undergoes glomerular filtration and is almost entirely re-absorbed in the renal tubules. Slightly increased albumin excretion which is still below the detection limit of classic dipsticks for urinary protein is called microalbuminuria. The definitions given in the literature vary, depending on the mode of urine collection and/or the reference quantity used (Table 8.1). Elevated rates of albumin excretion can be explained by extrarenal as well as renal factors (damage of renal architecture) (Table 8.2). Elevated albumin excretion which disappears after causal treatment is called "transient albuminuria" and is usually of no pathological consequence.

Table 8.1 Classification of albuminuria. normo-, micro- and macroalbuminuria

	Normoalbuminuria	Microalbuminuria	Macroalbuminuria
(a) Albumin excretion rate (mg/24 h)	< 30	30–300	> 300
(b) Albumin excretion rate (μg/min)	< 20	20–200	> 200
(c) Albumin concentration (mg/l, based upon normal fluid intake and approximately 1.5 l urine day)	< 20	20–200	> 200
(d) Albumino creatinine ratio (mg/g creatinine)			
Males	< 20	20–200	< 200
Females	< 30	30–300	< 300
(e) Albumino creatinine ratio (mg/mmol creatinine)			
Males	< 2.5	2.5–25	> 25
Females	< 3.5	3.5–35	> 35
(f) Albumino creatinine ratio, (mg/g creatinine)	< 30	30–300	> 300

From (2), modified according to (4).

(a,b) Albumin excretion rate (AER). The determination of AER is based on the albumin concentration, the duration of urine collection and the urine volume, and has therefore the advantage of giving results which are independent of the ingested fluid quantity. Therefore, AER is "the gold standard" for the diagnosis of microalbuminuria.

(c) Albumin concentration (AC) (c). The albumin concentration in the first morning urine which has been formed under resting conditions is a reliable screening parameter, if the fluid intake is generally normal.

(d–f) Albumin: creatinine ratio (ACR) (4). The creatinine quantity excreted is individually, but not intra-individually, rather constant and amounts to normally 1.0–1.5 g/24 h, so the creatinine concentration can be used as a measure of the urine osmolality. The ACR is therefore approximately independent of the fluid consumption or e.g. diuresis.

Table 8.2 Factors influencing albumin excretion

- Intense physical activity
- Urinary tract infections
- Decompensated diabetes mellitus
- Rising blood pressure
- "Non-dippers" in nocturnal blood pressure (7)
- Clinically overt heart failure
- Acute febrile infections or other acute illness
- Surgery
- Menstruation and vaginal discharge (5)
- Injection of dibasic amino acids, gentamycin, anaesthesia, large pharmacological doses of insulin) (5)
- Very low fluid consumption (for concentration-based screening)
- Use of non-steroidal anti-inflammatory drugs or ACE-inhibitors which alter protein excretion (6)
- Cigarette smoking (8)

Modified from (2).

WHO TO SCREEN

It is known from epidemiological studies that type 1 diabetic patients rarely develop MAU before puberty or within 5 years of onset of diabetes. However, patients with type 2 diabetes may excrete elevated levels of urinary albumin from onset (13). Therefore, from the point of view of cost effectiveness, screening for microalbuminuria is recommended in young diabetic patients from puberty, in adult patients with type 1 diabetes after more than 5 years' duration of the diabetes, and in adult patients with type 2 diabetes from diagnosis, once glycaemic control is stabilized and gross proteinuria excluded (2).

Patients with diabetes who fulfil these criteria should be screened where they are treated, that is in general practice, at diabetes clinics, in hospitals, by endocrinologists or nephrologists.

SAMPLE HANDLING

If urine cannot be examined immediately after voiding it can be stored refrigerated up to 2 weeks and up to 3 days at 20°C. While some authors did not find differences of albumin concentrations between fresh and frozen samples of identical urines, others report spuriously low results due to precipitation of albumin in urines with a pH below 5.5 (14).

Advantages and Disadvantages of Different Urine Samples

24 h urine collection for calculation of the albumin excretion rate within 24 h is regarded as the "gold standard" for diagnosis of MAU, as it gives the average albumin excretion during the hours of daily activity and also recumbency. However, it is cumbersome and inconvenient for the patient. Also, physical exercise cannot be excluded. Therefore, 24 h urine collection is not recommended as a first step in screening for MAU.

Timed overnight urine collection is a more convenient method of sampling for calculation of the albumin excretion rate in µg/min. Physical activity, which leads to an increase of urinary albumin independent of diabetes, can be ruled out. Critical factors are timing errors and also the inconvenience of urine collection.

Procedure (Example). At 10 p.m. the patient voids urine into the toilet and marks "10 p.m." on the label of a urine vessel of suitable size (usually 1 l). All further urine samples of that night, till rise at 7 a.m. (patient marks "7 a.m.") are collected in the vessel. The patient brings the vessel with the collected urine to the doctor's office, where the volume (0.51 l) and albumin concentration (49 mg/l or 49 000 µg/l) are measured, and the time period is calculated (9 hours or 540 min). The AER amounts to:

$$AER = AC(\mu g/l) \times U$$
$$- volume(l)/collection\ period(min), in\ the\ example\ here$$

$$AER = 49\,000\ \mu g/l \times 0.51\,l/540\ min = 46.3\ \mu g/min$$

An aliquot of *early morning urine* directly after rising is used for measurement of the albumin concentration which is not affected by physical exercise or fluid intake and correlates in 90% of all cases with the 24 h albumin excretion (15).

Determination of the *albumin: creatinine ratio* (ACR) in an aliquot of the morning urine is used to correct the albumin concentration for dilution or high concentration of urine. Suggestions to introduce sex- and age-specific limits for ACR (16) should improve differentiation between normo- and microalbuminuria; however, they may complicate the interpretation of the data.

Spot urine specimens can be obtained in the office. The creatinine concentration in such a sample should be used to correct the urine for dilution or concentration (ACR). However, quantitative measurements of the albumin and creatinine concentration in urine are necessary, and physical exercise, e.g. a brisk walk to the doctor's office, is not corrected by the creatinine and should therefore be ruled out.

SCREENING METHODS

The following considerations are important:

- Immunological methods are very suitable. They are highly sensitive, permitting detection of albumin concentrations of 20 mg/l or lower, and are specific for albumin.
- There should be no interference by urine pH, substances naturally occurring in urine or frequently used drugs and their metabolites.
- The method should allow screening of low or high numbers of samples in a short time, as single determinations as well as in series. Preferably the result should be available before consultation.
- For screening at the primary care level, any need for laboratory equipment would be an obstacle.
- Albumin excretion is subject to considerable biological day-to-day variation. Therefore, the diagnosis of "persistent microalbuminuria" or "incipient diabetic nephropathy" (IDN) should never be made on the basis of a single albumin measurement.

Table 8.3 shows recommendations for screening and confirmation of microalbuminuria and Figure 8.1 illustrates the screening procedure for IDN.

Methods for Screening for Microalbuminuria without Laboratory Equipment

Qualitative Methods

Micro-Bumintest® *(trademark of Bayer AG, Leverkusen, Germany)* This is a method using the chemical test principle of the protein error of pH indicators with bromophenol blue as indicator. One drop of urine is placed on the test tablet, allowed to soak in, and then washed out with two drops of distilled water. A colour change from yellow (negative) to blue-green (trace, +, ++, + + +) indicates albumin values above 15–30 mg/l. The reaction is not specific for albumin and may give false positive results if alkaline urine is examined or if other proteins or non-protein components react with the dye (17–20). While the sensitivity of the test is ≥ 90%, the specificity apparently varies between 35% and 95%, depending on the cutoff for positive and the composition and pH of samples (17, 20). The time needed to test 10 samples is 5 min (20).

Rapitex®-Albumin (trademark of Behringwerke AG, Marburg, Germany) The test principle is immunological latex agglutination of antibodies to human

Table 8.3 Recommendations for screening for and confirmation of microalbuminuria, 1993–1999

Source	Screening					Confirmation of positive screening result		
	Urine sample	Urine tested for	Parameter measured	Cut off	Repeated when −ve, +ve	Urine sample	Parameter	Cut-off
IDDM Consensus Guidelines, 1993 (9)	Spot urine	Micro-albuminuria	ACR, albumin conc	2.5 mg/mmol or 20 mg/l	If negative, yearly, if positive, at each consulation	Timed urine collection	ACR, AER (?)	2.5 mg/mmol, 20 µg/min or 30 mg/24h
NIDDM Desk Top Guide, 1993 (10)	Not specified	Proteinuria, micro-albuminuria	Protein by dipstick, albumin conc	Not specified	If negative, regularly retest	3 × overnight	AER, overnight	20 µg/min
St Vincent Declaration 1994 (11)	Early morning urine	Albumin	Albumin conc, ACR	20 mg/l or 2.5/ 3.5 mg/mmol	If negative, retest in 1 year	3 × timed urine sample (or ACR)	AER, ACR	20 µg/min or 30 mg/24h 2.5 (3.5) mg/mmol (f,m)
MAU in Diabetes Australia, 1994, (12)	Spot urine	Micro-albuminuria	Albumin conc (Micral.Test)	20 mg/l	Annual screening	2 × 24h urine collections in 6 weeks	AER	20 µg/min
National Kidney Foundation 1995 (6)	Preferably early morning urine	Albumin and creatinine	ACR	30 mg/g	If negative, repeat in 1 year	Twice in 3 months if positive	ACR	30 mg/g
German Diabetes Association, 1997 (2)	Early morning urine	Protein (test strip), albumin	Albumin conc	20 mg/l	2 × (+), confirmed; 2 × (−), retest in 1 year	Two timed urine collections (or 1 × if conc was 2 × clearly positive)	AER	20 µg/min

conc, concentration; ACR, albumino: creatinine ratio; AER, albumin excretion rate; f, female; m, male.

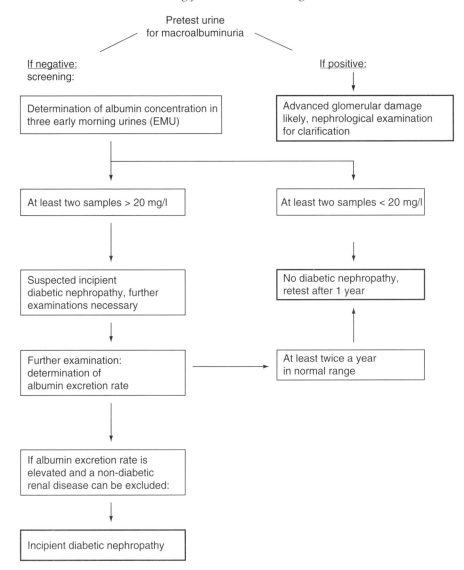

Figure 8.1 Screening procedure for incipient diabetic nephropathy

albumin in the presence of albumin in concentrations $\geq$ 18–20 mg/l. After dilution of the urine in the ratio 1:20, three segments of a test plate are treated with one drop of urine, saline or positive control, respectively, followed by buffer solutions and antibody–latex reagent for each segment. The plate has to be shaken for 2 min. The albumin concentration is estimated to be either normal or $\geq 20\,mg/l$ by comparison of the sample with the saline and positive controls. Sensitivity is 96%, specificity 94% (20). Semi-quantitative assessment of the albumin concentration is possible if the urine is diluted in a series of different ratios and determined again. Before testing with Rapitex®-Albumin, high albumin concentrations must be excluded, e.g. by a conventional test strip for proteinuria, as albumin concentrations > $1000\,mg/l$ may produce a false negative result (hook effect). The time needed to test 10 samples is 12 min (20).

Albusure™ *(trademark of Cambridge Life Sciences plc, Cambridge, UK)*   The test principle is immunological latex agglutination inhibition. The handling is similar to Rapitex®-Albumin. However, there is no predilution of the urine and, in contrast to Rapitex®-Albumin, albumin concentrations below $20\,mg/l$ produce agglutination, and the reaction mixture remains clear if the albumin concentration is $20\,mg/l$ or higher. There is no hook effect. Sensitivity is 90%, specificity 100% (20). The time needed to test 10 samples is 7 min (20).

Semiquantitative Method

Micral-Test® *II (trademark of a member of the Roche group: in USA, Chemstrip Micral*®*)*   This is an immunological test strip using gold-labelled anti-bodies to human albumin. A capture matrix containing immobilized albumin binds free antibodies without albumin. The strip is immersed in the urine up to the depth mark for 5 s to soak up enough fluid for chromatography, then laid down horizontally for chromatography. After 1 min the colour of the detection pad can be compared with the colour scale for negative, 20, 50 and 100 mg/l albumin. Reaction colours brighter than the 20 mg/l colour pad should be regarded as negative. Other substances in the urine (except oxytetracycline, which leads to darker reaction colour) or pH values between 4 and 10 do not interfere; however, if the urine was refrigerated the temperature should be allowed to reach at least 10°C before analysis, as otherwise lower results will be displayed. Strong disinfectants in the urine container may lead to underestimation. Samples can be determined with Micral-Test II as single determinations or in series. Dilution of urines with albumin concentrations of 100 mg/l or above can extend the range of differentiation. The overall sensitivity of Micral-Test II in two evaluations were in the range 93–97%, the specificity 71–93% (21,22). The time needed to test 10 urine samples is 5 min (own experiments).

WHEN IS A DIFFERENTIAL DIAGNOSIS NECESSARY?

In patients with type 1 diabetes, elevated albuminuria means usually IDN. However, in rare cases a non-diabetic nephropathy may be present. Indications of a non-diabetic nephropathy are:

- Signs of retinopathy are lacking (diabetic nephropathy and retinopathy in type 1 diabetes develop usually in parallel).
- Rapid increase of albumin excretion in spite of normotension or moderate hypertension and sufficient metabolic control (normal increase of AER in diabetics without intervention is 20% yearly).
- No improvement in albumin excretion despite blood pressure normalization and improved metabolic control.
- Rapid increase of serum creatinine.

In patients with type 2 diabetes, abnormal albuminuria may not be associated with retinopathy. Therefore, a non-diabetic cause of MAU should be excluded by history, by ordinary objective examination and measurement of serum creatinine.

CONCLUSION

Screening methods must select those patients with diabetes who need special care. A screening procedure should be easy to follow for patients, reliable and allow rapid screening of high numbers of samples. The result should be available immediately.

Aliquots of three early morning urines as sample material and immunological rapid tests can be recommended as a reliable first-step screening procedure. If spot urines are used, albumin and creatinine have to be measured quantitatively for the ACR in order to correct the result, e.g. for diuresis.

In the case of negative results, screening should be repeated 1 year later. Two or three positive results require further diagnostic examinations with timed urine collection and quantitative determination.

A flow diagram that combines easy and reliable screening and confirmation procedures has been worked out by the Diabetic Nephropathy Working Group of the German Diabetes Association (2) (Figure 8.1). It is expected that the need for regular screening and intervention will be increasingly recognized at the primary care level too and that, with a delay of some years, the high number of patients with diabetes entering endstage renal failure could be reduced to the figure targeted by the St Vincent Declaration in 1989—a reduction by at least one-third in 5 years (23).

REFERENCES

1. Sheth JJ. Diabetes, microalbuminuria and hypertension. *Clin Exp Hypertens* 1999; **21**: 61–8.
2. Hasslacher C, Danne T, Ganz M, Sawicki P, Walter H. Frühdiagnose der diabetischen Nephropathie—Stellungnahme der Arbeitsgemeinschaft "Diabetische Nephropathie". *Diabetol Informat* 1997; **4**: 268–73.
3. Schmitz A, Vaeth M. Microalbuminuria: a major risk factor in non-insulin dependent diabetes. A 10-year follow-up study of 503 patients. *Diabet Med* 1988; **5**: 126–34.
4. Mogensen CE, Keane WF, Bennet PH et al. Prevention of diabetic renal disease with special reference to microalbuminuria. In *The Kidney and Hypertension in Diabetes Mellitus*, 3rd edn., Mogensen CE (ed.). Boston: Kluwer Academic, 1994: 541.
5. Mogensen CE, Vestbo E, Poulsen PL et al. Microalbuminuria and potential confounders. *Diabet Care* 1995; **18**: 572–81.
6. Bennett PH, Haffner S, Kasiske BL et al. Diabetic renal disease recommendations: screening and management of microalbuminuria in patients with diabetes mellitus—recommendations to the scientific advisory board of the National Kidney Foundation from an *ad hoc* committee of the Council on Diabetes Mellitus of the National Kidney Foundation. *Am J Kidney Dis* 1995; **25**: 107–12.
7. Bianchi S, Bigazzi R, Baldari G et al. Diurnal variations of blood pressure and microalbuminuria in essential hypertension. *Am J Hypertens* 1994; **7**: 23–9.
8. Chase PH, Garg SK, Marshall G et al. Cigarette smoking increases the risk of albuminuria among subjects with type 1 diabetes. *J Am Med Assoc* 1991; **295**: (5).
9. European IDDM Policy Group. Renal, eye, and nerve disease and foot problems. In *Consensus Guidelines for the Management of Insulin-dependent (Type I) Diabetes*. Medicom Europe: Bussum, The Netherlands, 1993; 23.
10. European NIDDM Policy Group. Screening and management of diabetic nephropathy. In *a Desk Top Guide for the Management of Non-insulin-dependent Diabetes Mellitus (NIDDM)*, 2nd edn. Kirchheim: Mainz, 1993; 29.
11. Viberti GC, Mogensen CE, Passa P, Bilous R, Mangili R. St Vincent Declaration, 1994: guidelines for the prevention of diabetic renal failure. In *The Kidney and Hypertension in Diabetes Mellitus*, 2nd edn, Mogensen CE (ed.). Boston: Kluwer Academic, 1994; 519.
12. Jerums G, Cooper M, Gilbert R, O'Brien R, Taft J. Position statement: microalbuminuria in diabetes. *Med J Aust* 1994; **161**: 265–8.
13. Uusitupa M, Siitonen O, Penttila I, Antti A, Pyorala K. Proteinuria in newly diagnosed type II diabetic patients. *Diabet Care* 1987; **10**: 191–4.
14. Townsend JC, Sadler WA, Shanks GM. The effect of storage pH on the precipitation of proteins in deep-frozen urine samples. *Ann Clin Biochem* 1987; **24**: 111.
15. Hasslacher C. Microalbuminurie-Screening bei Diabetikern. *Dtsch Med Wschr* 1989; **114**: 980–82.
16. Bakker AJ. Detection of microalbuminuria: receiver operating characteristics curve analysis favors albumin-to-creatinine ratio over albumin concentration. *Diabet Care* 1999; **22**: 307–13.
17. Haas M, Besenthal I, Renn W et al. Mikroalbuminurie-Screening: Eine vergleichende Untersuchung von drei Schnelltests gegen ein nephelometrisches Verfahren. *Diabet Stoffwechsel* 1994; **3**: 61–5.

18. Jung K, Nickel E. Non-protein components of urine interfere with colorimetry of urinary albumin with bromphenol blue. *Clin Chem* 1989; **35**: 336–7.
19. Colwell M, Halsey JF. High incidence of false-positive results with the Micro-Bumintest. *Clin Chem* 1989; **35**: 1252.
20. Hasslacher C, Bostedt-Kiesel A. Screening auf Mikroalbuminurie: Die Schnelltests im Vergleich. *Med Tribune* 1992; **24** (14): 50–51.
21. Mogensen CE, Viberti GC, Peheim E et al. Multicenter evaluation of the Micral-Test II test strip, an immunological rapid test for the detection of microalbuminuria. *Diabet Care* 1997; **20**: 1642–6.
22. Gilbert RE, Akdeniz A, Jerums G. Detection of microalbuminuria in diabetic patients by urinary dipstick. *Diabet Res Clin Pract* 1997; **35**: 57–60.
23. Anon. Diabetes mellitus in Europe—a problem at all ages in all countries. *Giorn Ital Diabetol* 1989; **9**: 317.

9

Differential Diagnosis of Proteinuria in Diabetic Patients

DANIEL CORDONNIER, CLAIRE MAYNARD, NICOLE PINEL AND SERGE HALIMI

Centre Hospitalier Universitaire, Grenoble, France

Proteinuria is suspected in practical medicine by the use of dipsticks in patients free of urinary infection or haematuria; it is confirmed in the laboratory, where both quantity (more than $0.3\,g/day$) and quality (ratio of albumin: other proteins) should be assessed. Therefore, at least in theory, the term "macroalbuminuria", widely used by diabetologists in order to distinguish it from microalbuminuria, does not have exactly the same significance.

Proteinuria is the most common marker of kidney diseases but, except in relatively rare situations, this sign is of little help for diagnosing the precise nature of the renal lesion. In a diabetic patient, proteinuria usually means that he/she has an "overt" diabetic nephropathy, meaning diabetic glomerulosclerosis (DGS) from the pathological point of view, and evolution towards terminal renal failure in a median delay of 8 years from the clinical point of view. It also signifies that the patient is at high risk of cardiovascular event and death. However, it is now well established that not every diabetic patient with proteinuria has DGS. He/she can have every other nephropathy (or urological disorder with renal impact), either alone or superimposed on DGS. This is particularly true for type 2 diabetes mellitus but it is also possible in type 1.

Diabetic Nephropathy. Edited by C. Hasslacher.
© 2001 John Wiley & Sons, Ltd.

The aim of this chapter is to evaluate how important the problem is both for the individual patient and for public health. For the patient, detecting and treating a non-diabetic disease might greatly modify his/her future because the evolution could be drastically changed, either spontaneously or after therapy, but also because the diagnosis of the primary renal disease could be of importance for the management of a (potential) future pregnancy or renal transplantation.

For the health care providers and Public Health Managers, it could be questionable to expand investigations and their potential iatrogenic effects if there is no global benefit to be expected, in other words, no modification of incidence of endstage renal failure (ESRD) leading to renal replacement therapy (RRT). The growing ("epidemic") incidence, prevalence and cost of so-called "diabetic nephropathy" (in fact, a composite of diverse renal diseases in diabetic patients) in ESRD programmes worldwide makes this problem a real one and its evaluation mandatory.

MAGNITUDE OF THE PROBLEM

There is no registry concerning this matter. There are some reviews available, in fact giving different points of view, depending upon the medical speciality of the authors and usually limited to the results of angiographies or renal biopsies. It is reasonable to say that one type 2 diabetic patient in 10 with proteinuria has a non-diabetic disease; it might be three in 10 in some particular categories, such as elderly people or patients living in some developing countries. A list of renal diseases potentially associated to diabetes (or to DGS) is given in Table 9.1

Table 9.1 Differential diagnosis. The diagnosis listed below should be checked systematically in every patient with any atypical clinical history, *particularly in patients without diabetic retinopathy*

Renal artery stenosis	Patients with severe hypertension
	Patients whose creatininaemia and kalaemia increase under ACE-I
	Patients with asymmetrical kidneys and clinical signs of atheroma
Nephrosclerosis	Patients with long-lasting history of hypertension, hypertensive retinopathy and two symmetrical constricted kidneys
Crescentic glomerulonephritis	Patients with rapidly progressive renal disease
Glomerulonephritis (other)	Patients with microscopic haematuria, cylindruria or immunological disorder
Chronic pyelonephritis	Patients with long-lasting history of urinary infections and (or) papillary necrosis. Small or dilated kidneys with reflux or urinary obstacle

Urologic Apparatus

Two traditional complications of diabetes have considerably diminished in incidence and are only historical observations in medically well-developed countries: *papillary necrosis* (with the improvement of diabetes management) and *pyelonephritis* (with early referral of any urinary infections) (1). We do not know exactly what the impact is on the kidneys of the very frequent *"neurological bladder"*, clinically perceptible as a post-micturitional residue (2). More evident are the consequences of *prostatic pathologies* in male diabetics aged over 50, the frequency of which has not been systematically evaluated.

Vascular Apparatus

Vascular renal diseases are, with diabetes, the main cause of RRT worldwide. It is now very clear that some patients have both diabetes (mainly but not exclusively type 2) and vascular disease(s) located to the kidney macro- or microvasculature (3).

Diffuse Atheroma

Diffuse atheroma involving the aorta (with or without aortic aneurysm) and inferior limbs is often but not always associated with atheroma of the renal arteries.

Renal Artery Stenosis (RAS)

RAS is more frequent in diabetic than in non-diabetic persons in an autopsy series (8% vs. 4%) (4). There are some limited series showing clearly that 10–30% of type 2 diabetic patients with proteinuria and hypertension have a "significant" RAS ($\geq$ 50–70% of diameter depending on the series) (5). By contrast, in type 1 diabetic patients RAS is very rare. The practical implications of a RAS is not completely clear. There is no consensus on treatment.

Cholesterol Embolism

This is probably under-recognized and therefore under-reported in diabetic patients. Like cruoric embolisms, cholesterol embolism could be responsible for peripherical infarcts inducing cortical defects, either unique or multiple, responsible for an irregular pattern of the renal cortex. It is quite infrequent that both retinal (by fundoscopy) cutaneous (by biopsy) or nail embolism can be evidenced to assist the diagnosis. Reports of pathological proofs of such embolisms in the kidney arteries are rare.

Renal Cortex

Studies dealing with renal biopsies have clearly shown that not only the glomeruli are important but also the renal arterioles and interstitium.

Glomerular Lesions

One can consider the frequency of non-diabetic glomerular pathologies in checking two kinds of series. The first category deals with biopsies of patients presenting with nephrotic syndrome or (often) heavy proteinuria in a (usually) atypical context or with additional extra renal pathologies. The second category deals with biopsies of every new diabetic patients presenting with proteinuria or before enrolling them in therapeutic trials after careful clinical selection. This second category is obviously closer to the true incidence of non-diabetic glomerular diseases in diabetics carefully monitored for years.

Careful analysis of these series show that retinal status does not completely cover renal status. A diabetic retinopathy usually corresponds to DGS but some superimposed other glomerulopathies may coexist. On the other hand, absence of diabetic retinopathy usually corresponds to a non-diabetic nephropathy but can very well be seen in patients with mild proteinuria and true "early" DGS. However, these discrepancies are numerically low [see reviews in (6,7,8)]. Recently, the frequency of an association between type 2 diabetes and hepatitis C virus infection has been emphasized. HCV associated hepatitis and membranoproliferative glomerulonephritis may be treated and eradicated at least in part (see Figure 9.4) (19).

Microvascular Lesions

It is striking to see that, apart from glomerulonephritis, a consistent number of glomerular lesions can be said to be "ischaemic", which means related to microvascular atheroma. As a matter of fact, these lesions are different from those associated with the typical established DGS (Figure 9.1).

Interstitial Lesions

It is important to differentiate between three kinds of interstitial modification. The first is the consequence of glomerular lesions; it is now clear that this is of prognosic importance, since it leads to fibrosis and renal death. Furthermore, it can be modified by therapy (9). The second kind of

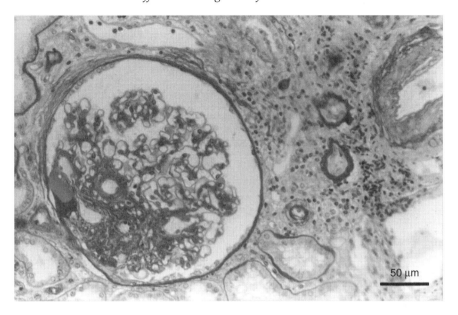

Figure 9.1 Fifty-six year-old male, type 2 diabetic patient for 14 years, hypertensive-treated for 12 years, microalbuminuric 3 years ago and presently proteinuric (1.54 g/24 h); GFR 105 ml/min/1.73 m². The patient had no diabetic retinopathy but hypertensive grade 2 retinopathy. *PAS staining*: glomerulus exhibits a focal multilayering of Bowman's capsule and a moderate shrinkage of the tuft. Mesangial sclerosis predominates at the vascular pole area. Interstitial connective tissue is enlarged, with some mononuclear inflammatory cells and atrophic tubules. Fibrous endarteritis of interlobular artery can be seen on the right. The diagnosis of ischaemic nephropathy was accepted

interstitial modifications that should be systematically searched for in the anamnesis are drug-induced tubular and interstitial lesions. As an example, it is very likely, but so far not clearly demonstrated, that chronic use of non-steroidal anti-inflammatory drugs is responsible for some part of these lesions. The third kind of interstitial lesions are the consequences of urinary abnormalities and infection. They are usually easy to recognize, thanks to the pleomorphic nature of the cellular infiltrate, which includes poly-morphic leucocytes.

PRACTICAL IMPORTANCE OF MAKING THE DIFFERENTIAL DIAGNOSIS IN DIABETIC PATIENT

Not every patient with a DGS at the stage of overt nephropathy evolves at the same pace (10). Those who evolve more slowly usually have a better glucose and blood pressure control and in general have been treated more intensively, e.g. with ACE inhibitors or angiotensin II receptors antagonists. In addition, however, the concept has emerged recently and arguments have been brought in favour of the genetic predisposition of patients both to evolve and to be resistant to the renoprotective effects of ACE inhibitors (11).

However, it is very clear that some patients will evolve at a slow and some at a rapid pace towards ESRD. The rate of decline of GFR, the rate of worsening of proteinuria, the importance of resistance of elevated blood pressure to antihypertensive drugs are not by themselves sufficient to give clear information concerning the nature of the underlying renal disease.

PRACTICAL MANAGEMENT

Even if the possibility is slim that proteinuria might be due entirely or partially to a non-diabetic renal disease, it should be evoked systematically in every patient, whatever the type of diabetes mellitus. The diagnostic process should be followed systematically (Figure 9.2) and should not be modified, except in the case of contraindication to some investigation.

Clinical History

Typical history has been established for type 1 diabetic-associated nephropathy in five sequential stages of known duration, proteinuria being the fourth after the hyperfiltration phase, the silent phase and microalbuminuria and occurring before uremia. In type 2 diabetes, this sequence is less clear, since the beginning of diabetes might go unrecognized for a long time, but it is generally admitted that the sequence of phases is very close to that in type 1. An isolated proteinuria occurring at the expected time, following a established phase of microalbuminuria and increasing regularly, is suggestive of DGS.

A proteinuria discovered in a patient who has no regular history of microalbuminuria, particularly if heavy, should be suspected of being due to another nephropathy. One should check the time of discovery of diabetes and proteinuria. When proteinuria precedes or occurs simultaneously with diabetes a non-diabetic nephropathy should be suspected. To have a family history of type 2 diabetes and nephropathy might help considerably. This favours the diagnosis of DGS.

Extra-renal and renal pathologies should be searched for carefully. Likewise, one should look for previous use of potentially nephrotoxic drugs, such as non-steroidal anti-inflammatory agents, analgesics, antibiotics and

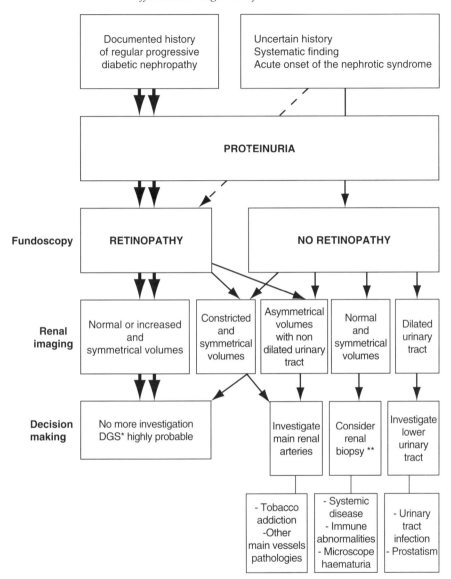

Figure 9.2 Practical diagnosis of proteinuria in a diabetic patient. *DGS: diabetic glomerulosclerosis. **Renal biopsy: consider only if blood pressure is controlled and if coagulation is normal

even angiotensin II converting enzyme inhibitors. Smoking is important to consider, both as a possible aetiologic factor (renal artery stenosis, ischaemic nephropathy) and as a marker for a quicker evolution.

Clinical Examination

Some points of particular interest should be focused upon:

- Ensure that the patient has no (partial) obstacle to urinary flow (pelvic examination; assess for neurologic bladder).
- Search for diffuse atheroma (peripheral and abdominal pulses).
- Search for a systemic disease, possibly involving the kidney.

Retinoscopy

This examination should be systematic in every diabetic, every year, whatever his/her renal status. For a proteinuric patient, not to have a diabetic retinopathy is very suggestive of a non-diabetic nephropathy (12,13), even if this is not completely true (14). The retinal status, provided that it is evaluated in an established fashion, will greatly help in management of the patient (see Table 9.1); the presence or absence of a peripheral neuropathy may also help.

Biology

Urinary Cells and Casts

Macro- or microscopic haematuria, particularly associated with normal-shaped red cells, with or without crystals or abnormal urinary cells, will lead to for a pyelography. Distorted red cells associated with casts are suggestive of glomerulonephritis. White cells alone (without infection and casts) should suggest the possibility of urinary tuberculosis. White cell cylinders are found in urinary centrifugates of proliferative glomerulonephritis.

Monoclonal Dysglobulinaemia

Discovering urinary monoclonal kappa chain dysglobulinuria does not necessarily mean that a diabetic patient has a dysglobulinaemia. In doubtful cases, however, a bone marrow examination should be performed.

Polyclonal Hyperglobulinaemia

This is very frequent in diabetes and does not help in practice. In particular hyper IgA globulinaemia usually linked to mesangial IgA glomerulonephritis in non diabetics is of little aid in diabetic patients (15,16) except when the level is particularly high (17) (Figure 9.3).

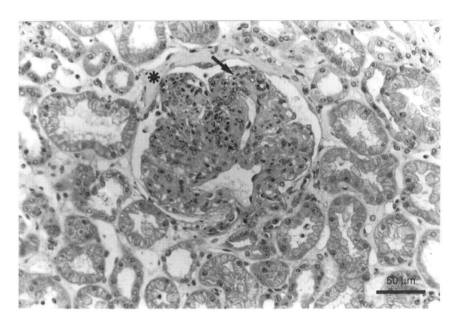

Figure 9.3 76 year-old male patient, referred for acute renal failure and type 2 diabetes known since 1963, treated with insulin since 1968; severe proliferative retinopathy and peripheral neuropathy (1978), proteinuria (detected in 1991), coronary bypass (1992), cardiac heart failure (1993, 1994, 1997) and benign IgG dysglobulinaemia (1997). In August 1997 he was admitted to an endocrinology unit for an infected wound of a toe. Despite antibiotic treatment, oedema with the nephrotic syndrome and oliguria developed when creatininaemia rose in 3 days from 101 to 365 µmol/l and in 7 days to 633 µmol/l. He then needed a transfer to a nephrology unit and five sessions of haemodialysis. Necrotic purpura of the limbs appeared. The C3 fraction of complement was very low and serum IgA level high (4.6 g/l N = 1–2 g/l). A biopsy was performed. *Masson's trichrome stain, renal biopsy*: global mesangial sclerosis with superimposed endocapillary cellular proliferation and inflammatory cell infiltration. Caryorhexis can be seen in different places (↓) and thickening of Bowman's capsule (*). Additional tubular lesions, probably related to aminoside treatment, are also present. There are diffuse membranous IgA deposits (not shown). *Evolution*: this very severe atypical glomerulonephritis related to a cutaneous infection and to a necrotic purpura was treated with antibiotics and corticosteroids. The patient was in good shape 4 months later with a controlled blood pressure, a proteinuria of 2.6 g/24 h and a creatininaemia of 159 µmol/l

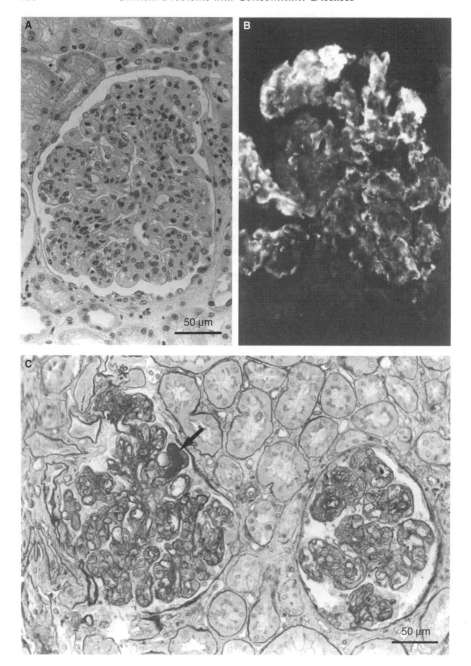

Hypocomplementemia

Idea to feature of hypocomplementemia is a useful first step, leading to a search for an acute diffuse glomerulonephritis, a lupus or a cryoglobulinaemia-associated glomerulonephritis or even to an idiopathic hypocomplementemic membranoproliferative glomerulonephritis (Figure 9.4).

Hyperuricaemia

This might testify to a gouty kidney, but also to hypertension-associated renal lesions (nephrosclerosis), or to diuretic-induced haemocontraction or, more simply, to an associated renal failure.

Hypokalaemia

With alkalosis, there can lead to the diagnosis of secondary hyperaldosteronism and specifically to renal artery stenosis.

Imaging

Both ultrasonography and Doppler ultrasonography are observer-dependent. They are good tools for detecting any abnormality, but further investigation will be needed, the nature of which will depend upon the level of renal function. If this is normal for age, contrast media could be used in a prudent manner (hyperhydratation, non-ionic agents, economy doses) in order to clearly evidence the renal arteries and the urinary tract; if renal function is altered (creatinine clearance $< 30\,\mathrm{ml/min}$) magnetic resonance imaging with gadolinium as a contrast medium should be considered (Figure 9.5).

Figure 9.4 71 year-old male type 2 diabetic patient with heavy proteinuria, renal insufficiency, no diabetic retinopathy, monoclonal IgM kappa peak, IgM κ-IgG cryoglobulinaemia, hypocomplementaemia (C4 + + +, C 3 +) and diffuse atheroma. *(A) Masson's trichrome. (B) Immunofluorescence, anti-C3. (C) PAS.* Glomeruli are enlarged and hypercellular with a lobular pattern. Expansion of the mesangium (cells and matrix) leads into compression of the vascular lumen. The peripheral glomerular basement membranes are irregularly thickened with a double contour or honeycomb. Amorphous masses are suggestive of a microthombus made of cryoglobulins precipitates ($\downarrow$). Coarse peripheral deposits of C3 (and IgM) outline the glomerular basement membranes: cryoglobulinemic mesangio-capillary glomerulonephritis. *Evolution*: Serology was stongly positive for hepatitis C. A liver biopsy was performed and treatment with interferon was conducted. Six months later the patient was in very good health, with a proteinuria of $0.16\,\mathrm{g/24\,h}$ and a creatininaemia of $105\,\mu\mathrm{mol/l}$

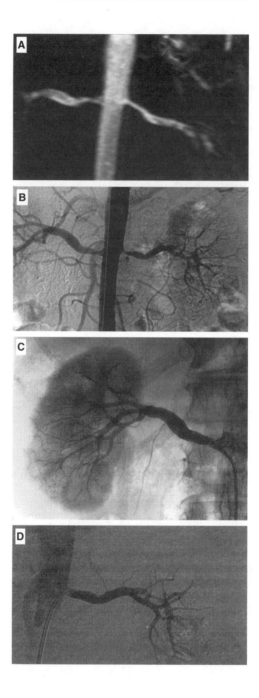

Renal biopsy

Renal biopsy should be considered if: (a) no urologic or vascular disease has been found; (b) no contraindication is present (very small or solitary kidney, coagulation trouble, uncontrollable elevated blood pressure); (c) the patient does not have a diabetic retinopathy; (d) nephrological (e.g. microscopic haematuria), systemic (e.g. cutaneous) or immunological (e.g. hypocomplementemia, dysglobulinemia) signs or symptoms are present.

The risks of a renal biopsy performed in a well-equipped centre by a highly skilled nephrologist, under ultrasonography with a gun-equipped needle, has become very low (18). When the patient has a typical diabetic retinopathy, it is acceptable not to perform a renal biopsy, assuming that it will show a DGS. However, renal biopsy should be considered if there is

CONCLUSION

Particularly in type 2 diabetes, urological, vascular and cortical (including glomerular) diseases can occur that are not due to diabetes. These represent up to 30% in some series.

Retinal status does not completely coincide with renal status. The differential diagnosis of proteinuria in a diabetic patient should not be resolved with this "tool" alone.

There are relatively few tools available for making the differential diagnostis of proteinuria, except for renal biopsy.

Prognosis, either spontaneously or via therapeutics, can be completely different depending upon the diagnosis. This is true both before

continues

Figure 9.5 Seventy-three year-old man with type 2 diabetes for 38 years and insulin treatment for 11 years; referred for renal insufficiency (creatininaemia = 163 μmol/l, creatinine clearance 30 ml/min), high blood pressure (normalized under furosemide 40 mg/day and a β-blocker) and proteinuria (0.9 g/24 h). The patient, a non-smoker, has been treated by laser therapy for a proliferative retinopathy. Two years ago he underwent a coronary bypass. The left pedal pulse was not found. Ultrasonography showed two kidneys of 9.5 cm and 10 cm length, with a cortex of 17 mm mean thickness. Magnetic resonance imaging showed (A) bilateral stenosis with post-stenosis dilatation. Both were confirmed by conventional arteriography (B) and were treated by endoluminal balloon angioplasty to the right artery (C). Nine months later, due to recurrence of left renal artery stenosis, an endovascular stent was introduced (D). No progression of renal insufficiency or proteinuria was observed within the following 36 months. Reproduced by courtesy of Dr Frederic Thony

continued

reaching ESRD (the pace of evolution could be strikingly distinct) and during the dialysis phase (patients with non-diabetic renal diseases will have fewer microvascular complications and will be more easily registered on transplantation waiting lists).

Prospective systematic studies in large cohorts of diabetic patients with proteinuria, with registries, should help to manage these diseases better.

any historical, anamnestic, clinical, biological or imaging abnormality suggestive of something unusual. It is also clear that renal biopsies are acceptable in well-designed trials for research purposes (18).

REFERENCES

1. Groop L, Laasonen L, Edgren J. Renal papillary necrosis in patients with IDDM. *Diabet Care* 1989; **12**: 198–202.
2. Frimodt-Moller C, Mortensen S. Treatment of diabetic cystopathy. *Ann Int Med*, 1980; **92**: 327–8.
3. Meyrier A, Hill GS, Simon P. Ischemic renal diseases: new insights into old entities. *Kidney Int* 1998; **54**: 2–13.
4. Sawicki PT, Kaiser S, Heinemann L, Frenzel H, Berger M. Prevalence of renal artery stenosis in diabetes mellitus—and autopsy study. *J Int Med* 1991; **229**: 489–92.
5. Courreges JP, Bacha J, Aboud E. Prevalence and profile of renovascular disease in diabetic type 2 with severe hypertension. *J Hypertens* 1997; **15**: 1348–52.
6. Cordonnier D. Glomerular involvement in type II diabetes. Is it all diabetic glomerulosclerosis? (editorial comments). *Nephrol Dialysis Transpl* 1996; **11**: 936–8.
7. Olsen S, Mogensen CE. How often is NIDDM complicated with non-diabetic renal disease? An analysis of renal biopsies and the literature. *Diabetologia* 1996; **39**: 1638–45.
8. Raine AEG, Bilous RW. End-stage renal disease in NIDDM: a consequence of microangiopathy alone? *Diabetologia* 1996; **39**: 1673–5.
9. Cordonnier D, Pinel N, Barro C et al. Expansion of cortical interstitium is limited by converting enzyme inhibition in type 2 diabetic patients with glomerulosclerosis. *J Am Soc Nephrol* 1999; **10**: 1253–63.
10. Biesenbach G, Janko O, Zazgornik J. Similar rate of progression in the predialysis phase in type I and type II diabetes mellitus. *Nephrol Dialysis Transpl* 1994; **9**: 1097–102.
11. Jacobsen P, Rossing K, Rossing P et al. Angiotensin converting enzyme gene polymorphism and ACE inhibition in diabetic nephropathy. *Kidney Int* 1998; **53**: 1002–6.

12. Christensen PK, Larsen S, Horn T et al. Causes of albuminuria in patients with type 2 diabetes without diabetic retinopathy *Kidney Int*, 2000; **58**: 1719–31.
13. Pinel N, Fadel B, Bilous RW et al. Renal biopsies in 30 micro- and macroalbuminuric non-insulin dependent (type 2) (NIDDM) patients: heterogeneity of renal lesions. *Nephrol Dialysis Transpl* 1995; **6**: 448 (abstr).
14. Kanauchi M, Kawano, Uyama H, Shiiki H, Dohi K. Discordance between retinopathy and nephropathy in type 2 diabetes. *Nephron* 1998; **80**: 171–4.
15. Claveyrolas-Bouillet L, Pinel N, Renversez JC, Halimi S, Cordonnier D. Elevation of seric IgA is of little diagnostic utility in patients with type 2 diabetes mellitus and nephropathy. *Nephron* 1999; **82**: 190 (letter).
16. Orfila C, Lepert JC, Modesto A, Pipy B, Suc JM. IgA nephropathy complicating diabetic glomerulosclerosis. *Nephron* 1998; **79**: 279–87.
17. Kawasaki I, Ishimura E, Shioi A et al. Renal dysfunction worsened by superimposition of IgA glomerulonephritis in a patient with overt diabetic nephropathy. *Nephron* 1998; **78**: 232–4.
18. Glassock RJ, Hirschmann GH, Striker GE. Workshop on the use of renal biopsy in research on diabetic nephropathy: a summary report. *Am J Kidney Dis* 1991; **18**: 589–92.
19. Soma J, Saito T, Taguma Y et al. High prevalence and adverse effect of hepatitis C virus infection in type 2 diabetic related nephropathy. *J Am Soc Nephrol* 2000; **11**: 690–99.

10

Hypertension in Diabetic Nephropathy

CHRISTOPH HASSLACHER

St Josefskrankenhaus, Heidelberg, Germany

Vascular hypertension is one of the most frequent concomitant diseases in patients with diabetes, and has a very unfavourable effect on the prognosis. Besides the deleterious effect on the development and progression of nephropathy and retinopathy, hypertensive diabetics show an excessive risk of cardiovascular complications, especially when proteinuria is present (see Chapter 16). According to the WHO's most recent hypertension and risk classification, diabetics with systolic blood pressure values in excess of 140 mmHg or diastolic values in excess of 90 mmHg are amongst the "high risk subjects" (1). When there are secondary diseases such as nephropathy, they belong to the "very high risk" class. "High risk" entails a 10 year risk of 20–30% and "very high risk" of more than 30% with regard to cardio-vascular incidents.

PREVALENCE

The time course and frequency of development of hypertension differ greatly in type 1 and type 2 diabetics. In type 1 diabetics with normal albumin excretion, the prevalence of hypertension is just as high as in the general population (2). With the occurrence of microalbuminuria, the blood pressure usually begins to rise, but initially it remains in the "normoten-sive" range (3). Only 3 years after the appearance of microalbuminuria,

Diabetic Nephropathy. Edited by C. Hasslacher.
© 2001 John Wiley & Sons, Ltd.

there is a somewhat higher blood pressure statistically. With the manifestation of macroalbuminuria, 60–70% of these patients have hypertension, and in the stage of renal failure practically all patients are hypertensive.

In patients with type 2 diabetes, arterial hypertension can already be demonstrated in a high percentage of cases at the time of diagnosis of diabetes. According to the results of the UKPDS Study, hypertension could be detected age-dependently in 33–55% in male diabetic patients as compared to 31–66% in female diabetic patients (4). Compared to the prevalence of hypertension in a metabolically healthy control group, this means that there is a 1.5–3 times higher prevalence of hypertension in type 2 diabetics. With occurrence of micro- or macroalbuminuria, the prevalence of hypertension shows a further (5) rise. In contrast to type 1 diabetes, isolated systolic hypertension is mainly found in type 2 diabetics. This is diagnosed when the systolic blood pressure is in excess of 140 mmHg (more than 160 mmHg in patients over 65 years old) and the diastolic blood pressure is below 90 mmHg.

PATHOGENESIS

The pathomechanism of the development of hypertension in patients with diabetes is complex and all its details are not yet known. Genetic factors are discussed in both type 1 and in type 2 diabetes. Table 10.1 shows typical changes of individual factors relevant to the development of hypertension in diabetics. Only a few factors can be referred to in this chapter.

Sodium Content and Extracellular Volume

In the pathogenesis of hypertension in diabetic patients, changes in the exchangeable sodium and the fluid volume play a major role. An elevation of body sodium could be detected in type 1 and type 2 diabetics irrespective

Table 10.1 Pathogenetic factors of hypertension: typical changes in diabetic patients with nephropathy

Exchangeable body sodium	Elevated
Plasma volume	Normal
Extracellular fluid volume	Elevated
Renin–angiotensin system	Inadequate suppressed
Plasma catecholamines	Normal
Plasma aldosterone	Normal/low
Atrial natriuretic peptide	Reduced renal effects
Vascular contractility	Enhanced
Vascular compliance	Reduced

of the presence of nephropathy by various authors (6,7,8). Several authors found a correlation between the exchangeable body sodium and the level of blood pressure in patients with micro- and macroalbuminuria (6,8). Investigations of the plasma volume mostly revealed normal values, whereas extracellular fluid volume was often found to be raised (8). In type 1 diabetics, a significant correlation between the level of blood pressure and the extracellular volume could be demonstrated. As a rule, the blood pressure is sensitive to salt in patients with type 1 and type 2 diabetes (9,10).

Effects of insulin on an intensified resorption of sodium are assumed to be the cause of the raised body sodium and the increased retention of water (11,12). Furthermore, it is known that glucose and ketone bodies are reabsorbed as sodium salts in co-transport in the renal tubules, so that an increased reabsorption of sodium occurs, especially when metabolic control is poor (13).

Vascular Resistance and Contractility

A raised peripheral resistance and an enhanced contractility of the smooth vascular musculature in response to vasopressor stimuli, such as noradrenaline or angiotensin II, are constant findings in hypertensive patients with diabetes (7,14). Alterations in the cation transport in the smooth musculature are discussed as the mechanism: these lead to a rise in free cytoplasmic calcium and thus to an enhanced vascular tonus. The raised contractility can be explained by the increased sodium content, since sodium sensitizes the vascular musculature to pressor effects. Furthermore, it is known that insulin stimulates the firing rate of the sympathetic nervous system. This is seen even under normoglycaemic conditions and is therefore not due to hypoglycaemia (15,16).

Renin–Angiotensin System (RAS)

Measurements of the RAS and aldosterone in patients with type 1 diabetes revealed divergent data which are based in part on individual differences with regard to metabolic status, therapy and duration (6,8,17,18). However, the results must be interpreted in connection with the sodium chloride volume status of the patients. Since as a rule body sodium and the extracellular volume are usually increased in patients with diabetes, especially when proteinuria is present, reduced activity of the RAS would actually be expected. An unchanged plasma renin activity therefore indicates inadequate suppression of this system, so that it is quite important for the pathogenesis of hypertension.

Renal Arterial Stenosis

The incidence of renal arterial stenosis as cause of hypertension, especially in type 2 diabetics, has not been meticulously investigated up to now. After an autopsy study, Sawicki et al (19) described a three-fold risk for the development of renal arterial stenosis in type 2 diabetics compared to non-diabetics. However, this investigation does not clearly show the extent to which the pathological and anatomical findings are of haemodynamic relevance. In a larger-scale angiographic study, a raised prevalence of renal arterial stenosis was not found in hypertensive diabetics (10 of 28 = 36%) compared to non-diabetics (50 of 104 = 48%) (20). In a further study on 117 hypertensive type 2 diabetics using magnetic resonance angiography, renal arterial stenosis was detected in 17% (21). The presence of a femoral bruit was a useful predictable clinical marker.

DIAGNOSIS OF HYPERTENSION

The definition and classification of blood pressure ranges of the WHO–IHS guidelines published in 1999 are given in Table 10.2. However, not only the blood pressure values, but of course other individual factors such as age, vascular status, clinical signs of organ damage due to hypertension, such as left ventricular hypertrophy, proteinuria, alterations in the fundus of the eye, etc., are crucial in establishing the individual indication for treatment.

Because of the pre-eminent importance of the blood pressure level for the development and progression of microangiopathy and macroangiopathy, the regular control of blood pressure is one of the most important parameters

Table 10.2 Definitions and classification of blood pressure levels (mmHg)

Category	Systolic	Diastolic
Optimal	< 120	< 80
Normal	< 130	< 85
High-normal	130–139	85–89
Grade 1 hypertension (mild)	140–159	90–99
Subgroup: borderline	140–149	90–94
Grade 2 hypertension (moderate)	160–179	100–109
Grade 3 hypertension (severe)	≥ 180	≥ 110
Isolated systolic hypertension	≥ 140	< 90
Subgroup: borderline	140–149	< 90

When a patient's systolic and diastolic blood pressures fall into different categories, the higher category should apply.
From (1).

in management of these patients. Since the blood pressure is affected by various factors, repeated measurements on different days must be available for diagnosis of hypertension. Some practical prerequisites for measurement of blood pressure (especially in patients with a type 2 diabetes) will be mentioned in Table 10.3.

Incorrect measurement of blood pressure may occur owing to pronounced vascular sclerosis. Pseudohypertension is an elevation of blood pressure which can be demonstrated in manometric measurement, but not in intra-arterial measurement. It must be suspected clinically when patients with blood pressure values that are still hypertensive when measured manometrically report states of collapse. If necessary, a direct measurement of blood pressure must be carried out.

In patients with autonomic neuropathy, orthostatic dysregulation may occur owing to a disturbed baroreceptor reflex arc. Normal or raised blood pressure values measured in the supine position (supine hypertension) fall substantially when the patient stands up (orthostatic hypotension). Hence, in diabetics blood pressure values should also be measured in the standing position, especially when there are relevant clinical symptoms.

Differential Diagnosis in Hypertension

In patients with type 1 diabetes and nephropathy, the cause of the hypertension is usually renal, so that detailed clarification of the causes is not required in most cases when there are no other clinical abnormalities.

In proteinuric patients with type 2 diabetes, the hypertension may be due to the nephropathy or only exacerbated by it, since hypertension is already present before development of nephropathy in the majority of patients. Depending on the clinical symptoms, other causes of hypertension should be clarified in the usual way in this group of patients.

A "white-coat hypertension" (WCH) appears to occur relatively often in patients with diabetes. There is WCH when blood pressure values of more than 140/90 mmHg are repeatedly measured in the doctor's office, whereas

Table 10.3 Some practical prerequisites for blood pressure measurement

- Allow the patient to sit for several minutes in a quite room before beginning blood pressure measurement
- Use a standard cuff with a bladder that measures 12–13 × 35 cm, with a larger bladder for fat arms and a smaller bladder for children
- Use phase V Korotkoff sounds (disappearance) to measure DBP
- Measure the blood pressure in both arms at the first visit if there is evidence of peripheral vascular disease
- Place the sphygmomanometer cuff at heart level, whatever the position of the patient

From (1).

daytime values of less than 135/80 mmHg are present in ambulant blood pressure monitoring (ABPM). Investigations in normoalbuminuric type 1 diabetics without a history of hypertension showed a WCH prevalence of 74% (22). The hypertension measured in the office corresponded to WHO stage I. In type 2 diabetics, the data vary between 23% and 62%, depending on the criteria used to evaluate ABPM (23,24). In an investigation on a general hypertensive population, Verdecchia et al (25) had measured a WCH prevalence of 19%. This rose to 33% when only patients with stage I hypertension were evaluated. These findings indicate that WCH is found more frequently in patients with less severe hypertension.

To avoid an unnecessary antihypertensive treatment, ABPM should be performed in all diabetic patients after diagnosis of office hypertension. However, the long-term prognostic significance of WCH is unclear as yet. In the study of Flores et al (22), type 1 diabetic patients with WCH showed a significantly higher systolic and diastolic blood pressure values during daytime and nighttime ABPM compared to normotensive type 1 diabetic patients without WCH. Moreover, patients with WCH presented higher levels of urinary albumin excretion than patients with normal office blood pressure, although they were in the normal range. Therefore, patients with WCH should probably not be considered as an absolutely "normal" patient group because they show several findings that may indicate an increased risk for the development of diabetic nephropathy.

Importance of the 24 Hour Measurement of Blood Pressure

ABPM is especially important, not only to rule out WCH in diabetic patients but also to monitor antihypertensive therapy and to detect the absence of nocturnal lowering of the blood pressure ("non-dipping") often observed in these patients. Non-dipping is commonly defined as a relative reduction of night blood pressure less than 10% of the day value for both systolic and diastolic blood pressure. The American Society of Hypertension Ad Hoc Panel has recently published recommendations on the classification of ABPM (26) (Table 10.4).

Various studies have shown that non-dipping is associated with increased level of albumin excretion in the 24 h urine in type 1 and type 2 diabetics. About 80–90% of patients with macroalbuminuria manifested this phenomenon, whereas it could be detected in 30–50% of patients with normal urinary albumin excretion in both type 1 and type 2 diabetes (27,28).

Poulsen et al (29) was also able to show that non-dipping is also associated with the manifestation of retinopathy in normoalbuminuric patients with type 1 diabetes. Non-dipping of blood pressure at night is regarded as the possible cause for the high cardiovascular mortality of diabetic patients

Table 10.4 Upper limits of normal of average ABP as recommended by the Ad Hoc Panel of the American Society of Hypertension, based upon observational data (22)

BP Measure	Probably normal	Borderline	Probably abnormal
Systolic average (mmHg)			
Awake	< 135	135–140	> 140
Asleep	< 120	120–125	> 125
24 h	< 130	130–135	> 135
Diastolic average (mmHg)			
Awake	< 85	85–90	> 90
Asleep	< 75	75–80	> 80
24 h	> 80	80–85	> 85

with microangiopathy or macroangiopathy (30). The nocturnal blood pressure characteristics should therefore be considered in the decision as to the hypertensive treatment to be administered (31).

The causes for the non-dipping of blood pressure have not been entirely elucidated. Besides the manifestation of autonomous neuropathy and disturbance of the water balance, new investigations show that this disorder already occurs at a very early stage in the development of diabetes (32).

REFERENCES

1. World Health Organization. International Society of Hypertension guidelines for the management of hypertension. *J Hypertens* 1999; **17**: 151–83.
2. Norgaard K, FeldtRasmussen B, Borch-Johnsen K. Prevalence of hypertension in type 1 (insulin-dependent) diabetes mellitus: *Diabetologia* 1990; **33**: 407–10.
3. Mathiesen ER, Rønn B, Jensen T, Storm B, Deckert T. Relationship between blood pressure and urinary albumin excretion in development of microalbuminuria. *Diabetes* 1990; **39**: 245–9.
4. United Kingdom Prospective Diabetes Study. Prevalence of hypotensive therapy in patients with newly diagnosed diabetes. *Hypertension* 1985; 7 (II): 8–13.
5. Tarnow L, Rossing P, Gall MA, Nielsen FS, Parving HH. Prevalence of arterial hypertension in diabetic patients before and after the JNC-V. *Diabet Care* 1994; **17**: 1247–51.
6. O'Hare JA, Ferriss JB, Brady D, Twomey B, O'Sullivan DJ. Exchangeable sodium and renin in hypertensive diabetic patients with and without nephropathy. *Hypertension* 1985; 7 (II): 43–8.
7. Weidmann P, Beretta-Piccoli C, Trost BN. Pressor factors and responsiveness in hypertension accompanying diabetes mellitus. *Hypertension* 1985; 7 (II): 33–42.
8. Feldt-Rasmussen B, Mathiesen ER, Deckert T. Central role for sodium in the pathogenesis of blood pressure changes independent of angiotensin, aldosterone and catecholamines in type 1 (insulin dependent) diabetes mellitus. *Diabetologia* 1987; **30**: 620.
9. Strojek K, Grzeszcak W, Lacka B, Gorska J, Keller CK, Ritz E. Increased prevalence of salt sensitivity of blood pressure in IDDM with and without microalbuminuria. *Diabetologia* 1995; **38**: 1443–8.

10. Tuck M, Corry D, Trujillo A. Salt-sensitive blood pressure exaggerated vascular reactivity in the hypertension of diabetes mellitus. *Am J Med* 1990; **88**: 210–16.
11. DeFronzo RA, Cooke CR, Andres R, Faloona GR, Davis PJ. The effect of insulin and renal handling of sodium, potassium, calcium and phosphate in man. *J Clin Invest* 1975; **55**: 845–55.
12. Trevisan R, Fioretto P, Semplicini A et al. Role of insulin and atrial natriuric peptide in sodium retention in insulin-treatment IDDM patients during isotonic volume expansion. *Diabetes* 1990; **39**: 289–98.
13. Ferrari P, Weidmann P. Insulin, insulin sensitivity and hypertension. *J Hypertens* 1990; **8**: 491–500.
14. Drury P, Smith PLGM, Ferriss JB. Increased vasopressor responsiveness to angiotensin II in type 1 (insulin-dependent) diabetic patients without complications. *Diabetologia* 1984; **27**: 174–9.
15. Lembo G, Napoli R, Capaldo B et al. Abnormal sympathetic overactivity evoked by insulin in the skeletal muscle of patients with essential hypertension. *J Clin Invest* 1992; **90**: 24–9.
16. Julius S. Autonomic nervous dysfunction in essential hypertension. *Diabet Care* 1991; **14**: 249–59.
17. Drury PL, Bodansky HJ, Oddie CJ, Edwards CRW. Factors in the control of plasma renin activity and concentration in type 1 diabetics. *Clin Endocrinol* 1984; **20**: 607–18.
18. Van Dyk DJ, Erman A, Erman T et al. Increased serum angiotensin vomnverting enzyme activity in type T insulin-dependent diabetes mellitus: ist relation to metabolic control and diabetic complications. *Eur J Clin Invest* 1994; **24**: 463–7.
19. Sawicki PT, Kaiser S, Heinemann L et al. Prevalence of renal artery stenosis in diabetes mellitus—an autopsy study. *J Int Med* 1991; **229**: 489–92.
20. Munichoodappa C, Délia JA, Libertino JA et al. Renal artery stenosis in hypertensive diabetics. *J Urol* 1979; **121**: 555.
21. Valabhji J, Robinson S, Poulter C et al. Prevalence of renal artery stenosis in subjects with type 2 diabetes and coexistent hypertension. *Diabet Care* 2000; **23**: 539–43.
22. Flores L, Recasens, Gomis R, Esmatjes E. White coat hypertension in type 1 diabetic patients without nephropathy. *American Journal of Hypertention* 2000; **13**: 560–63.
23. Nielsen F, Gaede P, Vedel P et al. White coat hypertension in NIDDM patients with and without incipient and overt diabetic nephropathy. *Diabet Care* 1997; **20**: 859–63.
24. Burgess E, Mather K, Ross S, Josefsberg Z. Office hypertension in type 2 (non-insulin-dependent) diabetic patients. *Diabetologia* 1991; **34**: 684–5.
25. Verdecchia P, Schillaci G, Boldrini F et al. Variability between current definitions of "normal" ambulatory blood pressure, implications in the assessment of while coat hypertension. *Hypertension* 1992; **20**: 555–62.
26. Pickering T, for an American Society of Hypertension ad hoc panel. Recommendations for the use of home (self) and ambulatory blood pressure monitoring. *Am J Hypertens* 1996; **9**: 1–11.
27. Equiluz-Bruck S, Schnack C, Kopp HP, Schernthaner G. Non-dipping of nocturnal blood pressure is related to urinary albumin excreation rate in patients with type 2 diabetes mellitus. *Am J Hypertens* 1996; **9**: 1139–43.
28. Poulsen PL, Ebbehoi E, Hansen KW, Mogensen CE. 24 hour pressure and autonomic function is related to albumin excretion within the normoalbuminuric range in IDDM patients. *Diabetologia* 1997; **40**: 718–25.

29. Poulsen PL, Beck T, Ebberhoi, Hansen KW, Mogensen CE. 24-h ambulatory blood pressure and retinopathy in normoalbuminuric IDDM patient. *Diabetologia* 1998; **41**: 105–110.
30. Nakano S, Fukuda M, Hotta F et al. Reversed circadian blood pressure rhythm is associated with occurrences of both fatal and non-fatal vascular events in NIDDM subjects. *Diabetes* 1998; **47**: 1501–6.
31. Myers MG, Haynes RB, Rabkin SW. Canadian hypertension society guidelines for ambulatory blood pressure monitoring. *Am J Hypertens* 1999; **12**: 1149–57.
32. Chen JW, Jen SL, Lee WL et al. Differential glucose tolerance in dipper and non-dipper essential hypertension. *Diabet Care* 1998; **21**: 1743–8.

11

Cardiovascular Complications in Proteinuric Diabetic Patients

PETER T. SAWICKI

St Franziskus Hospital, Cologne, Germany

PROGNOSTIC IMPACTS OF ELEVATED URINARY ALBUMIN EXCRETION

Non-diabetic Subjects

Although excretion of small but abnormally elevated quantities of albumin in the urine may be an early feature of diabetic glomerular disease, it is also found in non-diabetic subjects. In an investigation of healthy, normotensive, untreated factory workers with a mean age of 50 years the prevalence of microalbuminuria (albumin excretion $> 20\,\mu g/min$) was 2.2% (1). In the Islington Diabetes Survey, including random patients selected from general practice, microalbuminuria was found in 9.4% non-diabetic subjects and in 23% of newly diagnosed diabetic patients (2). In this study there was a significant correlation between the albumin excretion rate and both systolic and diastolic blood pressure values. The higher prevalence of microalbuminuria in non-diabetic patients with essential hypertension has been repeatedly described. A survey of patients from general practice found a prevalence of microalbuminuria of 10% in hypertensive patients compared to 4% in normotensives and 23% of diabetic patients (3). Among a hospitalized group of nearly 400 hypertensive non-diabetic patients the prevalence of microalbuminuria was 27% (4). In this study the albumin excretion rate was

---

Diabetic Nephropathy. Edited by C. Hasslacher.
© 2001 John Wiley & Sons, Ltd.

significantly correlated not only with 24 h systolic and diastolic blood pressure values but was also higher in patients with hypertensive retinopathy, cardiac ventricular hypertrophy and reduced glomerular filtration rate. In obese subjects, elevated urinary albumin excretion is not only associated with hypertension and body mass index, but seems also to depend upon waist to hip circumferences, reflecting the fat distribution of the body (5).

In the Framingham study, a cohort aged 50–62 years at entry was followed up for 16 years (6); proteinuria above 200 mg/l was associated with a three-fold increase in mortality. In a 4 year follow-up study of non-diabetic subjects, albuminuria, independently of other cardiovascular risk markers, strongly predicted death, coronary heart disease and peripheral vascular disease (2). The analysis of a 6 years follow-up study of subjects aged 60–74 years showed that three times as many people whose albuminuria was equal to or above the median (7.5 μg/min) died, compared to those who had rated below the median.

Different mechanisms could be involved in an elevated urinary albumin excretion. Such mechanisms include renal haemodynamic changes, secondary to the direct transmission of raised systemic pressure to the glomerular arteriolar network (7). Also, direct effects of endothelial damage and/or permselectivity changes of the glomerular filtering barrier and/or altered tubular albumin reabsorption and structural damage to the glomerulae and arterioles are likely to play a role in the amount of albumin found in the urine (8).

Insulin-dependent Diabetes

Several studies from all over the world show that patients with insulin-dependent diabetes (type 1) exhibit an dramatic excess in mortality compared to non-diabetic subjects. While acute, metabolic complications dominate the causes of death in patients with short diabetes duration, the long-term excess in mortality is restricted nearly totally to those patients who develop diabetic nephropathy during the course of the disease. In his study of excess mortality in a representative sample of type 1 diabetic patients, Borch-Johnsen found a very high excess mortality only in those patients who developed persistent proteinuria (i.e. clinical diabetic nephropathy), while patients with normal proteinuria had a mortality rate very similar to the non-diabetic population, Figure 11.1 (9). However, nephropathy is not the direct cause of this increased mortality risk. Despite the fact that the risk of progression to renal failure is very high in type 1 diabetic patients with macroalbuminuria, in Europe only few type 1 diabetic patients will die a renal death, because renal replacement therapy is offered to nearly to all type 1 diabetic patients with end stage renal failure. Instead, cardiovascular events represent the main cause of death in patients with nephropathy. Due to yet unknown factors, the incidence of coronary heart disease starts to

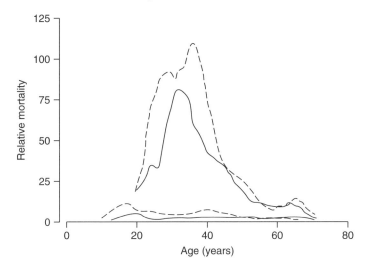

Figure 11.1 Relative mortality among patients with persistent proteinuria (upper curves) and without proteinuria (lower curves) as a function of current age; – – – – women; — men. From (9), © 1985 Springer-Verlag, with permission

rise soon after development of overt proteinuria, Figure 11.2 (10). This is very different from the situation in non-insulin-dependent-diabetes (type 2), in these patients coronary heart disease and elevated albumin excretion in urine often precede the development of diabetes. In two long-term follow-up trials we have described the causes of death in 85 type 1 diabetic patients with overt diabetic nephropathy (11) and in 216 consecutive type 2 diabetic patients (12). Cardiac mortality was the leading cause of death in both type 1 and type 2 diabetic patients. The distribution of the different causes of death in both groups is shown in Table 11.1.

Non-insulin-dependent Diabetes

Several reports have shown that microalbuminuria is already present before or very early in the course of type 2 diabetes. Non-diabetic subjects with impaired glucose tolerance or a parental history of diabetes already have an increased risk of microalbuminuria (13). Elevated albumin excretion is associated with insulin resistance (14,15) and hence, microalbuminuria precedes the development of type 2 diabetes (16). This comes as no surprise, since in non-diabetic subjects microalbuminuria is associated with high blood pressure, high insulin concentrations, low high-density lipoprotein cholesterol concentrations and high triglyceride concentration, a cluster of risk markers typical for prediabetic subjects. In the Kuopio study, including more than 1000 participants (aged 65–74 years), as many as 30% of normoglycaemic

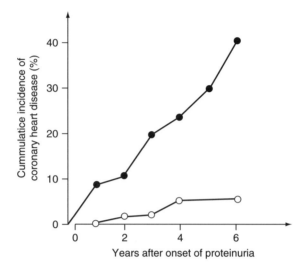

Figure 11.2 Cumulative incidence of coronary heart disease in insulin-dependent diabetic patients, with (•—•) and without (o—o) proteinuria. From 10, © 1987 Springer-Verlag, with permission

Table 11.1 Causes of death over a period of 9 years in 85 patients with insulin-dependent diabetes mellitus (IDDM) and overt diabetic nephropathy (11) and over a study period of 15 years in 216 patients with non-insulin-dependent diabetes mellitus (NIDDM) (12)

Causes of death during follow-up	IDDM patients with diabetic nephropathy (%)	NIDDM patients (%)
Cardiovascular	52	46
Cerebrovascular	18	15
Septicaemia	9	11
Malignoma	0	8
Hypoglycaemia	6	0
Other	15	20

subjects had microalbuminuria (16). During the follow-up of 3.5 years 69 non-diabetic subjects developed diabetes and 70% of those already had elevated albumin excretion at entry into the study.

Most importantly, the nature of albuminuria in type 2 diabetic patients is heterogeneous. This is very different from patients with type 1 diabetes in whom, in most cases, microalbuminuria hallmarks the presence of glomerular lesions typical for diabetic nephropathy. While microalbuminuria predicts overt proteinuria in 80% of type 1 diabetic patients, only 20% of microalbuminuric type 2 diabetic patients will progress to overt nephropathy (17). In kidney biopsy studies of unselected microalbuminuric type 2 diabetic patients, only about 30% have glomerular changes typical for diabetic nephropathy, while 30% have non-specific histological kidney lesions and the rest have a normal renal structure (18). Hence, despite the presence of microalbuminuria, a substantial proportion of type 2 diabetic patients do not have any renal disease. In addition, in those with histological renal alterations, microalbuminuria is associated with elevated markers of endothelial dysfunction, such as von Willebrand factor (19). This indicates that some of the renal structure abnormalities in microalbuminuric type 2 diabetic patients are consequent to endothelial dysfunction rather than being a sign of typical renal disease.

Since albuminuria is associated with several markers of widespread endothelial dysfunction in type 2 diabetes, it should also in univariate analyses predict mortality and cardiovascular morbidity. However, several studies in type 2 diabetic patients have unanimously suggested that micro-albuminuria, independently of other known cardiovascular risk markers, predicts all-cause mortality mainly by increasing the risk for cardiovascular events. In a 3.4 year follow-up study, microalbuminuric type 2 diabetic patients showed highly significant excess mortality, chiefly from cardiovas-cular causes, being 28% compared to those without microalbuminuria of 4% only; in this study 50% of deaths were caused by cardiovascular events (20). The higher the albumin excretion rate, the higher the risk of death: in a 3 year follow-up study, type 2 diabetic patients with normoalbuminuria had a 5% risk of death compared to 10% in those with microalbuminuria and 26% in macroalbuminuric patients (21). Similar results were obtained in an 8-year follow-up trial, where mortality was 32% in initially normoalbuminuric type 2 diabetic patients and increased to 56% in those with elevated albuminuria (22). Deaths due to cardiovascular disease occurred in 7% of patients with normoalbuminuria and in 26% of patients with micro- or macroalbuminuria. Only two patients died due to renal causes. Microalbuminuria nearly doubles the risk of dying of a cardiovascular cause, while the risk of dying due to a large vessel disease is about 70% (23). Interestingly, Stehouwer found that microalbuminuria in type 2 diabetic patients was associated with an increased risk of new cardiovascular events only in the presence of endothe-lial dysfunction, as indicated by elevated von Willebrand factor (24). It seems clear that elevated urinary albumin excretion represents a powerful predi-ctor of cardiovascular mortality in type 2 diabetic patients; however, the mechanisms of the pathophysiological link between both are mainly unclear.

ALBUMINURIA AND VENTRICULAR ARRHYTHMIAS

Both type 1 and type 2 diabetic patients with micro- and macroalbuminuria have an increased risk of dying from sudden death, which is presumed to be caused in most cases by fatal ventricular arrhythmia. We have looked on the causes of death in 85 type 1 diabetic patients with hypertension and diabetic nephropathy who were followed for a mean period of 9 years (11). The total mortality was nearly 40%; there were no renal deaths but over 60% of the patients who died, died due to cardio- or cerebrovascular causes (Table 11.1). Sudden and unexpected deaths occurred only in patients with a maximum QT interval duration in the ECG of $\geq 450\,ms^{1/2}$; 30% of mortality was attributed to sudden or unexpected death in this group. In the life table analysis, the group of patients with the longest maximal QTc period, which was arbitrary defined as $>470\,ms^{1/2}$, had a considerably higher mortality risk (Figure 11.3). QT prolongation is has also been correlated with nephropathy and ischaemic heart disease in the EURODIAB Study (25). In this study the prevalence of prolonged QT interval was 11% in males and 21% in females. Most interestingly, the length of the QT interval increased with higher albumin excretion in the urine.

QT prolongation predisposes to ventricular arrhythmias in patients with and without diabetes, presumably by increasing the risk of ventricular re-entry tachycardias and ventricular fibrillation. Most patients with diabetic nephropathy exhibit some degree of autonomic neuropathy (26), resulting in a reduced vagal activity, which can lead to alteration on the QT interval and increase the risk of sudden death (27). In young type 1 diabetic patients, elevated albumin excretion rates and autonomic nerve function deficits are

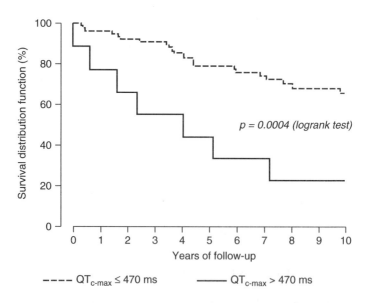

Figure 11.3   Kaplan-Meier curves of survival over the study period of 5–13 years of 85 patients with insulin-dependent diabetes mellitus (IDDM) and overt diabetic nephropathy and maximal QTc intervals $> 470\,ms^{1/2}$ and $\leq 470\,ms^{1/2}$ at baseline $p = 0.0004$ (log rank test). From 11, © 1996 Springer-Verlag, with permission

closely related (28). However, QT prolongation may not only result from decreased parasympathetic cardiac nerve activity but may be directly due to myocardial cell defects (29), which lead to a reduced electrical stability and also predispose to ventricular arrhythmia. Such cell defects may, for example, be caused by (silent) ischaemia and/or myocardial fibrosis in patients with coronary artery disease. In addition, volume overload and/or hypertension can reduce the threshold for arrhythmia through an increased ventricular wall stress. Also, renal failure, diuretic treatment and treatment with angiotensin-converting enzyme inhibitors (ACEIs) can induce electrolyte imbalances, leading to reduced myocardial stability. Furthermore, patients with diabetic nephropathy have an increased risk of severe hypoglycaemia. Prolongation of the QT interval occurs during very low blood glucose concentrations and may increase the risk of arrhythmic death in predisposed patients (30). In patients with newly diagnosed type 2 diabetes the cumulative incidence of sudden death after 4.5 years is about 10% of all fatal events (31). Patients with impaired glucose tolerance and type 2 diabetic patients with long QT intervals have been found to have an increased risk of sudden death (32), caused by torsade de points and ventricular fibrillation (33). Recently, an increased sympathetic activity during sleep was described in proteinuric type 2 diabetic patients (34). Such alterations in the sympathetic activity may contribute to the QT interval and alteration in type 2 diabetic patients and lead to an increased risk of sudden death in these patients.

We have followed 216 unselected consecutive type 2 diabetic patients for a period of 15 years to delineate the impact of the QT interval duration on total and cardiac mortality (12). During the follow-up period 158 patients (73%) died. In the final model, independent predictors of total mortality were the length of QT dispersion corrected for heart rate (QTc dispersion), age, male sex, systolic blood pressure, total cholesterol, HDL cholesterol, presence of diabetic retinopathy and micro- or macroproteinuria. Of the 108 patients with a QTc dispersion above the median of $0.0686\,s^{1/2}$, 101 died during the follow-up period as compared to 57 of those with a lower/equal length of QTc dispersion, Figure 11.4. There was a continuous increase in the mortality risk with prolongation of the QTc dispersion.

In non-diabetic patients a prolonged QTc interval and/or QTc dispersion were described as mortality risk markers in chronic heart failure, hypertrophic cardiomyopathy, coronary heart disease, peripheral artery disease and after myocardial infarction (12). Such co-morbidity is particularly frequent in type 2 diabetic patients and contributes to the higher mortality risk. Disturbed glucose metabolism of the heart may directly contribute to an impaired myocardial electrical stability. In a recent report of the Zutphen Elderly Study, QTc duration was associated with levels of insulin and glucose tolerance (35). Hence, reduced myocardial glucose uptake may be involved in impaired cardiac repolarization, as indicated by a prolongation of the QT interval. As in type 1 and type 2 diabetic patients, QT dispersion

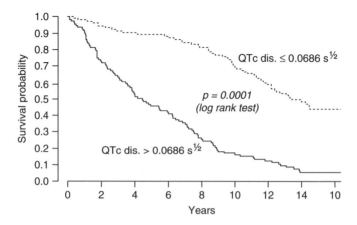

Figure 11.4 Kaplan–Meier curves of survival over the study period of 15–16 years of 216 patients with non-insulin-dependent diabetes mellitus and a QTc dispersion at baseline below and above the median of $0.0686\,\mathrm{s}^{1/2}$; $p = 0.0001$ (log rank test). From (12) with permission

prolongation may also result from cardiac adrenergic dysinervation with altered balance of sympathetic and parasympathetic cardiac nerve activity and lead to a reduced electrical stability (27,36,37). Regional myocardial hypoxia and dysinervations may lead to focal QT prolongation, increasing the QT dispersion (38). Such prolonged QTc dispersion indicates the presence of electrical myocardial inhomogenity, which may be expected to create a potential difference during repolarization and generate an excitatory current of a sufficient magnitude to re-excite the fibres with a shorter action potential duration and consecutively lead to re-entry arrhythmias (39). Likewise, blockade of adenosine triphosphate-sensitive potassium channels by sulphonylurea drugs is known to lengthen re-polarization and produce early afterdepolarizations, which can cause triggered activity in the hypoxic myocardium and lead to fatal ventricular tachyarrhythmias (40–42).

Hence, oral agents with ATP-channel-blocking properties may be of particular danger in proteinuric type 2 diabetic patients and β blocking agents may offer protection against sudden death.

GLYCAEMIC CONTROL, ORAL ANTIDIABETIC AGENTS AND INSULIN

In type 1 diabetic patients maintenance of near-normoglycaemic control has been convincingly shown to prevent the development of microangiopathic complications, i.e. diabetic nephropathy, retinopathy and neuropathy (43). This may also apply in some extent to younger type 2 diabetic patients (44,45). Since the reduction of life expectancy in type 1 diabetic patients is restricted to those patients who develop diabetic nephropathy (9) (Figure 11.1), it can be assumed that prevention of diabetic nephropathy by near-normoglycaemia will dramatically reduce the incidence of cardiovascular complications in type 1 diabetic patients. In fact, such a trend has already been described in a large intervention trial in type 1 diabetic patients (43). However, there is no evidence that normoglycaemia will have a direct beneficial effect on the macrovascular coronary disease (46–48). The perpetuation of the causal link between hyperglycaemia and coronary heart disease is mainly based on studies suggesting an increasing gradient of cardiovascular risk with decreasing glucose tolerance, increasing glycaemia and glycosylated haemoglobin. However, a review of several epidemiological studies found only a small and inconsistent effect of mild hyperglycaemia on cardiovascular disease risk, especially after adjustment for other known cardiovascular risk markers. In addition, there is no intervention study showing any direct effect of blood glucose lowering treatment on the development or progression of coronary artery disease.

The only prospective randomized study that claims an impact of blood glucose lowering on cardiovascular events is the diabetes mellitus, Insulin Glucose Infusion in Acute Myocardial Infarction (DIGAMI) study, which has been presented in a series of original publications (49–51). In this trial a total of 620 diabetic patients with acute myocardial infarction were randomized either to an acute treatment with glucose–insulin infusion followed by multidose subcutaneous insulin for more than 3 months, or to a control group, which was treated with diet or oral hypoglycaemic medication. After a follow-up of 12 months, 18.6% of insulin-treated patients and 26.1% of the control patients had died, resulting in a significant reduction of relative mortality with insulin of 29%. During the first years of treatment the number of fatal reinfarctions was significantly reduced from 45% in the control group to 28% in the insulin group. After a mean follow-up of 3.4 years there were 33% of deaths in the insulin group compared to 44% in the control group. This substantial difference in mortality can hardly be due to long-term differences in the degree of metabolic control: HbA_{1c}-levels at 3 months were 7.1% compared to 7.5% and at 1 year 7.3% compared to 7.6%. This insignificant difference is most unlikely to result in a clinically apparent change of the prognosis of the diabetic patients following myocardial infarction (52). Much rather, the difference in the mortality rate between the groups can be probably explained by the insulin–glucose infusion in the intervention group (53) and a higher proportion of patients treated with sulphonylurea drugs in the control group (52).

ANTIHYPERTENSIVE TREATMENT IN HIGH RISK DIABETIC PATIENTS

There is no doubt that antihypertensive treatment reduces mortality and morbidity in type 1 and type 2 diabetes. This beneficial effect has been shown for thiazide diuretics, β-blockers and ACE Inhibitors (54–60) However, there is still a controversy about whether some antihypertensive agents are superior to others.

Until recently no mortality endpoint data were available for the treatment with calcium channel blockers in diabetic patients. Nevertheless, these agents have been widely recommended for antihypertensive treatment in diabetic patients, despite the fact that they have repeatedly been shown to increase mortality in patients with coronary heart disease in randomized controlled trials (61,62). Recently, evidence has accumulated from three randomized prospective studies that treatment of diabetic patients with calcium channel blockers results in an increase of cardiovascular morbidity and mortality when compared to other antihypertensive agents. In the MIDAS study, the calcium channel blocker isradipine was compared with the diuretic hydrochlorothiazid: isradipine leads to an increased risk of cardio- and cerebrovascular events, especially in patients with raised glycosylated haemoglobin levels (63). In the ABCD trial in hypertensive type 2 diabetic patients, treatment with nisoldipine resulted in a five-fold increased risk for fatal and non-fatal myocardial infarction when compared to enalapril (25/235 vs. 5/235) (64). In the FACET study, amlodipine doubled the risk of cardio- and cerebrovascular events as compared to fosinopril (27/191 vs. 14/189) (64). In a meta-analysis of intervention studies comparing different antihypertensive agents in patients with coronary heart disease, treatment with β-blockers resulted in a 24% reduction of cardiac morbidity mortality risk, while calcium channel blockers increased this risk by 63% (64). Recently, in the Syst Eur trial (65), antihypertensive treatment with nitrendipine, enalapril and hydrochlorothiazid reduced the risk of mortality, cardiovascular events and stroke in hypertensive diabetic patients. Comparing the effects in diabetic and non-diabetic hypertensive patients, this study also confirms previous results that the relative benefit of antihypertensive treatment increases with higher baseline risk. However, this trial does not answer the question of whether nitrendipine-based antihypertensive treatment is equal, better or worse than conventional antihypertensive medication with diuretics and/or β-blockers. Based upon a comparison between the relative risk reductions in the Syst Eur trial and the SHEP study (66), the authors claim that long-acting dihydropyridines may provide a better cardiovascular protection than low-dose thiazides. However, the SHEP study included patients with diastolic blood pressure (BP) values below 90 mmHg, while this limit was 95 mmHg in the Syst Eur trial, which resulted in approximately 10 mmHg higher diastolic BP in the in the Syst Eur trial. As shown in the HOT study (67), in diabetic patients even a smaller difference in diastolic BP within the normotensive range has a major impact on the risk of cardiovascular events. Hence, the Syst Eur trial included patients with a higher risk at baseline and this is likely to be responsible for the greater relative risk reduction in the Syst Eur trial when compared to the SHEP study. The WHO definition of isolated systolic hypertension is: "systolic BP values above 140 and diastolic BP below 90 mmHg without antihypertensive medication". However, the Syst Eur trial included patients with diastolic BP below 95 mmHg, of whom nearly half were already on antihypertensive medication at the time of baseline examination. Hence, the Syst Eur study also included a substantial number of patients with diastolic and systolic hypertension. Therefore, the authors should also have compared their results with the effect of thiazide-based antihypertensive treatment in trials including older hypertensive patients with any form of hypertension. The numbers needed to treat to prevent one death per year were 286 in the Syst Eur, 294 in the diuretic arm of the MRC and 66 in the STOP trials. Clearly, any valid conclusions with regard to the different effects of antihypertensive drugs on morbidity and mortality can only come from randomized direct comparison trials. Hence, when compared to conventional antihypertensive agents, calcium channel blockers can increase cardiovascular mortality and morbidity and should be used only very restrictively in diabetic patients.

The two major aims of antihypertensive treatment in hypertensive type 1 diabetic patients with diabetic nephropathy are the prevention of dialysis and the reduction of the severely increased risk of cardiovascular mortality. Often an antihypertensive therapy is changed despite optimal blood pressure control because of a postulated specific nephroprotective effect of ACE inhibitors. However, a careful review of the controlled intervention trials aiming at valid clinical end-points does not indicate a specific, i.e. blood pressure independent, nephroprotective effect of ACE inhibitors.

In nephropathic insulin-dependent diabetic patients, treatment with ACE inhibitors was associated in two studies with a slower loss of kidney function as compared to placebo (68) or to a betablocker (69). However, in both studies blood pressure values were significantly lower with the ACE inhibitor treatments when compared to the respective control groups (70, 71). It is of note, that in other randomized intervention studies, in which blood pressure control was kept comparable between the study groups, there was no difference in the decline on GFR when comparing ACE inhibitors to placebo (72) or a betablocker (73). In metaanalyses including controlled and uncontrolled studies ACE inhibitors have been reported to be more effective than other antihypertensive agents with regard to the reduction of albuminuria and proteinuria (74), but equally effective with regard to their influence on the decline of glomerular filtration rate (GFR) in diabetic nephropathy (75). These results have been attributed to the effect of ACE inhibitors on the charge of the glomerular basement membrane which influences glomerular albumin leakage; this action is, however, without impact on the progression of glomerular histopathological changes and, hence, on the decline of GFR (76). In nephropathic type 1 diabetic patients, the ACE inhibitor lisinopril was reported to reduce albuminuria, but to result in a faster loss of GFR when compared to the calcium channel blocker nisoldipine (77). Thus, there is still no evidence for a specific, i.e. blood pressure independent, beneficial effect of any antihypertensive agent including ACE inhibitors on the progression of diabetic nephropathy as measured by the progression to renal replacement therapy or by the decline of GFR. Recently, we have shown, that it is possible over a period of two years to achieve a stabilization of glomerular filtration rate in type 1 diabetic patients with already impaired renal function due to diabetic nephropathy, if the goals of intensified antihypertensive treatment have been reached (78). The antihypertensive drug therapy was based on a random allocation to an open treatment either with an ACEI, a calcium channel blocker or a cardio-selective betablocker. As assessed by inulin clearance, we have found no differences between the investigated drugs with regard to the percentage of patients with stable renal function and the course of GFR.

Hence, when blood pressure is well controlled with conventional anti-hypertensive therapy in nephropathic diabetic patients, there is no need to switch to ACE inhibitors.

IMPROVEMENT OF ANTIHYPERTENSIVE CARE IN DIABETIC PATIENTS

The main problem in antihypertensive care of diabetic patients is the fact that, despite antihypertensive treatment, hypertension remains uncon-trolled in the vast majority of these patients. Even in specialized diabetes centres, only about 11% of hypertensive type 1 diabetic patients had blood pressure values within the target range (79).

Recently, we have investigated the effects of improved antihypertensive treatment strategies in a high-risk group of type 2 diabetic patients, all of whom were hypertensive and micro- or macroproteinuric and nearly all of them insulin-treated (80). All patients were treated for hypertension and half of them participated, in addition, in an ambulatory hypertension treat-ment and teaching programme aimed at improving patients' compliance to pharmacological and non-pharmacological therapy. Participation in this programme resulted in a major improvement in the quality of blood pressure control. After a mean follow-up of 4 years, the combined incidence of cardio- and cerebrovascular events was reduced from 26% in the control group to 14% in the intervention group, Figure 11.5.

In a further long-term prospective 10 year intervention study we have demonstrated that such an intensification of antihypertensive treatment in type 1 diabetic patients with diabetic nephropathy is associated with a major improvement in life expectancy (Figure 11.6) (81). The major causes of

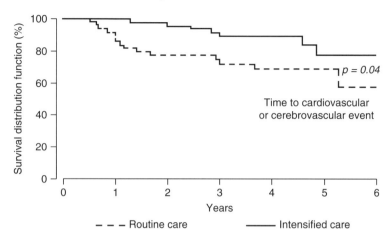

Figure 11.5 Kaplan–Meier curves of survival in non-insulin-dependent diabetic patients with micro- or macroproteinuria until a cardiovascular or cerebrovascular event treated according to an intensified antihypertensive therapy regimen ($n = 50$) and in the routine antihypertensive therapy group ($n = 50$). From (90) with permission

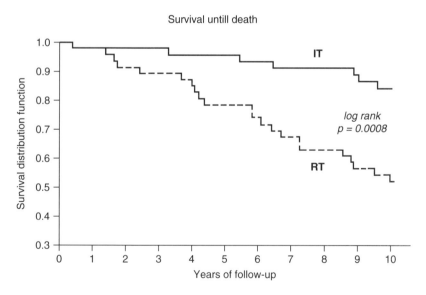

Figure 11.6 Kaplan–Meier curves of patients' survival in hypertensive insulin-dependent diabetic patients with diabetic nephropathy, treated according to an intensified antihypertensive therapy regimen ($n = 45$) and in the routine antihypertensive therapy group ($n = 46$). From (91) with permission

death were cardiovascular. As compared to routine antihypertensive therapy, intensified antihypertensive treatment based on a structured teaching and treatment programme reduced the risk of death, dialysis, amputation and blindness (Table 11.2).

NICOTINE REPLACEMENT THERAPY

Several large prospective cohort studies have shown that diabetic patients who smoke have an approximately two-fold increased mortality risk, with the main cause of death being cardiovascular (82–84). Smoking increases blood pressure in patients with diabetic nephropathy (85) and may contribute to the progression of diabetic nephropathy (86). Patients with endstage renal disease who smokerun a particularly high mortality risk (87).

Programmes to help diabetic patients to stop smoking have so far been unsuccessful (88). Even an extensive behaviour therapy anti-smoking intervention programme's outcome was as poor as a single unstructured anti-smoking advice given by a physician (89): only 11% agreed to participate in a "stop smoking programme" and 6 months after the intervention non-smoking was confirmed in only 5% of the behavioural therapy group and 16% of the physician's advice group. However, since nicotine replacement therapy has been shown to double the success of smoking cessation in non-diabetic patients (90), such intervention is worth while trying, even though studies showing satisfactory smoking cessation rates in diabetic patients are still lacking.

CHOLESTEROL-LOWERING THERAPY

Total serum cholesterol has been shown to be a predictor of cardiovascular mortality and morbidity in middle-aged type 2 diabetic patients. Until recently, evidence about the effects of cholesterol lowering on morbidity and mortality in diabetic patients was lacking. A subgroup analysis of the

Table 11.2 Significant reduction of the primary and secondary study endpoints during the follow-up of 10 years or until death in the intensified antihypertensive therapy and routine antihypertensive therapy groups

Study endpoints (cumulative prevalence after a follow-up of 10 years)	Intensified antihypertensive therapy $n = 45$ (%)	Routine antihypertensive therapy $n = 46$ (%)
Death	16	48
Dialysis	26	46
Amputation	7	25
Blindness	14	35

From (91) with permission.

Helsinki Heart Study (91), using gemfibrocil as the lipid-lowering drug, described a 5 year incidence of major cardiovascular events in type 2 diabetic patients of 3.4% in the intervention and 10.5% in the placebo group; however, this difference was not statistically significant ($p = 0.19$). In a double-blind 5 year study in patients with myocardial infarction, which included 3573 non-diabetic and 582 diabetic patients with plasma total cholesterol levels below 240 mg/dl, treatment with pravastatin, an inhibitor of 3-hydroxy-3-hydroxymethyl co-enzyme A reductase (statin), resulted in a 23% ($p = 0.001$) reduction in major coronary events in non-diabetic patients and in a 25% reduction ($p = 0.05$) in diabetic patients (92). Recently, sub-group analyses of the 4S-Study in type 2 diabetic patients and patients with impaired glucose levels with previous myocardial infarction or angina pectoris have been published (93,94). In these studies, simvastatin significantly reduced major coronary events by revascularizations and total and coronary mortality. In the CARE study treatment with pravastatin in diabetic and glucose-intolerant myocardial infarction survivors reduced the total number of coronary events, the risk for revascularization (95).

Given these new results, it seems reasonable to treat diabetic patients under 65 years of age with signs of coronary artery disease with a statin when total serum cholesterol concentrations exceed 200 mg/dl, or low density lipoprotein concentrations exceed 130 mg/dl.

ASPIRIN

In an overview of published intervention studies in nearly 47 000 patients (including 10% of diabetic patients), aspirin given in doses of 100–400 mg/ day has been shown to reduce the risk of myocardial infarction and stroke in patients with high risk of such events (96). In this analysis, diabetic patients on aspirin had 17% fewer vascular events, whereas relative risk reduction was 22% in non-diabetic patients. Overall, aspirin treatment resulted in an about 30% reduction in the risk of myocardial infarction. In the Veterans Administration study, including 231 diabetic men with limb gangrene or recent amputation, aspirin and dipyridamole did not reduce the incidence of cardiovascular events (97). In the early treatment of retinopathy study, diabetic patients treated with 650 mg aspirin/day had a 13% lower risk for cardiovascular death when compared to placebo (98). Hence, available evidence suggests treatment with low-dose aspirin in diabetic patients with coronary heart disease (99).

REFERENCES

1. Zavaroni I, Bonini L, Gasparini P et al. Dissociation between urinary albumin excretion and variables associated with insulin resistance in a healthy population. *J Int Med* 1996; **240**: 151–6.

2. Yudkin JS, Forrest RD, Jackson CA. Microalbuminuria as a predictor of vascular disease in non-diabetic subjects. *Lancet* 1988; **ii**: 530–33.
3. Höhner D, Fliser D, Klimm HP, Ritz E. Albuminuria in normotensive and hypertensive individuals attending offices of general practitioners. *J Hypertens* 1996; **14**: 655–60.
4. Cerasola G, Cottone S, Mule G et al. Microalbuminuria, renal dysfunction and cardiovascular complication in essential hypertension. *J Hypertens* 1996; **14**: 915–20.
5. Basdevant A, Cassuto D, Gibault T, Raison J, Guy-Grand B. Microalbuminuria and body fat distribution in obese subjects. *Int J Obesity* 1994; **18**: 806–11.
6. Kannel WB, Stampfer MJ, Castelli WP, Verter J. The prognostic significance of proteinuria: the Framingham study. *Am Heart J* 1994; **108**: 1347–52.
7. Brenner B, Meyer TW, Hostetter TH. Dietary protein intake and the progressive nature of kidney disease: the role of hemodynamically mediated glomerular injury in the pathogenesis of progressive glomerular sclerosis in ageing, renal ablation and intrinsic renal disease. *N Engl J Med* 1982; **307**: 652–9.
8. Sawicki PT, Berger M. Measuring progression of diabetic nephropathy. Review. *Eur J Clin Invest* 1994; **24**: 651–5.
9. Borch-Johnsen K, Andersen PK, Deckert T. The effect of proteinuria on relative mortality in type 1 (insulin-dependent) diabetes mellitus. *Diabetologia* 1985; **28**: 590–96.
10. Jensen T, Borch-Johnsen K, Kofoed-Enevoldsen A, Deckert T. Coronary heart disease in young type 1 (insulin-dependent) diabetic patients with and without nephropathy: Incidence and risk factors. *Diabetologia* 1987; **30**: 144–8.
11. Sawicki PT, Dähne R, Bender R, Berger M. Prolonged QT interval as a predictor of mortality in diabetic nephropathy. *Diabetologia* 1996; **39**: 77–81.
12. Sawicki PT, Kiwitt S, Bender R, Berger M. The value of QT interval dispersion for identification of total mortality risk in non insulin dependent diabetes mellitus. *J Intern Med* 1998; **243**: 49–56.
13. Haffner SM Gonzáles C, Valdez RA et al. Is microalbuminuria part of the prediabetic state? The Mexico City Diabetes Study. *Diabetologia* 1993; **36**: 1002–6.
14. Groop L, Ekstrand A, Forsblom C et al. Insulin resistance, hypertension and microalbuminuria in patients with type II (non-insulin-dependent) diabetes mellitus. *Diabetologia* 1993; **36**: 642–7.
15. Niskanen L, Laakso M. Insulin resistance is related to microalbuminuria in patients with type II (non-insulin-dependent) diabetes mellitus. *Metabolism* 1993; **42**: 1541–5.
16. Mykkänen L, Haffner SM, Kuusisto J, Pyörälä K, Laakso M. Microalbuminuria precedes the development of diabetes. *Diabetes* 1994; **43**: 552–7.
17. Mogensen CE. Microalbuminuria as a predictor for clinical diabetic nephropathy. *Kidney Int* 1987; **31**: 673–89.
18. Fioretto P, Mauer M, Brocco E et al. Patterns of renal injury in NIDDM patients with microalbuminuria. *Diabetologia* 1996; **39**: 1569–76.
19. Fioretto P, Stehouwer CDA, Mauer M et al. Heterogeneous nature of microalbuminuria in NIDDM: studies of endothelial function and renal structure. *Diabetologia* 1998; **41**: 233–6.
20. Mattock MB, Morrish NJ, Viberti CG et al. Prospective study of microalbuminuria as predictor of mortality in NIDDM. *Diabetes* 1992; **41**: 736–41.
21. Stiegler H, Standl E, Schulz K, Roth R, Lehmacher W. Morbidity, mortality, and albuminuria in type 2 diabetic patients: a three-year prospective study of a random cohort in general practice. *Diabet Med* 1992; **9**: 646–53.
22. Neil A, Hawkins M, Potok M et al. A prospective population-based study of microalbuminuria as a predictor of mortality in NIDDM. *Diabet Care* 1993; **16**: 996–1003.

23. MacLeod JM, Lutale J, Marshall SM. Albumin excretion and vascular deaths in NIDDM. *Diabetologia* 1995; **38**: 610–16.
24. Stehouwer CDA, Nauta JJP, Zeldenrust GC et al. Urinary albumin excretion, cardiovascular disease and endothelial dysfunction in non-insulin-dependent diabetes mellitus. *Lancet* 1992; **340**: 319–23.
25. Veglio M, Borra M, Stevens LK et al. and the Eurodiab IDDM Complications Study Group. *Diabetologia* 1999; **42**: 68–75.
26. Molgaard H, Christensen PD, Hermansen K et al. Early recognition of autonomic dysfunction in microalbuminuria: significance for cardiovascular mortality in diabetes mellitus? *Diabetologia* 1994; **37**: 788–96.
27. Tentolouris N, Katsilambros N, Papazachos G et al. Corrected QT interval in relation to the severity of diabetic autonomic neuropathy. *Eur J Clin Invest* 1997; **27**: 1949–54.
28. Clarke CF, Eason M, Reilly A, Boyce D, Werther GA. Autonomic nerve function in adolescents with type 1 diabetes mellitus: relation to microalbuminuria. *Diabet Med* 1999; **16**: 550–54.
29. Towbin JA. New revelations about the long-QT syndrome. *N Engl J Med* 1995; **333**: 384–5.
30. Marques JLB, George E, Peacey SR, Harris ND, Macdonald IA, Cochrane T, Heller. Altered ventricular repolarisation during hypoglycaemia in patients with diabetes. *Diabet Med* 1997; **14**: 648–54.
31. The Hypertension in Diabetes Study Group. Hypertension in Diabetes Study (HDS): II. Increased risk of cardiovascular complications in hypertensive type 2 diabetic patients. *J Hypertens* 1993; **11**: 319–25.
32. Curb JD, Rodrigues BL, Burchfiel CM et al. Sudden death, impaired glucose tolerance, and diabetes in Japanese-American men. *Circulation* 1995; **91**: 2591–5.
33. Abo K, Ishida Y, Yoshida R et al. Kazumi T. Torsade de point in NIDDM with long QT intervals. *Diabet Care* 1996; **19**: 1010.
34. Nielsen FS, Hansen HP, Jacobsen P et al. Increased sympathetic activity during sleep and nocturnal hypertension in type 2 diabetic patients with diabetic nephropathy. *Diabet Med* 1999; **16**: 555–62.
35. Dekker JM, Feskens EJM, Schouten EG et al. QTc duration is associated with levels of insulin and glucose tolerance. *Diabetes* 1996; **45**: 376–80.
36. Bellavere F, Ferri M, Guarini L et al. Prolonged QT period in diabetic autonomic neuropathy: a possible role in sudden cardiac death. *Br Heart J* 1988; **59**: 379–83.
37. Shimabukuro M, Chibana T, Yoshida H et al. Increased QT dispersion and cardiac adrenergic dysinervation in diabetic patients with autonomic neuropathy. *Am J Cardiol* 1996; **78**: 1057–9.
38. Turpeinen AK, Vanninen E, Kuikka JT, Uusitupa MIJ. Demonstration of regional sympathetic denervation of the heart in diabetes. *Diabet Care* 1996; **19**: 1083–90.
39. Kuo CS, Munakata K, Reddy P, Surawicz R. Characteristics and possible mechanism of ventricular arrhythmia dependent on the dispersion of action potential durations. *Circulation* 1983; **67**: 1356–67.
40. Zipes DP. The long QT interval syndrome. A Rosetta Stone for sympathetic related ventricular tachyarrythmias. *Circulation* 1991; **84**: 1414–19.
41. Yang T, Roden DM. Extracellular potassium modulation of drug block of I_{Kr}: implications for torsade de points and reverse use-dependence. *Circulation* 1996; **93**: 407–11.
42. Nichols CG, Lederer WJ. Adenosine triphosphate-sensitive potassium channels in the cardiovascular system. *Am J Physiol* 1991; **261**: H1675–86.
43. The Diabetes Control and Complications Trial Research Group. The effect of intensive treatment of diabetes on the development and progression of long-term complications in insulin-dependent diabetes mellitus. *N Engl J Med* 1993; **329**: 977–86.

44. Ohkubo Y, Kishikawa H, Araki E et al. Intensive insulin therapy prevent the progression of diabetic microvascular complications in Japanese patients with non-insulin-dependent diabetes mellitus: a randomized prospective 6-year study. *Diabet Res Clin Pract* 1995; **28**: 103–17.

45. UKPDS Group. Intensive blood-glucose control with sulfonylureas or insulin compared with conventional treatment and risk of complications in patients with type 2 diabetes (UKPDS 33). *Lancet* 1998; **352**: 837–953.

46. Barrett-Connor E. Does hyperglycemia really cause coronary heart disease? *Diabet Care* 1997; **20**: 1620–23.

47. McCormack J, Greenhalgh T. Seeing what you want to see in randomised controlled trials: versions and perversions of UKPDS data. *Br Med J* 2000; **320**: 1720–23.

48. University Group Diabetes Programme. A study of the effects of hypoglycemic agents on vascular complications in patients with adult onset diabetes. *Diabetes* 1976; **25**: 1129–53.

49. Malmberg K, Rydén L, Effendic S et al. Randomised trial of insulin-glucose infusion followed by subcutaneous insulin treatment in diabetic patients with acute myocardial infarction (DIGAMI Study): effects on mortality at 1 year. *J Am Coll Cardiol* 1995; **26**: 57–65.

50. Malmberg K, Rydén L, Hamsten A et al on behalf of the DIGAMI study group. Effects of insulin treatment on cause-specific one-year mortality and morbidity in diabetic patients with acute myocardial infarction. *Eur Heart J* 1996; **17**: 1337–44.

51. Malmberg K. For the DIGAMI Study Group. Prospective randomised study of intensive insulin treatment on long-term survival after acute myocardial infarction in patients with diabetes mellitus. *Br Med J* 1997; **314**: 1512–15.

52. Mühlhauser I, Sawicki PT, Berger M. Possible risk of sulfonylureas in the treatment of non-insulin-dependent diabetes mellitus and coronary artery disease. *Diabetologia* 1997; **40**: 1492–3.

53. Farth-Ordoubadi F. Glucose-insulin-potassium therapy for treatment of acute myocardial infarction. An overview of randomised placebo-controlled trials. *Circulation* 1997; **96**: 1152–6.

54. SHEP Cooperative Research Group. Prevention of stroke by antihypertensive drug treatment in older persons with isolated hypertension. *J Am Med Assoc* 1991; **265**: 3255–64.

55. Dahlöf B, Lindholm LH, Hansson L et al. Morbidity and mortality in Swedish trial in old patients with hypertension. *Lancet* 1991; **338**: 1281–5.

56. Medical Research Council Working Party. MRC trial of treatment of hypertension in older adults. *Br Med J* 1992; **304**: 405–12.

57. Curb JD, Pressel SL, Cutler JA et al for the Systolic Hypertension in the Elderly Program Cooperative Research Group. Effect of diuretic-based antihypertensive treatment on cardiovascular disease risk in older diabetic patients with isolated systolic hypertension. *J Am Med Assoc* 1996; **276**: 1886–92.

58. Moser M, Ross H. The treatment of hypertension in diabetic patients. *Diabet Care* 1993; **16**: 542–7.

59. UKPDS Group. Efficacy of antenolol and cptopril in reducing risk of macrovascular and microvascular complications in type 2 diabetes: UKPDS 39. *Br Med J* 1998; **317**: 713–20.

60. HOPE Study Investigators. Effects of ramipril on cardiovascular and microvascular outcomes in people with diabetes mellitus: results of the HOPE study and MICRO-HOPE substudy. *Lancet* 2000; **355**: 253–9.

61. Lichtlen PR, Hugenholtz PG, Rafflenbeul W et al, on behalf of the INTACT Group. Retardation of angiographic progression of coronary artery disease by nifedipine: results of the International Nifedipine Trial on Antiatherosclerotic Therapy (INTACT). *Lancet* 1990; **335**: 1109–13.

62. Goldbourt U, Behar S, Reicher-Reis H et al., for the SPRINT Study Group. Early administration of nifedipine in suspected acute myocardial infarction: the Secondary Prevention of Reinfarction Israel Nifedipine Trial 2 Study. *Arch Intern Med* 1993; **153**: 345–53.
63. Byington RP, Craven TE, Furberg CD, Pahor M. Isradipine, raised glycosylated haemoglobin, and risk of cardiovascular events. *Lancet* 1997; **350**: 1075–6.
64. Alderman M, Madhavan S, Cohen H. Calcium antagonists and cardiovascular events in patients with hypertension and diabetes. *Lancet* 1998; **351**: 216–17.
65. Tuomilehto J, Rastenyte D, Birkenhäger WH et al. fects of calcium-channel blockade in older patients with diabetes and systolic hypertension. *N Engl J Med* 1999; **340**: 677–84.
66. Curb JD, Pressel SL, Cutler JA et al. for the Systolic Hypertension in the Elderly Program Cooperative Research Group. Effect of diuretic-based antihypertensive treatment on cardiovascular disease risk in older diabetic patients with isolated systolic hypertension. *J Am Med Assoc* 1996; **276**: 1886–92.
67. Hansson L, Zanchetti A, Carruthers SG et al. Effects of intensive blood-pressure lowering and low-dose aspirin in patients with hypertension: principal results of the Hypertension Optimal Treatment (HOT) randomised trial. *Lancet* 1998; **351**: 1755–62.
68. Lewis EJ, Hunsicker LG, Bain RP et al. The effect of angiotensin-converting-enzyme inhibition on diabetic nephropathy. *N Engl J Med* 1993; **329**: 1456–62.
69. Björck S, Mulec H, Johnsen SA et al. Renal protective effect of enalapril in diabetic nephropathy. *Br Med J* 1992; **304**: 339–42.
70. Sawicki PT, Mühlhauser I, Berger M. Captopril, blood pressure, and diabetic nephropathy. *JAMA* 1994; **272**: 1005.
71. Sawicki PT, Berger M. Renal protective effect of enalapril in diabetic nephropathy. *Br Med J* 1992; **304**: 841–2.
72. Bauer JH, Reams GP, Hewett J et al. A randomised, double-blind, placebo-controlled trial to evaluate the effect of enalapril in patients with clinical diabetic nephropathy. *Am J Kidney Dis* 1992; **20**: 443–57.
73. Elving LD, Wetzels JMF, van Lier HJJ et al. Captopril and atenolol are equally effective in retarding progression of diabetic nephropathy. *Diabetologia* 1994; **37**: 604–9.
74. Weidmann P, Boehlen M, de Courten M. Effects of different antihypertensive drugs on human proteinuria. *Nephrol Dial Transplant* 1993; **8**: 582–4.
75. Parving HH, Rossing P. The use of antihypertensive agents in prevention and treatment of diabetic nephropathy. *Curr Opinion Nephrol Hypertension* 1994; **3**: 292–300.
76. Sawicki PT, Berger M. Measuring progression of diabetic nephropathy. Review. *Europ J Clin Invest* 1994; **24**: 651–5.
77. Rossing P, Tarnow L, Boelskifte S et al. Differences between nisoldipine and lisinopril on glomerular filtration rates and albuminuria in hypertensive IDDM patients with diabetic nephropathy during the first year of treatment. *Diabetes* 1997; **46**: 481–7.
78. Sawicki PT. Stabilisation of glomerular filtration rate over two years in patients with diabetic nephropathy and intensified therapy regimes. *Nephrol Dial Transplant* 1997; **12**: 1890–99.
79. Collado-Mesa F, Colhoun HM, Stevens LK et al and the Eurodiab Type 1 Complications Study Group. Prevalence and management of hypertension in type 1 diabetes mellitus in Europe: the Eurodiab IDDM Complications Study. *Diabet Med* 1999; **16**: 41–9.
80. Sawicki PT, Mühlhauser I, Didjurgeit U et al. Mortality and morbidity in treated hypertensive type 2 diabetic patients with micro-or macroproteinuria. *Diabet Med* 1995; **12**: 893–8.

81. Trocha AK, Schmidtke C, Didjurgeit U et al. Intensified antihypertensive treatment in diabetic nephropathy: mortality and morbidity results of a prospective controlled 10 years study. *J Hypertens* 1999; **17**: 1497–1503.
82. Moy CS, LaPorte RE, Dorman JS et al. Insulin-dependent diabetes mellitus mortality. The risk of cigarette smoking. *Circulation* 1990; **82**: 37–43.
83. Morrish NJ, Stevens LK, Head J et al. A prospective study of mortality among middle-aged diabetic patients (the London cohort of the WHO multinational study of vascular disease in diabetics) II: associated risk factors. *Diabetologia* 1990; **33**: 542–8.
84. Ford ES, DeStefano F. Risk factors for mortality from all causes and from coronary heart disease among persons with diabetes. Findings from the National Health and Nutrition Examination Survey I. Epidemiological follow-up study. *Am J Epidemiol* 1991; **133**: 1220–30.
85. Sawicki PT, Mühlhauser I, Bender R et al. Effects of smoking on blood pressure and proteinuria in patients with diabetic nephropathy. *J Intern Med* 1996; **239**: 345–52.
86. Sawicki PT, Didjurgeit U, Mühlhauser I et al. Smoking is associated with progression of diabetic nephropathy. *Diabet Care* 1994; **17**: 126–31.
87. Stegmayr B, Lithner F. Tobacco and end stage diabetic nephropathy. *Br Med J* 1987; **295**: 581–2.
88. Mühlhauser I. Smoking and diabetes. *Diabet Med* 1990; **7**: 10–15.
89. Sawicki PT, Didjurgeit U, Mühlhauser I, Berger M. Behaviour therapy versus doctor's anti-smoking advise in diabetic patients. *J Intern Med* 1993; **234**: 407–9.
90. Henningfield JE. Nicotine medications for smoking cessation. *N Engl J Med* 1995; **333**: 1196–203.
91. Koskinen P, Mänttäri M, Manninen V et al. Coronary heart disease incidence in NIDDM patients in the Helsinki Heart Study. *Diabet Care* 1992; **15**: 820–25.
92. Sacks FM, Pfeffer MA, Moye LA et al for the Cholesterol and Recurrent Events Trial investigators. The effect of pravastatin on coronary events after myocardial infarction in patients with average cholesterol levels. *N Engl J Med* 1996; **335**: 1001–9.
93. Pyörälä K, Pedersen TR, Kjekshus J et al. The Scandinavian Simvastatin Survival Study (4S) Group. Cholesterol lowering with simvastatin improves prognosis of diabetic patients with coronary heart disease. *Diabet Care* 1997; **20**: 614–20.
94. Haffner SM, Alexander CM, Cook TJ et al. Reduced coronary events in simvastatin-treated patients with coronary heart disease and diabetes or impaired fasting glucose levels. *Arch Intern Med* 1999; **159**: 2661–7.
95. Goldberg RB, Mellies MJ, Sacks FM et al. Cardiovascular events and their reduction with pravastatin in diabetic and glucose-intolerant myocardial infarction survivors with average cholesterol levels. *Circulation* 1998; **98**: 2513–19.
96. Antiplatelet Trialists' Collaboration. Collaborative overview of randomised trial of antiplatelet therapy, I: prevention of death, myocardial infarction, and stroke by prolonged antiplatelet therapy in various categories of patients. *Br Med J* 1994; **308**: 81–106.
97. Colwell JA, Bingham SF, Abreira C et al and the Cooperative Study Group. Veterans Administration cooperative study on antiplatelet agents in atherosclerotic vascular diseases rates. *Diabet Care* 1986; **9**: 140–48.
98. Early Treatment of Retinopathy Study Investigators. Aspirin effects on mortality and morbidity in patients with diabetes mellitus. Early treatment diabetic retinopathy study report 14. *J Am Med Assoc* 1992; **268**: 1292–300.
99. Yudkin J. Which diabetic patients should be taking aspirin? *Br Med J* 1995; **311**: 641–2.

12

Lipid Disorders in Diabetic Nephropathy

CHRISTOPH WANNER, JOSEF ZIMMERMANN
AND THOMAS QUASCHNING
University Hospital, Würzburg, Germany

INTRODUCTION

Diabetes mellitus is a major risk factor for cardiovascular disease in both type 1 and type 2 diabetes (1, 2). There is growing consensus that most patients with diabetes mellitus, especially those with type 2 diabetes, belong in a category of patients with high short-term risk. Therefore, diabetic nephropathy is a special case in risk assessment. Diabetic nephropathy with incipient microalbuminuria or proteinuria greatly enhances the absolute risk. When the risk factors of diabetic patients are summed, their risk already approaches that of patients with established coronary heart disease (CHD) (3). The absolute risk of patients with type 2 diabetes and nephropathy usually exceeds all known risk scores, including the Framingham score for hyperglycaemia, because multiple risk factors almost always coexist. Another reason to elevate the patient with diabetic nephropathy to the highest-ever established risk category, as suggested by Consensus Conference and Task Force guideline scoring, is the poor prognosis of these patients once they develop coronary heart disease (4). These factors point to the need to intensify the management of coexisting risk factors in patients with diabetic nephropathy, including aggressive management of diabetic dyslipidaemia (5).

Diabetic Nephropathy. Edited by C. Hasslacher.
© 2001 John Wiley & Sons, Ltd.

ATHEROGENIC DYSLIPIDAEMIA

Diabetic dyslipidaemia is often called atherogenic dyslipidaemia. Athero-genic dyslipidemia is characterized by three lipoprotein abnormalities: elevated VLDL, small LDL particles and low HDL cholesterol. This type of dyslipidaemia occurs frequently in patients with premature CHD and appears to be an atherogenic lipoprotein phenotype independent of elevated LDL cholesterol (6). Most patients with atherogenic dyslipidaemia are insulin-resistant (7, 8). Many patients with atherogenic dyslipidaemia also have an elevated serum total apolipoprotein B (9). Growing evidence suggests that all of the components of this type of dyslipidaemia are independently atherogenic. Together they represent a set of lipoprotein abnormalities, apart from elevated LDL cholesterol, that promote athero-sclerosis.

DIABETIC NEPHROPATHY AND DYSLIPIDAEMIA: WHEN DOES IT AGGRAVATE?

Besides hypertension, glycaemic control and genetic predisposition, diabetic dyslipidaemia plays an important role in the pathophysiology and progression of vascular disease and probably diabetic nephropathy as well (10). Diabetic nephropathy *per se*, in additional to diabetes, impairs lipid metabolism (11) mainly, but not exclusively, via urinary protein excre-tion. Already in early (GFR < 70 ml/min), but also in advanced stages of diabetic nephropathy, diabetes-, proteinuria- and uraemia-associated dyslipidaemia can be diagnosed (6). However, it is rather difficult to distin-guish are from the other. Lipid metabolism in diabetes mellitus is further altered when renal replacement therapy is instituted.

PATTERNS OF DYSLIPIDAEMIA IN NIDDM

In type 2 diabetes, moderate hypertriglyceridaemia associated with reduced levels of HDL cholesterol is common (12). When glycaemia is well controlled, serum triglycerides in NIDDM patients can be normalized (12). Since glycaemia control is often insufficient, serum triglycerides in type 2 diabetic patients typically are elevated (13) up to three-fold of normal. A correlation of hypertriglyceridaemia can be found with both glycaemic control (14) and obesity (15). Diabetic hypertriglyceridaemia is based on enhanced hepatic VLDL secretion and diminished VLDL and chylomicron clearance (16). Because of their cholesterol content, increase in triglyceride-rich lipoproteins leads to mild elevation in total serum cholesterol (17). When glycaemic control is poor, total serum cholesterol in type 2 diabetes can be significantly enhanced due to the additional accumulation of LDL. Distinct quantitative and qualitative alterations of lipoproteins are present in NIDDM patients. They have been outlined in several reviews (18, 19) and will be described in detail below.

Chylomicrons and VLDL

NIDDM patients, especially when glycaemic control is poor, often express hyperchylomicronaemia (20), which is mainly based on a retarded clearance for apoB in chylomicrons (21). Reduced activity of lipoprotein lipase was suggested to be the underlying mechanism (22). Enhancement of chylomicrons contributes, besides the enhancement of VLDL, to the typical hypertriglyceridaemia of diabetic patients. The rise in serum triglycerides is also due to an elevation of triglycerides in VLDL. The insulin-resistant state impairs the normal suppression of fatty-acid release from adipose tissue in the postprandial state (23). Acute hyperinsulinaemia, such as after a meal, suppresses the production of large, buoyant VLDL particles in the liver in non-diabetic subjects but not in type 2 diabetic patients (24). Furthermore, there is overwhelming evidence that insulin resistance and compensatory hyperinsulinaemia lead to enhanced hepatic VLDL triglyceride secretion. One important reason for retarded VLDL clearance is the decrease of lipoprotein lipase activity in NIDDM. Lipoprotein lipase activity is low in untreated or poorly controlled NIDDM and increases with improved glycaemic control. Biochemical examination of VLDL in type 2 diabetes has revealed large, triglyceride-rich particles. Their apolipoproteins might undergo glycation, dependent on the quality of glycaemic control, similar to what has been shown for LDL. VLDL particles in type 2 diabetes have a high triglyceride:apoB ratio and exhibit an increase in apoE (25).

IDL Metabolism

Only little attention has be paid to IDL metabolism in type 2 diabetes. Joven et al (25) demonstrated an increase in both cholesterol and triglyceride concentrations of IDL in type 2 diabetic patients with renal disease. It has been hypothesized that enhancement of IDL might play a role in the progression of renal failure (26), independent of the origin of renal disease.

The Impact of Triglycerides on LDL Composition, Structure and Metabolism

Type 2 diabetic patients with good or reasonable glycaemic control have normal LDL cholesterol concentration. Nevertheless, LDL catabolism is impaired in patients with moderately severe diabetes, resulting in an increased proportion of triglycerides. The increase in the concentration of small, dense LDL (27) in serum, their glycation and oxidative modification (28) contribute to the increase of total serum LDL in poorly controlled diabetic subjects. The size and density of LDL is considerably influenced by changes in triglyceride content. Under conditions of poor glycaemic control, LDL of type 2 diabetic patients contain an elevated proportion of triglycerides, mostly at the expense of cholesterol (29, 30). Triglyceride enrichment in LDL is even more pronounced in obese type 2 diabetic patients with elevated total serum triglycerides. Since triglyceride enrichment in LDL modulates particle size and density, small dense and triglyceride-rich LDL subfractions are found to be elevated in type 2 diabetes (31). Diabetic hyperinsulinaemia based on insulin resistance might further promote the formation of small, dense LDL. Finally, small dense LDL subfractions exhibit enhanced susceptibility for oxidation (32), which again enhances modification. Alterations in the lipid composition or size of LDL-particles have consequences for their binding to lipoprotein receptors: triglyceride-rich and small, dense LDL show reduced cellular uptake via the LDL-receptor (29), leading to accumulation of LDL in the vascular system.

Glycation of LDL and Advanced Glycation Endproducts (AGE)

In diabetes mellitus, glucose is bound non-enzymatically to lysine residues in a variety of proteins. Since modification influences the function of lipoproteins (33), glycation of apoB alters its biological activity: it reduces its affinity to the LDL receptor and interferes with its metabolism (34). It therefore tends to accumulate in the circulation. The condensation reaction between reducing sugars and reactive amino groups produces Schiff base intermediates that undergo Amadori rearrangement, resulting in the irreversible development of AGE (35). It has been suggested that they accelerate the loss of renal function in the development of diabetic nephropathy (36). Furthermore, AGE-modified proteins (AGE–ApoB) additionally impair LDL metabolism by several mechanisms (37). In addition, collagen modified by AGE is capable of trapping lipoproteins and induces further glycoxidative changes.

Oxidative Modification of LDL

The vascular risk in patients with diabetic nephropathy is inadequately explained by increases in the concentrations of total or LDL cholesterol, hypertension or smoking. The glycation of LDL is closely connected with their oxidation: the lysine groups of the apoproteins are oxidized through free oxygen radicals from carbohydrate molecules. In addition, the charge of LDL particles is altered. Oxidative modification is accompanied, similar to the effects of glycation, by impaired receptor-specific binding and elevation of lipoprotein half-life. Some authors have even introduced the term "glycoxidation". It has been proposed that glycated LDL of diabetic subjects are more susceptible to oxidative modification.

Additionally, LDL oxidation is significantly correlated with plasma triglyceride levels. Small dense LDL, as present in type 2 diabetes, have even shown enhanced susceptibility to oxidation (38). Oxidatively modified lipoproteins are thought to be direct mediators of glomerular injury and hence might promote diabetic nephropathy. Furthermore, several groups have suggested that lipid modification and peroxidation are important for the development of atherosclerosis (30). Already in relatively young type 1 diabetic patients with average normal concentrations of LDL cholesterol, the ratio of autoantibodies against oxidized vs. native LDL is increased by 50% (39).

HDL Metabolism

A decrease in HDL cholesterol up to 20% in type 2 diabetic patients has often been reported in combination with altered composition of HDL (19). Similar to VLDL and LDL, HDL particles contain an increased proportion of triglycerides. Triglyceride-rich HDL show a faster catabolic rate than normal HDL, followed by a decreased number of circulating HDL particles. A decrease in the activity of lipoprotein lipase limits the cholesterol transfer from VLDL to HDL particles. Besides triglyceride enrichment, HDL in type 2 diabetes exhibit an increased ratio of cholesterol to protein and a depletion of apoAI (40). The decrease of HDL in type 2 diabetes is mostly accounted for by the decrease in the HDL_2 subfraction, whereas concentrations of small dense HDL_3 are relatively high (18). Since average particle size in HDL is related to serum triglyceride levels, HDL metabolism might additionally be influenced by alterations in the size of HDL.

Apolipoproteins

During hyperglycaemia, apoproteins undergo non-enzymatic glycation involving their lysine residues. Glycation could be demonstrated for apoAI, ApoAII, ApoB, ApoCI and ApoE. In particular, the glycation of apoB is of major importance in the impairment of LDL metabolism. In addition, triglyceride-rich lipoprotein levels, apoB and apoCII, as well as the apoCIII: CII ratio, are enhanced (41). No significant changes were found for apoAII, CII and E. Since apoCII is an activator of lipoprotein lipase and apoCII inhibits lipoprotein lipase and hepatic chylomicron uptake (42), apolipoprotein findings are consistent with impaired chylomicron and VLDL metabolism. Some authors additionally describe depletion of apoAI (42) and an increased ratio of cholesterol to protein.

Lipoprotein(a)

Patients with type 1 diabetes exhibit elevated serum lipoprotein(a) [Lp(a)] concentrations, especially when they present with overt nephropathy (43). In contrast, serum Lp(a) seems not to be increased in type 2 diabetes (44), even though an elevation of Lp(a) levels would be expected as a consequence of proteinuria. Some authors describe even reduced Lp(a) levels in type 2 diabetes, in combination with enlargement of Lp(a) particles. However, there is no reason why diabetic patients should have high Lp(a) levels, as long as their renal function is not affected. Contradictory results might result from studies performed with an inappropriately small number of patients and without consideration for the different behaviour of the various Lp(a) isoforms.

CLINICAL SIGNIFICANCE OF DYSLIPIDAEMIA IN TYPE 2 DIABETIC NEPHROPATHY

An elevated concentration of serum LDL cholesterol is a major risk factor for CHD (45). In fact, some elevation of LDL cholesterol appears to be necessary for the initiation and progression of atherosclerosis. In populations having very low LDL cholesterol levels, clinical CHD is relatively rare, even when other risk factors—hypertension, cigarette smoking and diabetes—are common (46). In contrast, severe elevations in LDL cholesterol can produce full-blown atherosclerosis and premature CHD in the complete absence of other risk factors. The view has been expressed that most patients with diabetes do not have an elevated serum LDL cholesterol; if not, a high LDL serum cholesterol would not be a common risk factor in patients with diabetes. It is true that most patients who have diabetes do not have marked elevations of LDL cholesterol, but these patients nonetheless carry high enough levels to support the development of atherosclerosis (e.g. 100–130 mg/dl small dense LDL).

Dyslipidaemia and Cardiovascular Disease

Death from cardiovascular disease is two to three times more common in diabetic patients than in the non-diabetic population (47). The development of nephropathy accelerates vascular damage and is strongly related to early cardiovascular morbidity and mortality in type 1 and type 2 diabetic patients (48).

Prospective studies have shown that the major risk factors for myocardial infarction in non-diabetic subjects also operate in type 2 diabetes (49). Unfortunately, there is a complex interrelationship between many risk factors in diabetic patients, especially in those suffering from diabetic nephropathy. Thus, it is difficult to establish the relative importance of a single risk factor. The described abnormalities of lipid and lipoprotein concentrations and composition in diabetic nephropathy may contribute to the increased risk of coronary heart disease.

The Multiple Risk Factor Intervention Trial (MRFIT) has demonstrated that high serum cholesterol confers a two–four-fold higher risk in diabetic patients for developing cardiovascular events than in non-diabetic subjects (50). The role of hypertrigyceridaemia as an independent risk factor for CHD has ceased to be the subject of dispute. Several studies, cross-sectional and prospective, have clearly demonstrated a relationship between hyper-triglyceridaemia and vascular disease in diabetic patients (51). Uusitupa et al (52) were able to demonstrate that, besides serum total triglycerides, the compositional abnormalities of lipoproteins, evidently associated with disturbed catabolism of VLDL, were related to cardiovascular mortality.

The adverse effect of low HDL cholesterol concentrations on cardiovascular risk in patients with type 2 diabetes was demonstrated by the study of Laakso et al (53), who prospectively followed 313 type 2 diabetic patients for up to 7 years. Lehto et al (54) recently demonstrated that low HDL cholesterol, high serum triglycerides and poor glycaemic control were the strongest predictors of coronary heart disease in 1059 type 2 diabetic patients during a follow-up of 7 years.

A role for LDL in hyperglycaemic patients became apparent in recent clinical trials, e.g. the Scandinavian Simvastatin Survival Study (4S) (55), the Cholesterol and Recurrent Events (CARE) trial (56) and the Long-term Intervention with Pravastatin in Ischaemic Disease (LIPID) trial (57). In all of these trials, aggressive LDL-lowering therapy reduced recurrent CHD events in patients with diabetes. In the 4S-study, a *post hoc* subgroup analysis of 202 diabetic patients revealed that the absolute clinical benefit achieved by cholesterol-lowering therapy was greater in diabetic than in non-diabetic patients with pre-existing coronary artery disease. During the 5.4 year median follow-up period, the relative risks of total mortality (0.57 vs. 0.71), as well as major CHD events (0.45 vs. 0.68) and any atherosclerotic events (0.63 vs. 0.74), were significantly lower in diabetic patients than in non-diabetic patients on simvastatin therapy (55).

A clinical benefit was also achieved by cholesterol lowering therapy in diabetic patients from the CARE study. Therapy with pravastatin reduced the risk of recurrent vascular events, even in patients with normal or mild elevated LDL cholesterol serum levels (115–174 mg/dl). However, the risk reduction was similar in the subgroup of diabetic patients ($n = 586$) compared to non-diabetics (56).

DYSLIPIDAEMIA AND THE PROGRESSION OF DIABETIC NEPHROPATHY

In experimental animal models, hyperlipidaemia has been implicated in causing direct renal injury. In animal models, treatment of hyperlipidaemia has led to an improvement of glomerular injury in non-diabetic as well as diabetic renal disease. It has been shown that altered serum lipoproteins interact with structures of the glomerulus. LDL particles modified by glycosylation and oxidation exhibit enhanced binding to glycosaminoglycans of the glomerular basement membrane, causing increased permeability of the basement membrane. In addition, the deposition of modified altered LDL particles in the mesangium may induce chemotactic signals for macrophages and stimulate mesangial cell proliferation. The preferential scavenger receptor-mediated uptake of modified LDL by monocytes/macrophages has recently been considered to cause the formation of glomerular and mesangial foam cells (58). Other mechanisms include mesangial expansion by accumulation of apoB and apoE leading to a reduction in glomerular filtration surface area, an alteration in renal cortical tissue lipids, alterations in membrane fluidity and function induced by disturbances in fatty acid concentrations, and alterations in glomerular haemodynamics.

In humans with diabetic nephropathy, hyperlipidaemia has been identified as a risk factor for a more rapid rate of decline in GFR and increased mortality (59). Especially, an increased plasma concentration of triglyceride-rich apoB-containing lipoproteins has been found to be linked to a more rapid decrease in renal function and the combination of dyslipoproteinaemia and hypertension appears to act synergistically to indicate a more rapid decline of renal function. Type I diabetics with cholesterol serum levels above 7 mmol/l (270 mg/dl) show a more rapid decline of glomerular filtration rate than patients with plasma cholesterol below 7 mmol/l. In a follow-up study, multivariate analysis revealed that ACE inhibition, associated with lower serum cholesterol concentrations, was superior to metoprolol therapy associated with higher cholesterol concentrations in preventing the deterioration of renal function in type 1 patients with diabetic nephropathy (60). Recently, high triglycerides and low HDL cholesterol could be identified as strong predictors of more rapid progression of microalbuminuria in type 2 diabetic patients with well-controlled blood pressure.

Several uncontrolled preliminary studies in small numbers of patients with diabetes and proteinuria have suggested that treatment with a statin stabilizes or improves renal function. Further prospective long-term studies involving a large number of patients are required to prove or disprove the relevance of cholesterol-lowering therapy in retarding the progression of diabetic nephropathy.

MANAGEMENT OF LIPID DISORDERS IN TYPE 2 DIABETIC NEPHROPATHY

Because hyper- and dyslipidaemia are so closely related to the progression of cardiovascular disease, treatement is warranted irrespective of their potential beneficial effect on diabetic nephropathy. Since the risk for CHD is excessive in diabetic patients, recommendations of an aggressive lowering of LDL cholesterol levels, given for patients with established CHD, can also be extended to diabetic patients. The US Adult Treatment Panel II of the National Cholesterol Education Program (61) recommended that the target level of LDL cholesterol should be less than 2.6 mmol/l (100 mg/dl), whereas the European goal (Recommendations of the Second Joint Task force of European and other Societies on Coronary Prevention) proposed an LDL-C < 3.0 mmol/l (115 mg/dl). Lipid-lowering drug therapy should be initiated if the LDL cholesterol concentration is greater than 3.4 mmol/l (135 mg/dl). In a recent consensus conference, the American Diabetes Association recommended an identical threshold for drug therapy (62). With regard to the potential benefits of lowering serum triglycerides in diabetic patients, much less information is available from clinical trials. Nevertheless, the American Diabetes Association recommended drug therapy for triglyceride levels greater than 4.5 mmol/l (400 mg/dl). In the presence of a further CHD risk factor, pharmacological therapy should be considered if triglyceride concentrations exceed 2.3 mmol/l (200 mg/dl) in diabetic patients with clinical vascular disease, if the triglyceride concentrations exceed 1.7 mmol/l (150 mg/dl). Since diabetic patients with overt nephropathy (microalbumuinuria or proteinuria) exhibit an even higher cardiovascular risk, we recommend treating these patients using guidelines of secondary prevention. Thus, LDL cholesterol target levels should be 2.6 mmol/l (100 mg/dl) and optimal triglyceride levels should be 1.7 mmol/l (150 mg/dl). (Table 12.1).

Table 12.1 Treatment goals of lipid-lowering in diabetic nephropathy

LDL cholesterol	< 2.6 mmol/l (100 mg/dl)[1]
	< 3.0 mmol/l (115 mg/dl)[2]
HDL cholesterol	> 1.1 mmol/l (42 mg/dl)
Triglyceride	> 1.7 mmol/l (150 mg/dl)

[1]NCEP goal; [2]European goal.

However, no definite target levels are given for the concentration of HDL cholesterol and triglycerides, but an unfavourable condition is present when HDL cholesterol is lower than 40 mg/dl or serum triglyceride is > 200 mg/dl). The results of the VA-HIT study (Veterans Affairs High-density Lipoprotein Cholesterol Intervention Trial) encourage the use of gemfibrocil in those with hypertriglyceridaemia and low HDL cholesterol. The data show that a decrease of serum triglyceride (−31%) and a rise of HDL cholesterol by +6% in the presence of unchanged values for LDL cholesterol—a reduction of myocardial events (non-fatal myocardial infarction or coronary death)—was achieved by 22% (63).

NON-PHARMACOLOGICAL LIPID LOWERING

Dietary Advice

Generally, in patients with diabetic nephropathy, the optimum lipid-modifying diet remains to be determined. The goals of dietary counselling have to be defined on an individual basis, with regards to excessive weight, hypertension or severe renal insufficiency. Diet should also help to achieve near-normoglycaemia. A prudent recommendation for all diabetic patients with dyslipidaemia is to reduce dietary fat to 30% or less of total energy intake, the intake of saturated fat to no more than one-third of total fat intake, with an increase in the use of mono-unsaturated and polyunsaturated fats (64). In insulin-resistent type 2 diabetic patients, the traditional high-carbohydrate, low-fat diet may have an adverse effect on dyslipidaemia. In these patients an alternative approach is a low carbohydrate diet enriched with mono-unsaturated fatty acids (65). A practical recommendation for all diabetic patients, including those with diabetic nephropathy, is the use of a Mediterranean diet enriched in fresh fruit and vegetables.

Physical Activity

All patients should be professionally encouraged and supported to increase their physical activity safely to a level associated with the lowest risk of vascular disease. Aerobic exercise (e.g. walking, swimming or bicycling) for 20–30 min four or five times a week is recommended. Physicians should emphasize the importance of physical activity in giving the patient a sense of well-being. Being physically active helps to reduce weight (together with a Mediterranean diet), increase HDL cholesterol and lower triglycerides and the propensity to thrombosis. The family is important in supporting an active lifestyle.

Glycaemic Control

Primarily, attention should be directed to improving glycaemic control. In general, a tightening of blood glucose control with either oral hypoglycae-mic agents or insulin results in a reduction of plasma triglyceride levels. The findings with regard to total and LDL cholesterol are not as consistent, with some studies showing decreases and others no change. HDL cholesterol levels tend to increase with improved blood glucose control, but in general this takes some weeks to be apparent (66). In addition, optimizing glycaemic control by insulin therapy reduces small dense LDL particles in diabetic patients. Several oral antidiabetic drugs, such as biguanides and acarbose, impair insulin sensitivity, resulting in an improvement of dyslipidaemia (67). Treatment with glibenclamide had only marginal effects on lipoprotein metabolism in type 2 diabetic patients. Recently, it has been shown that troglitazone, a new oral antidiabetic agent, can reduce *in vitro* HDL and LDL oxidation. Therefore, the class of glitazones may be helpful to slow the progression of atherosclerotic lesions in diabetic patients.

LIPID-LOWERING DRUGS

Treatment with hypolidaemic drugs (Table 12.2) should be considered if amelioration of blood glucose control and dietary measures do not achieve the appropriate goals. The most useful hypolipidamic drug classes for use in

Table 12.2 Lipid-lowering drugs in diabetic nephropathy

Fibric acid derivatives	Gemfibrozil	900 mg/day
HMG-CoA reductase inhibitors	Lovastatin	10–80 mg/day
	Simvastatin	10–40 mg/day
	Pravastatin	10–40 mg/day
	Fluvastatin	10–40 mg/day
	Cerivastatin	100–300 μg/day
	Atorvastatin	10–80 mg/day
Nicotinic acid derivatives	Acipimox	3 × 250 mg/day
Fish oil		6–12 capsules/day

both the diabetic population and patients with chronic renal failure are fibric acid derivatives and HMG-CoA reductase inhibitors (statins). Since nicotinic acid aggravates insulin resistance, leading to a deterioration in glycaemic control, and bile acid binding resins tend to increase serum triglyceride concentration, these drugs are not recommended in diabetic patients. However, acipimox may overcome these effects, being useful in diabetic patients with hypertriglyceridaemia (Table 12.3).

Statins

This class of agents are preferred in patients with elevated LDL cholesterol. These drugs were shown to be highly effective in reducing LDL cholesterol concentrations in both diabetic and non-diabetic patients with chronic renal failure, including patients with diabetic nephropathy. Statins also lower high levels of atherogenic IDL (68). In severe renal insufficiency, therapy with statins appears to be safe, but experience is limited and maximal doses should be used with caution. The most important but rare side-effect is rhabdomyolysis, with muscle pain and an increase in creatine kinase. The risk for developing rhabdomyolysis usually is low, but is high in those receiving additional drug therapy, particularly cyclosporin and gemfibrozil. Therefore patients should be advised to present when myositis develops, and statins should be withdrawn when creatine kinase levels reach 10 times normal values.

Fibric Acid Derivatives

Fibric acid derivaties have been shown to improve lipoprotein lipase activity and inhibit hepatic synthesis of VLDL cholesterol, resulting in a reduction of triglycerides and an increase in HDL cholesterol. Fibrate drugs do not adversely affect glycaemic control and some also reduce plasma fibrinogen levels. In principle, they appear to be suitable lipid-lowering

Table 12.3   Choice of hypolipidaemic drugs in diabetes mellitus

Isolated hypercholesterolaemia	
Mild/moderate/severe	Statins
Mixed hyperlipidaemia*	
Predominant hypercholesterolaemia	Statins
Predominant hypertriglyceridaemia	Fibric acid derivatives
Hypertriglyceridaemia	
Moderate (2.3–4.5 mmol/l)	Fibric acid derivatives
Severe (> 4.5 mmol/l)	Fibric acid derivatives + acipimox
Hyperchylomicronaemia (> 11 mmol/l)	Fibric acid derivatives + acipimox + fish oil

*The combination of statins and fibrates is possible in low doses, but bears a high risk of rhabdomyolysis.

agents in patients with diabetic nephropathy. However, fibrates are primarily excreted by the kidney and accumulate in advanced renal insufficiency. The risk of side-effects, mainly rhabdomyolysis, is increased. Therefore, in severe renal failure clofibrate and fenofibrate should not be used. The dose of bezafibrate has to be reduced to 200–400 mg/week. Among the second generation of fibric acid analogues, gemfibrozil has been found to be the drug of choice in patients with renal insufficiency. Low to moderate dosages of gemfibrozil (< 900 mg/day) are well tolerated in these patients.

Fish Oil

In excessive hypertriglyceridaemia (> 1000 mg/dl), fish oil effectively reduces serum triglyceride levels in combination with a fibric acid derivatives or acipimox, a nicotinic acid derivative. However, the amount of drug that has to be ingested (6–12 capsules/day) is unlikely to be tolerated over time.

ACE Inhibitors

In a prospective trial, Ravid et al (69) could demonstrate that treatment of normotensive type 2 diabetic patients with enalapril over a 5 year period reduces microalbuminuria as well as serum cholesterol, LDL cholesterol and triglycerides. The authors stated that, besides proteinuria, hypercholesterolaemia should be regarded as an independent risk factor for the impairment of kidney function. Jerums et al (70) observed that an increase in proteinuria is associated with an elevated serum concentration of lipoprotein(a). As expected, reduction of proteinuria by ACE inhibition improved the serum lipid profile and decreased serum levels of lipoprotein(a).

ONGOING TRIALS

There are several trials under way that aim to prove the value of lipid lowering in subjects with diabetes mellitus: The HPS (Heart Protection Study) is a placebo-controlled trial investigating simvastatin effects in 20 000 patients, of whom approximately 6000 will be diabetics. The ASPEN study as well investigates the effect of atorvastatin on the prevention of coronary heart disease endpoints in 2300 type 2 diabetic patients without coronary heart disease. The CARDS (Collaborative Atorvastatin Diabetes Study) is conducted in 1800 UK diabetics and is characterized by a design similar to ASPEN. The LDS (Lipids in Diabetes Study) will enroll approximately 5000 patients with diabetes and investigate cardiovascular endpoints using fenofibrat or placebo in comparison to cerivastatin or placebo. Studies are also under way investigating the influence of micronized fenofibrate on the catabolism of triglyceride-rich lipoproteins and on mortality in diabetic patients with normal kidney function [the FIELD study and the Diabetes Atherosclerosis Intervention Study (*DAIS*)].

SUMMARY

Type 2 diabetic patients are at high risk of vascular disease, especially those with signs of nephropathy. Since dyslipidaemia is so closely related to the progression of cardiovascular disease, aggressive lipid-lowering therapy is recommended, irrespective of its potential beneficial effect on diabetic nephropathy. The initial management should involve attempts to improve glycaemic control, weight reduction and a Mediterranean diet. Hypolipidaemic drugs are necessary if these measures fail to achieve the treatment goals of current guidelines.

REFERENCES

1. Lloyd EC, Kuller LH, Ellis D et al. Coronary artery disease in IDDM: gender differences in risk factors but not risk. *Arterioscler Thromb Vasc Biol* 1996; **16:** 720–26.
2. Wilson PW. Diabetes mellitus and coronary heart disease. *Am J Kidney Dis* 1998; **32:** S89–100.
3. Haffner SM, Lehto S, Ronnemaa T, Pyörälä K, Laakso M. Mortality from coronary heart disease in subjects with type 2 diabetes and in non-diabetic subjects with and without prior myocardial infarction. *N Engl J Med* 1998; **339:** 229–34.
4. MILIS Study Group; Stone PH, Muller JE, Hartwell T et al. The effect of diabetes mellitus on prognosis and serial left ventricular function after acute myocardial infarction: contribution of both coronary disease and diastolic left ventricular dysfunction to the adverse prognosis: the MILIS Study Group. *J Am Coll Cardiol* 1989; **14:** 49–57.
5. Management of dyslipidemia in adults with diabetes: American Diabetes Association. *Diabet Care* 1998; **21:** 179–82.
6. Samuelsson O, Attman PO, Knight-Gibson C et al. Lipoprotein abnormalities without hyperlipidaemia in moderate renal insufficiency. *Nephrol Dialysis Transplant* 1994; **9:** 1580–85.
7. Attman PO, Samuelsson O, Alaupovic P. Diagnosis and classification of dyslipidemia in renal disease. *Blood Purif* 1996; **14:** 49–57.
8. Attman PO, Samuelsson O, Alaupovic P. Lipoprotein metabolism and renal failure. *Am J Kidney Dis* 1993; **21:** 573–92.
9. Attman PO, Nyberg G, William-Olsson T, Knight-Gibson C, Alaupovic P. Dyslipoproteinemia in diabetic renal failure. *Kidney Int* 1992; **42:** 1381–9.

10. Austin MA, King M-C, Vranizan KM, Krauss RM. Atherogenic lipoprotein phenotype: a proposed genetic marker for coronary heart disease risk. *Circulation* 1990; **82:** 495–509.
11. Austin MA, Edwards KL. Small, dense low density lipoproteins, the insulin resistance syndrome and non-insulin dependent diabetes. *Curr Opin Lipidol* 1996; **7:** 167–71.
12. Betteridge DJ. Diabetic dyslipidaemia: treatment implications. *J Intern Med* 1994; **736** (suppl): 47–52.
13. Betteridge DJ. Diabetic dyslipidemia. *Am J Med* 1994; **96:** 25–31S.
14. Laakso M, Sarlund H, Mykkanen L. Insulin resistance is associated with lipid and lipoprotein abnormalities in subjects with varying degrees of glucose tolerance. *Arteriosclerosis* 1990; **10:** 223–31.
15. Laakso M, Pyorala K. Adverse effects of obesity on lipid and lipoprotein levels in insulin dependent and non-insulin dependent diabetes. *Metabolism* 1990; **39:** 117–22.
16. Koschinsky T, Gries FA. Dyslipoproteinemia and diabetes mellitus. *Horm Metab Res* 1992; **26** (suppl): 76–84.
17. Betteridge D. Cholesterol is the major atherogenic lipid in NIDDM. *Diabet Metab Rev* 1997; **13:** 99–104.
18. Taskinen MR, Lahdenpera S, Syvanne M. New insights into lipid metabolism in non-insulin dependent diabetes mellitus. *Ann Med* 1996; **28:** 335–40.
19. Taskinen MR. Quantitative and qualitative lipoprotein abnormalities in diabetes mellitus. *Diabetes* 1992; **41** (2): 12–17.
20. Chait A, Robertson HT, Brunzell JD. Chylomicronemia syndrome in diabetes mellitus. *Diabet Care* 1981; **4:** 343–8.
21. Haffner SM, Foster DM, Kushwaha RS, Hazzard WR. Retarded chylomicron apolipoprotein-B catabolism in type 2 diabetic subjects with lipaemia. *Diabetologia* 1984; **26:** 349–54.
22. Nikkila EA, Huttunen JK, Ehnholm C. Postheparin plasma lipoprotein lipase and hepatic lipase in diabetes mellitus. *Diabetes* 1977; **26:** 11–21.
23. Frayn KN. Insulin resistance and lipid metabolism. *Curr Opin Lipidol* 1993; **4:** 197–204.
24. Malmstrom R, Packard CJ, Caslake M et al. Apolipoprotein 13. Defective regulation of triglyceride metabolism by insulin in the liver in NIDDM. *Diabetologia* 1997; **40:** 454–62.
25. Joven J, Vilella E, Costa B et al. Concentrations of lipids and apolipoproteins in patients with clinically well-controlled insulin-dependent and non-insulin-dependent diabetes. *Clin Chem* 1989; **35:** 813–16.
26. Samuelsson O, Attman P-O, Knight-Gibson C et al. Complex apolipoprotein-B-containing lipoprotein particles are associated with a higher rate of progression of human chronic renal insufficiency. *J Am Soc Nephrol* 1998; **9:** 1482–8.
27. Feingold KR, Grunfeld C, Pang M, Doerrler W, Krauss RM. LDL subclass phenotypes and triglyceride metabolism in non-insulin dependent diabetes. *Arterioscler Thromb* 1992; **12:** 1496–502.
28. Brownlee M, Vlassara H, Cerami A. Nonenzymatic glycosylation and the pathogenesis of diabetic complications. *Ann Int Med* 1984; **101:** 527–37.
29. Krämer-Guth A, Quaschning T, Galle J et al. Structural and compositional modifications of diabetic LDL influence their receptor mediated uptake by hepatocytes. *Eur J Clin Invest* 1997; **27:** 460–68.
30. Krämer Guth A, Quaschning T, Greiber S, Wanner C. Potential role of lipids in the progression of diabetic nephropathy. *Clin Nephrol* 1996; **46:** 262–5.

31. Krauss RM. Low density lipoprotein subclasses and risk of coronary heart disease. *Curr Opin Lipidol* 1992; **2**: 248–52.
32. de Graaf J, Hak-Lemmers HL, Hectors MP et al. Enhanced susceptibility to *in vitro* oxidation of the dense low density lipoprotein subfraction in healthy subjects. *Arterioscler Thromb* 1991; **11**: 298–306.
33. Vlassara H. Protein glycation in the kidney: role in diabetes and aging. *Kidney Int* 1996; **49**: 1795–804.
34. Lopes-Virella MF, Klein RL, Lyons TJ, Stevenson HC, Witztum JL. Glycosylation of low-density lipoprotein enhances cholesteryl ester synthesis in human monocyte-derived macrophages. *Diabetes* 1988; **37**: 550–57.
35. Makita Z, Radoff S, Rayfield EJ et al. Advanced glycosylation end products in patients with diabetic nephropathy. *N Engl J Med* 1991; **325**: 836–42.
36. Vlassara H. Advanced glycation in diabetic renal and vascular disease. *Kidney Int* 1995; **51** (suppl): S43–4.
37. Bucala R, Makita Z, Vega G et al. Modification of low density lipoprotein by advanced glycation end products contributes to the dyslipidemia of diabetes and renal insufficiency. *Proc Natl Acad Sci USA* 1994; **91**: 9441–5.
38. Chait A, Brazg RL, Tribble DL, Krauss RM. Susceptibility of small, dense, low-density lipoproteins to oxidative modification in subjects with the atherogenic lipoprotein phenotype, pattern B. *Am J Med* 1993; **94**: 350–56.
39. Mäkimattila S, Luoama JS, Ylä-Herttuala S et al. Autoantibodies against oxidized LDL and endothelium-dependent vasodilation in insulin-dependent diabetes mellitus. *Atherosclerosis* 1999; **147**: 115–22.
40. Schernthaner G, Kostner GM, Dieplinger H. Apolipoproteins (A-I, A-II, B), Lp(a) lipoprotein and lecithin: cholesterol acyltransferase activity in diabetes mellitus. *Atherosclerosis* 1983; **49**: 277–93.
41. Breckenridge WC, Little JA, Steiner G, Chow A, Poapst M. Hypertriglyceridemia associated with deficiency of apolipoprotein C-II. *N Engl J Med* 1978; **298**: 1265–73.
42. Ginsberg HN, Le NA, Goldberg IJ et al. Apolipoprotein B metabolism in subjects with deficiency of apolipoproteins CIII and AI. Evidence that apolipoprotein CIII inhibits catabolism of triglyceride-rich lipoproteins by lipoprotein lipase *in vivo*. *J Clin Invest* 1986; **78**: 1287–95.
43. Csaszar A, Dieplinger H, Sandholzer C, Karadi I, Juhasz E, Drexel H. Plasma lipoprotein (a) concentration and phenotypes in diabetes mellitus. *Diabetologia* 1993; **36**: 47–51.
44. Haffner SM, Morales PA, Stern MP, Gruber MK. Lp(a) concentrations in NIDDM. *Diabetes* 1992; **41**: 1267–72.
45. Expert Panel on Detection and Treatment of High Blood Cholesterol in Adults, National Cholesterol Education Program. Second report of the Expert Panel on Detection, Evaluation, and Treatment of High Blood Cholesterol (Adult Treatment Panel II). *Circulation* 1994; **89**: 1333–445.
46. Grundy SM, Wilhelmsen L, Rose G, Campbell RWF, Assman G. Coronary heart disease in high-risk populations: lessons from Finland. *Eur Heart J* 1990; **11**: 462–71.
47. Panzram G. Mortality and survival in type 2 (non-insulin-dependent) diabetes mellitus. *Diabetologia* 1987; **30**: 123–31.
48. Messent JW, Elliott TG, Hill RD, Jarrett RJ, Keen H, Viberti GC. Prognostic significance of microalbuminuria in insulin-dependent diabetes mellitus: a 23 year follow-up study. *Kidney Int* 1992; **41**: 836–9.

49. Koskinen P, Mänttäri M, Manninen V et al. Coronary heart disease incidence in NIDDM patients in the Helsinki Heart Study. *Diabet Care* 1992; **15:** 820–25.
50. Stamler J, Vaccaro O, Neaton J, for the Multiple Risk Factor Intervention Trial Research Group. Diabetes, other risk factors, and 12-year cardiovascular mortality for men screened in the multiple risk factor intervention trial. *Diabet Care* 1993; **16:** 434–9.
51. Hanefeld M, Fischer S, Julius U et al, the DIS Group. Risk factors for myocardial infarction and death in newly detected NIDDM: the Diabetes Intervention Study, 11-year follow-up. *Diabetologia* 1996; **39:** 1577–83.
52. Uusitupa MIJ, Niskanen LK, Siitonen O, Voutilainen, E, Pyörälä K. Ten-year cardiovascular mortality in relation to risk factors and abnormalities in lipoprotein composition in type 2 (non-insulin-dependent) diabetic and nondiabetic subjects. *Diabetologia* 1993; **36:** 1175–84.
53. Laakso M, Lehto S, Penttilä I, Pyörälä K. Lipids and lipoproteins predicting coronary heart disease mortality and morbidity in patients with non-insulin-dependent diabetes. *Circulation* 1993; **88:** 142–3.
54. Lehto S, Ronnemaa T, Haffner SM et al. Dyslipidemia and hyperglycemia predict coronary heart disease events in middle-aged patients with NIDDM. *Diabetes* 1997; **48:** 1354–9.
55. Pyörälä K, Pedersen TR, Kjekshus J et al. Cholesterol lowering with simvastatin improves prognosis of diabetic patients with coronary heart disease. *Diabet Care* 1997; **20:** 14–62.
56. Goldberg RB, Mellies MJ, Sacks F et al, for the CARE investigators. Cardiovascular events and their reduction with pravastatin in diabetic and glucose-intolerant myocardial infarction survivors with average cholesterol levels: subgroup analyses in the cholesterol and recurrent events (CARE) trial. *Circulation* 1998; **98:** 2513–19.
57. The Long-Term Intervention with Pravastatin in Ischemic Disease (LIPID) Study Group. Prevention of cardiovascular events and death with pravastatin in patients with coronary heart disease and a broad range of initial cholesterol levels. *N Engl J Med* 1998; **339:** 1349–57.
58. Schlöndorff D. Cellular mechanisms of lipid injury in the glomerulus. *Am J Kidney Dis* 1993; **22:** 279–85.
59. Samulsson O, Aurell M, Knight-Gibson C, Alaupovic P, Attman P-O. Apolipoprotein-B-containing lipoproteins and the progression of renal insufficiency. *Nephron* 1993; **63:** 279–85.
60. Mulec H, Johnson SA, Wiklund O, Bjorck S: Cholesterol: a renal risk factor in diabetic nephropathy? *Am J Kidney Dis* 1993; **22:** 196–201.
61. Expert Panel on Detection, Evaluation and Treatment of High Blood Cholesterol in Adults. Summary of the Second Report of the National Cholesterol Education Program (NCEP) Expert Panel on Detection, Evaluation, and Treatment of High Blood Cholesterol in Adults (Adult Treatment Panel II). *J Am Med Assoc* 1993; **269:** 3015–23.
62. Consensus Statement. Detection and management of lipid disorders in diabetes. *Diabet Care* 1993; **16:** 106–12.
63. Bloomfield Rubins H, Robins SJ et al, for the Veterans Affairs High-density Lipoprotein Cholesterol Intervention Trial Study Group. Gemfibrozil for the secondary prevention of coronary heart disease in men with low levels of high-density lipoprotein cholesterol. *N Engl J Med* 1999; **341:** 410–18.

64. Wood D, De Backer G, Faergeman O et al, and members of the Second Joint Task Force of European and other Societies on Coronary Prevention. Prevention of coronary heart disease in clinical practice. *Eur Heart J* 1998; **19:** 1434–503.
65. Garg A, Grundy SM, Unger RH. Comparison of effects of high and low carbohydrate diets on plasma lipoproteins and insulin sensitivity in patients with mild NIDDM. *Diabetes* 1992; **41:** 1278–85.
66. Garg A, Bonanome A, Grundy SM, Zhang ZY, Unger RH. Comparison of a high carbohydrate diet with a high mono-unsaturated fat diet in patients with non-insulin dependent diabetes mellitus. *N Engl J Med* 1988; **319:** 829–34.
67. DeFronzo RA, Goodman AM. Efficacy of metformin in patients with non-insulin dependent diabetes mellitus. The Multicenter Metformin Study Group. *N Engl J Med* 1995; **333:** 541–9.
68. Nishizawa Y, Shoij T, Emoto M et al. Reduction of intermediate density lipoprotein by pravastatin in hemo-and peritoneal dialysis patients. *Clin Nephrol* 1995; **43:** 268–77.
69. Ravid M, Neumann L, Lishner M. Plasma lipids and the progression of nephropathy in diabetes mellitus II: effect of ACE inhibitors. *Kidney Int* 1995; **47:** 907–10.
70. Jerums G, Allen TJ, Tsalamandris C et al. Relationship of propressively increasing albuminuria to apoprotein(a) and blood pressure in type 2 (non-insulin dependent) and type 1 (insulin dependent) diabetic patients. *Diabetologia* 1993; **36:** 1037–44.

13

Eye Complications in Diabetic Nephropathy

MASSIMO PORTA

Diabetic Retinopathy Centre, University of Turin, Italy

That diabetic retinopathy and nephropathy are intimately related in both their epidemiology and their pathogenesis has been long considered a matter of fact. In his seminal report on the relationships between long-term metabolic control and the development of complications, Pirart (29) proposed the term "diabetic triopathy" to include retinal, renal and periph-eral nervous system alterations. The links between these complications are, however, rather more complicated. The pathogenesis of neuropathy is con-sidered by most to depend more on metabolic than a vascular determinants and it is known that, while nearly all patients with kidney involvement also have retinopathy, the reverse is not necessarily true and proliferative lesions are often present in people without clinically apparent renal damage. In this chapter the natural history of diabetic retinopathy (DR) will be briefly summarized, followed by a review of current evidence for its association and pathogenic pathways in common with nephropathy (DN). Finally, eye care in diabetes will be discussed, with special emphasis on patients with nephropathy.

NATURAL HISTORY OF DR

Clinical DR is a disease of the retinal capillaries, which undergo closure, hyperpermeability and, later on, new vessel proliferation (23). Occlusion of

Diabetic Nephropathy. Edited by C. Hasslacher.
© 2001 John Wiley & Sons, Ltd.

small vessels is accompanied by focal and generalized dilatation of the remaining vessels and progressive retinal non-perfusion. Focal dilatation is evident as microaneurysms, discernible at the ophthalmoscope as red dots, typically surrounding non-perfused areas. Dilatation of longer segments results in wider but fragile capillaries which bleed easily, producing microhaemorrhages and larger blot haemorrhages, and lose their barrier selectivity, leading to the deposition of lipoproteins and cholesterol in bright yellow deposits within the nerve layers known as "hard exudates". Ischaemic infarcts in larger areas of non-perfusion produce localized swelling of the retinal nerve fibres and accumulation of material of axonic transport, taking the appearance of whitish-greyish ill-delineated lesions, known as cotton-wool spots. Some or all of the above lesions indicate non-proliferative (formerly known as "background") DR, which is divided into mild, moderate and severe (formerly pre-proliferative) (Figure 13.1). Other abnormalities of severe non-proliferative DR include venous irregularities, such as dilatation, beading, reduplication and loop formation, and intraretinal microvascular abnormalities (IRMA), which are dilated, convoluted capillaries often difficult to discriminate from intraretinal new vessels.

Characteristically, non-proliferative DR does not cause visual symptoms, and must therefore be searched for through an active screening procedure in order to diagnose early the sight-threatening forms of DR. Edema,

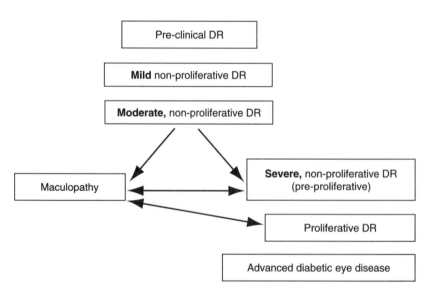

Figure 13.1 Stages of diabetic retinopathy

haemorrhages and hard exudates developing in the proximity of the macula, the centre of detailed vision, lead to diabetic maculopathy, which can be classified as edematous, exudative or ischaemic but is more often a combination of them all. Proliferative DR develops once extensive retinal ischaemia has caused new vessels to grow from the optic disc and/or the periphery in an inappropriate attempt to re-perfuse the retina. It can cause irreversible sight loss because new vessels bleed easily, causing pre-retinal haemorrhages, and stimulate the proliferation of fibrous tissue, anchored at different points of the retina. Tractional detachment, caused by progressive contraction of the fibrovascular membranes over large areas of vitreo-retinal adhesion, may be the cause of irreversible damage.

Detachment is a feature of advanced diabetic eye disease, in which neo-vascularization may extend to the anterior segment of the eye, involving the iris (*rubeosis iridis*) and leading ultimately to thrombotic, or neovascular, glaucoma.

ASSOCIATION BETWEEN DIABETIC RETINOPATHY AND NEPHROPATHY

Proteinuria is not considered in most reports to be an independent predictor for the incidence of new retinopathy, although its presence may predict progression of existing lesions to proliferative retinopathy. In fact, while virtually all patients with nephropathy also have retinopathy (17,26), often in its proliferative form, about one-third of patients with proliferative lesions do not have microalbuminuria (14). In patients with IDDM, DR is present in 85–99% of cases with persistent proteinuria, although only in 47–63% of cases with NIDDM (27,32), suggesting that about 30% of protein-uria in NIDDM is not diabetic in pathogenesis. A practical consequence of this is that absence of retinopathy may constitute an indication to renal biopsy in confirmed proteinuria, as it strongly suggests that kidney lesions are not due to diabetic microangiopathy.

Incidences of the two complications are rather different. Retinopathy tends to increase progressively with duration of diabetes, so that after 15–30 years the cumulative prevalence reaches nearly 100% of patients, while the incidence of nephropathy rises sharply between 5 and 15 years duration and then declines over the subsequent years, so that only about one-third of all patients ever develop the complication (25). On the other hand, if one considers only proliferative as opposed to any stage of retino-pathy, then both incidence and cumulative prevalence behave similarly to those of nephropathy, suggesting that this is where pathogenic analogies should be sought. A study carried out at the Joslin Clinic (24) showed that

80% of diabetic patients with persistent proteinuria had proliferative DR, as opposed to 25% of those without proteinuria. Incidence of new proliferative DR is less than 1% per year among diabetic patients without proteinuria but rises to 10–15% per year in the presence of proteinuria. Interestingly, incidence rates start to increase 3–4 years before the onset of nephropathy and retinal lesions then tend to deteriorate more rapidly.

Stephenson et al (33) with the EURODIAB cross-sectional study of 3250 patients with IDDM, introduced elements of further complexity, because the correlation between albuminuria and blood pressure abnormalities was only confirmed in patients with concomitant retinopathy, independently of glycaemic control or duration of diabetes, suggesting that the presence of even mild retinopathy and increased blood pressure is an important risk factor for the progression of nephropathy. Presumably, the relationship between microalbuminuria and retinopathy is compounded by the fact that the former is a strong predictor of macrovascular disease, which in turn is more frequent in patients with severe retinopathy.

Blindness due to proliferative retinopathy and diabetic maculopathy is particularly frequent among patients with end-stage renal disease. In 1985, 35% of diabetic people on renal replacement therapy in the UK were blind (19). Progress in laser photocoagulation therapy and vitreo-retinal surgery have presumably helped to reduce the incidence of sight loss, although indications from recent surveys suggest that prolongation of life expectancy may have actually increased the incidence of both end-stage renal disease and new blindness secondary to diabetes. Scatter photocoagulation has, however, helped to minimize the risk of vitreous haemorrhage consequent to heparin use during haemodialysis.

COMMON PATHOGENIC MECHANISMS

Retinopathy and nephropathy are two manifestations of diabetic microangiopathy thought to share common pathogenic mechanisms, even though common pathways of capillary damage may lead to rather different histological and clinical manifestations because of the different structure and function of the organs involved. Much data has accumulated but it is still difficult to identify a unifying pathogenic hypothesis. An attempt can be made to reconstruct the development of retinal and renal lesions in diabetes if one starts from the few accepted ubiquitous functional abnormalities of the microcirculation in diabetes.

Capillary blood flow is known to increase in the retina before the appearance of clinically detectable lesions (18), while increased renal flow and filtration pressure are reported in pre-microalbuminuria (28). Capillary flow is known to rise with hyperglycaemia and to decrease when blood sugar returns to normal levels (1). Endothelium reacts to increased shear stress on the vessel wall, as brought about by high blood flow, by releasing vasodilators such as nitric oxide (NO) and perhaps prostacyclin, while decreasing at the same time the synthesis of vasoconstrictors such as endothelin (16). Circulating levels of endothelin (35) may be increased and stable by-products of prostacyclin decreased (10) in diabetes. Endothelial ability to synthesize NO from externally administered precursors may be reduced in diabetes (37). Keen and Chlouverakis (21) had reported that excess production of lactate, resulting from increased glucose utilization, may effect vasodilatation and that early explanation remains a plausible one. Intracapillary pressure is increased in IDDM in the nailfold capillaries (31) and may be similarly higher in the retinal and renal microcirculation. Tension receptors on endothelium promote the generation of vasoconstrictors, matrix components and mitogenic factors (36) and chronic hypertension produces narrower vessels with a thicker wall. *In vitro*, high glucose has been shown to increase endothelial synthesis of matrix components, such as types IV and VI collagen and fibronectin (5), and to decrease that of glycosaminoglycans, such as heparan sulphate (34). Enzymes that degrade the matrix, in turn, are controlled by endothelial-produced protease inhibitors, one of which, plasminogen activator inhibitor-1 (PAI-1), is notably oversynthesized by diabetic endothelium (20). Diabetes produces qualitative and quantitative changes in the composition of the capillary basement membrane and this altered material undergoes accelerated glycosylation and further rearrangement to form advanced glycosylation endproducts (AGE), which stimulate protein synthesis (9), further decrease degradability of the basement membrane (3), increase its permeability (13) and impair NO-induced vasodilatation (4). The histological correspondent of these changes is easily recognized as thickening of the capillary basement membrane in retinopathy and accumulation of mesangial material in diabetic glomeruli. Leukocytes have recently been indicated as a possible mechanism of capillary occlusion. White blood cells usually adhere to the vessel wall, where they constitute the "marginated pool". Since their diameter is larger than that of the smallest vessels, white cells slow down further when they reach the capillaries and may temporarily block them. Increased levels of adhesion molecules were reported in the plasma of people with diabetes, suggesting that capillary plugging by leukocytes may occur in the retina. Involvement of the clotting system had been advocated earlier than that of white cells. Endothelium synthesizes and regulates factors that promote or inhibit several mechanisms of platelet activation, plasma coagulation and fibrinolysis. In physiological conditions, the balance tilts towards prevention of thrombus formation, whereas under the effect of injury, endotoxins or some cytokines, clot-promoting activities prevail (30).

EYE CARE IN PATIENTS WITH DIABETIC NEPHROPATHY

Clarifying its pathogenesis would undoubtedly help in developing a rationale for the medical treatment of DR. At present, medical approaches are aimed at reducing incidence of new retinopathy and progression of existing lesions by optimized control of blood sugar levels and blood pressure. The Diabetic Control and Complications Trial (DCCT) (6) has shown that, in people with type 1 diabetes, 7.5 years of optimized metabolic control (meaning average levels of glycated haemoglobin at around 7%, as opposed to 9% in patients on conventional treatment) reduce the onset of new retinopathy by 76%, progression of mild non-proliferative DR by 54%, development of severe non-proliferative DR and of PDR by 47%, development of macular oedema by 26% and the need for laser treatment by 51%. However, strict metabolic control, as obtained in the DCCT, increases body weight and the risk of severe hypoglycaemia is difficult to achieve and maintain and is costly and possibly not so rewarding in the longer term. Projections based on the data of the DCCT (7) suggest that optimized control may result, over a lifetime span, in 3.8 years free from non-proliferative DR (from 23.7 years on conventional treatment to 27.5 years on intensified treatment), 14.7 years free from PDR (from 39.1 to 53.9), 8.2 years free from macular edema (from 44.7 to 52.9), and just 7.7 years free from blindness (from 49.1 to 56.8).

The UKPDS (38) has shown similar results in people with type 2 diabetes. Progression of retinopathy over 12 years was reduced by 21%, and that of albuminuria by 33%, with a reduction in HbA_{1c} of 0.9%. There were, however, increased body weight and incidence of severe hypoglycaemia. Even more striking were the results of blood pressure control UKPDS (39). Average reduction by 10 mmHg systolic and 5 mmHg diastolic pressure reduced the risks of retinopathy progression by 34% and deterioration of vision by 47% (this includes effects on cataract).

However, optimized metabolic and blood pressure control can only delay but not avoid retinopathy. Detailed knowledge of its natural history is extremely useful, at least in indicating when to intervene with the only effective treatment available: laser photocoagulation. The Diabetic Retinopathy Study (DRS) (8), Early Treatment of Diabetic Retinopathy Study (ETDRS) (11) and Diabetic Retinopathy Vitrectomy Study (DRVS) (12) have conclusively shown that:

- Focal photocoagulation prevents moderate visual loss (defined as doubling of the visual angle) by 50% at 3 years in clinically significant macular edema.
- Panretinal photocoagulation reduces severe visual loss (5/200 or worse on two consecutive visits 4 months apart) by 60% at 3 years in all levels of high-risk PDR.

- Panretinal photocoagulation applied to developing high-risk PDR reduces severe visual loss at 3 years by 87%, bilateral severe visual loss at 3 years by 97%, and legal blindness at 5 years by 90%.
- Vitrectomy applied to severe PDR and severe vitreous haemorrhage increases by 60% the chances of preserving 20/40 vision after 2 years.
- Vitrectomy in severe PDR with vision 10/200 or better (type 1 diabetes only) increases by 34% the chances of preserving 20/40 vision after 2 years.

Since DR can be delayed but not prevented by medical treatment, and since the best chances of preserving vision are obtained when photocoagulation is applied to high-risk DR before it has caused symptoms, organized screening for sight-threatening lesions remains the only option to prevent blindness.

The *Field Guidebook* to screening for retinopathy (22) has been independently validated (15) and its application has resulted in the only evidence available today, albeit indirect, of achieving the Saint-Vincent target of reducing incident blindness in one region of Europe by more than one-third over 5 years (2).

According to all recommendations, pupils should be dilated prior to fundus examination. Ophthalmoscopy, if possible, should be complemented by colour photography. The use of digital imaging has proved superior to traditional photographic film because it allows immediate quality checks, more practical data storage and telemedicine procedures, and will probably become the procedure of choice in the near future. Although most authors agree that patients without retinopathy at the previous screening could safely be seen every other year, annual examination is definitely more practical to organize and easier to comply with. Patients with diabetic renal disease, in particular, should be seen even more frequently, every 4–6 months, according to the European screening protocols. This is because they are more likely to have severe DR, which might be missed at periodic visits, and because retinopathy may progress more rapidly. Fluorescein angiography is not considered a screening test because it is not as fast, cheap, repeatable and harmless to the patients as the above procedures. Since sodium fluorescein is excreted by the kidneys, patients with renal impairment should not be subjected to the procedure unless specific diagnostic circumstances (usually to assess laser treatment of maculopathy) strongly require it. In such case, reduced amounts of the dye should be administered.

In summary, patients with overt diabetic nephropathy are almost certain to have retinopathy and very likely to have, or have had, sight-threatening retinopathy. Although procedures for its detection and treatment are not qualitatively different from those applied in the absence of renal complications, with the possible exception of an even more prudent use of fluorescein angiography, retinopathy should definitely be searched, with special attention and readiness to intervene.

REFERENCES

1. Atherton A, Hill DW, Keen H, Young S, Edwards EJ. The effect of acute hyperglycaemia on the retinal circulation of the normal cat. *Diabetologia* 1980; **18**: 233–7.
2. Backlund LB, Algvere PV, Rosenqvist U. New blindness in diabetes reduced by more than one-third in Stockholm Country. *Diabetic Med* 1997; **14**: 732–40.
3. Brownlee M, Cerami A, Vlassara H. Advanced glycosylation end-products in tissue and the biochemical basis of diabetic complications. *N Engl J Med* 1988; **318**: 1315–21.
4. Bucala R, Tracey KJ, Cerami A. Advanced glycosylation products quench nitric oxide and mediate defective endothelium-dependent vasodilatation in experimental diabetes. *J Clin Invest* 1991; **87**: 432–8.
5. Cagliero E, Roth T, Roy S, Lorenzi M. Characteristics and mechanisms of high-glucose-induced overexpression of basement membrane components in cultured human endothelial cells. *Diabetes* **40**: 102–10.
6. Diabetes Control and Complications Trial Research Group. The effect of intensive treatment of diabetes on the development and progression of long-term complications in insulin dependent diabetes mellitus. *N Engl J Med* 1993; **329**: 977–986.
7. Diabetes Control and Complications Trial Research Group. Lifetime benefits and costs of intensive therapy as practiced in the Diabetes Control and Complications Trial. *J Am Med Assoc* **276**: 1409–15.
8. Diabetic Retinopathy Study Research Group. Photocoagulation treatment of proliferative diabetic retinopathy: the second report of DRS findings. *Ophthalmology* 1978; **85**: 82–106.
9. Doi T, Vlassara H, Kirstein M et al. Receptor specific increase in extracellular matrix production in mouse mesangial cells by advanced glycosylation end products is mediated via platelet derived growth factor. *Proc Natl Acad Sci USA* 1992; **89**: 2873–7.
10. Dollery CT, Friedman LA, Hnsby CN et al. Circulating prostacyclin may be reduced in diabetes. *Lancet* 1979; **ii**: 1365.
11. Early Treatment Diabetic Retinopaty Study Research Group. Early photocoagulation for diabetic retinopathy: ETDRS report No. 9. *Ophthalmology* 1991; **98**: 766–85.
12. Diabetic Retinopathy Vitrectomy Study Research Group. Early vitrectomy for severe proliferative diabetic retinopathyin eyes with useful vision: results of a randomized trial: DRVS report No. 3. *Ophthalmology* 1978; **95**: 1307–20.
13. Esposito C, Gerlach H, Drett J, Stern D, Vlassara H. Endothelial receptor-mediated binding of glucose modified albumin is associated with increased monolayer permeability and modulation of cell surface coagulant properties. *J Exp Med* 1992; **170**: 1387–407.
14. Feldman JN, Hirsch SR, Beyer MB et al. Prevalence of diabetic nephropathy at time of treatment for diabetic retinopthy. In *Diabetic Renal–Retinal Syndrome*,

Vol. 2, Friedman EA, L'Esperance FA (eds). Grune and Stratton: New York; 9–20.

15. Gibbins RL, Owens DR, Allen JC, Eastman L. Practical application of the European Field Guide in screening retinopathy by using ophthalmoscopy and 35 mm retinal slides. *Diabetologia* **41**: 59–64.

16. Gibbons GH, Dzau VJ. The emerging concept of vascular remodelling. *N Engl J Med* 1994; **330**: 1431–7.

17. Grenfell A, Watkins PJ. Clinical diabetic nephropathy. Natural history and complications. *Clin Endocrinol Metab* 1986; **15**: 783–805.

18. Grunwald JE, Riva CE, Baine J, Brucker AJ. Total retinal volumetric blood flow rate in diabetic patients with poor glycemic control. *Invest Ophthalmol Vis Sci* 1992; **33**: 356–63.

19. Joint Working Party on Diabetic Renal Failure. Treatment and mortality of diabetic renal failure patients identified in the 1985 UK survey. *Br Med J* **299**: 1135–6.

20. Juhan-Vague I, Alessi MC, Vague P. Increased plasma plasminogen activator inhibitor 1 levels: a possible link between insulin resistance and atherothrombosis. *Diabetologia* 1991; **34**: 457–62.

21. Keen H, Chlouverakis C. Metabolic factors in diabetic retinopathy. In *Biochemistry of the Retina*, Graymore CN (ed.). Academic Press: London; 123–8.

22. Kohner EM, Porta M. *Screening for Diabetic Retinopathy in Europe: A Field Guidebook*. World Health Organization: Regional Office for Europe, Copenhagen; 1–51.

23. Kohner EM. The lesions and natural history of diabetic retinopathy. In *Chronic Complications of Diabetes*, Pickup JC, Williams G (eds). Blackwell: Oxford; 63–76.

24. Krolewski AS, Warram JH, Rand LI et al. Risk of proliferative diabetic retinopathy in juvenile-onset type I diabetes: a 40-year follow-up study. *Diabet Care* 1986; **9**: 443–52.

25. Krolewski AS, Warram JH, Rand LI, Kahn CR. Epidemiologic approach to the etiology of type I diabetes mellitus and its complications. *N Engl J Med* 1987; **317**: 1390–98.

26. Parving H-H, Hommel E, Mathiesen E et al. Prevalence of microalbuminuria, arterial hypertension, retinopathy and neuropathy in patients with insulin-dependent diabetes. *Br Med J* **296**: 156–60.

27. Parving H-H, Gall M-A, Skott P et al. Prevalence and causes of albuminuria in non-insulin dependent diabetic NIDDM patients. *Kidney Int* 1990; **37**: 243.

28. Paulsen EP, Pauly FL, Croft BY, Teates CD. Simultaneous measurement of glomerular filtration rate and effective renal plasma flow reveals increased glomerular capillary pressure among teenage diabetic subjects. *Contrib Nephrol* 1990; **79**: 52–7.

29. Pirart J. Diabète et complications dégénératives. Présentation d'une étude prospective portant sur 4400 cas observés entre 1947 et 1973. *Diabèt Metabol* 1977; **3**: 97–107, 173–82, 245–56.

30. Porta M. Endothelium: the main actor in the remodelling of the retinal microvasculature in diabetes. *Diabetologia* 1996; **39**: 739–744.

31. Sandeman DD, Shore AC, Tooke JE. Relation of skin capillary pressure in patients with insulin-dependent diabetes mellitus to complications and metabolic control. *New Engl J Med* 1992; **327**: 760–64.

32. Schmitz A, Vaeth M. Microalbuminuria: a major risk factor in non-insulin dependent diabetes. A 10-year follow-up study of 503 patients. *Diabet Med* **5**: 126–34.

33. Stephenson JM, Fuller JH, Viberti GC et al; the EURODIAB IDDM Complications Study Group. Blood pressure, retinopathy and urinary albumin excretion in IDDM: the EURODIAB IDDM Complications Study. *Diabetologia* 1995; **38:** 599–603.
34. Tamsma TT, van den Born J, Bruijn JA et al. Expression of glomerular extracellular matrix components in human diabetic nephropathy: decrease of heparan sulphate in the glomerular basement membrane. *Diabetologia* 1994; **37:** 313–20.
35. Takahashi K, Ghatei MA, Lam HC, O'Halloran DJ, Bloom SR. Elevated plasma endothelin in patients with diabetes mellitus. *Diabetologia* 1990; **33:** 306–10.
36. Tozzi CA, Pojani GJ, Haranzogo AM, Boyd CD, Riley DJ. Pressure-induced connective tissue synthesis in pulmonary artery segments is dependent on intact endothelium. *J Clin Invest* 1989; **84:** 1005–12.
37. Tesfamariam B, Brown ML, Cohen RA. Elevated glucose impairs endothlium-dependent relaxation by activating protein kinase C. *J Clin Invest* 1991; **87:** 1643–8.
38. UK Prospective Diabetes Study (UKPDS) Group. Intensive blood glucose control with sulphonylureas or insulin compared with conventional treatment and risk of complications in patients with type 2 diabetes (UKPDS 33). *Lancet* 1998a; **352:** 837–53.
39. UK Prospective Diabetes Study (UKPDS) Group. Tight pressure control and risk of macrovascular and microvascular complications in type 2 diabetes. *Br Med J* 1998b; **317:** 703–13.

14

Pregnancy and Diabetic Nephropathy

ALASDAIR MACKIE

Northern General Hospital, Sheffield, UK

INTRODUCTION

Women with type 1 diabetes mellitus without nephropathy can anticipate an outcome of pregnancy approaching those without diabetes mellitus, providing they achieve good glycaemic control (19). Moreover, those with microalbuminuria, or proteinuria with preserved renal function, share the expectation of a successful maternal and foetal outcome (21,42). Greater uncertainty exists for women with impaired renal function. Whereas a favourable outcome was noted in early studies (34,50), recent observations (32,48) suggest that a more cautious approach should be adopted.

Around 3% of pregnancies in diabetes mellitus are reported in women with nephropathy (11). Few diabetologists, obstetricians and paediatricians outwith tertiary referral centres gain significant experience in the management of such pregnancies. To date, fewer than 400 cases with diabetic nephropathy have been reported. The case-mix of the series published is variable, ranging from those with proteinuria and normal renal function to those who commence renal replacement therapy (RRT) shortly after, or occasionally before, delivery. Furthermore, there are often limited data on pre-pregnancy renal function. Both factors potentially can lead to differences in interpretation of the influence of pregnancy on outcome.

This chapter discusses renal function in normal pregnancy and highlights the differences seen in uncomplicated diabetes and in nephropathy. The

Diabetic Nephropathy. Edited by C. Hasslacher.
© 2001 John Wiley & Sons, Ltd.

main section is devoted to the consequences of pregnancy in women with nephropathy, concentrating upon the progression of nephropathy, together with a review of the factors affecting the short- and long-term outcome for the foetus. The issue of pre-eclampsia and diabetic nephropathy is also addressed. Brief consideration will be given to the outcome of pregnancy in women on dialysis or in receipt of a renal, or combined renal–pancreas, transplant.

RENAL CHANGES IN NORMAL AND UNCOMPLICATED DIABETIC PREGNANCY

Dilatation of the renal collecting system is almost universal in pregnancy, beginning in many in the first trimester and present in over 90% by delivery (49). Serial renal ultrasound examinations confirm that kidney volume, too, increases during pregnancy in both non-diabetic (9) and diabetic subjects (39). In the rat, Davison and Lindheimer (14) established that this volume increase is fluid, whilst Christiansen and colleagues (8) confirmed these findings, again in the rat, using magnetic resonance imaging (MRI) techniques.

Glomerular filtration rate (GFR) and effective renal plasma flow (ERPF) increase significantly during pregnancy. Dunlop (17) demonstrated the latter to increase by 80% by the second trimester, and that it remained 60% above the non-pregnant state by the end of the third trimester. More recent studies by Sturgiss et al (58) indicate that these changes are well established by the 12th week of pregnancy. GFR, estimated by creatinine clearance, rises by up to 25% within 4 weeks of fertilization, attains a peak value of 20–80% (mean 45%) above non-pregnant levels by the end of the first trimester and decreases towards normal as delivery approaches (15). A small increment in creatinine clearance (CrCl) may be seen in the initial post-partum period. The limited evidence from inulin clearance studies fails to substantiate the notion of a pre-delivery decline in CrCl, although studies have not been extended beyond 37 weeks. Increased GFR is, in part, responsible for the doubling of protein excretion from $\sim$ 100 to 180 mg/day from the first to the third trimester observed in non-diabetic pregnancy. For a more detailed review of this subject see Davison and Lindheimer (16).

THE RENIN–ANGIOTENSIN SYSTEM IN NORMAL PREGNANCY

There is a net daily increment in sodium of 2–6 mmol during pregnancy, leading to an accumulation of around 900 mmol. Volume expansion exceeds

7 l, of which 1–1.5 l is intravascular. This increase is due primarily to plasma water and, to a lesser degree, red cell mass. These increments commence within the first trimester, reach a maximum by week 32 and remain elevated until delivery. Whilst the physiological significance of the volume expansion is uncertain, sub-maximal increments have been associated with a poorer outcome of pregnancy. Foetal growth is linked to plasma volume expansion, with intra-uterine growth retardation evident in sub-normal volume expansion.

All components of the renin–angiotensin (RA) system increase in pregnancy. In early gestation, aldosterone levels rise in greater proportion to renin, reflecting additional non-angiotensin stimulation, e.g. by ACTH and progesterone, and may exceed those observed in primary aldosteronism. Angiotensin II (AII) levels are raised in line with increased renin. It is uncertain whether the changes seen in the RA system are due to, or cause, the differences observed in volume homeostasis in pregnancy. There are no specific studies of the RA system in diabetic nephropathy. A detailed review of the renin–angiotensin system in pregnancy can be found in Lindheimer and Katz (40) and aldosterone metabolism in August and Sealey (2). Paradoxically, pre-eclampsia, a state associated with volume contraction and vasoconstriction, is associated with reduced renin, AII and aldosterone levels compared to normal pregnancy. GFR is often reduced in pre-eclamptic toxaemia (7).

CLINICAL IMPLICATIONS OF ALTERED RENAL HAEMODYNAMICS IN NORMAL AND DIABETIC PREGNANCY

The increased plasma clearance of creatinine leads to a progressive reduction of serum creatinine through pregnancy, from 73 μmol/l in the pre-pregnant period to 65, 51 and 47 μmol/l, respectively for the 1st, 2nd, and 3rd trimesters (59). Therefore, women with non-pregnant levels of serum creatinine should alert the obstetrician or physician to possible underlying renal disease. Errors in measuring creatinine clearance may occur in women with diabetic cystopathy and be introduced by the "dead-space" volume of the dilated pelvi-calyceal systems.

Hyperfiltration is regarded by some as central to the initiation and progression of renal disease in diabetes mellitus (24). In pregnancy it may, in theory, accelerate the process of glomerulosclerosis and contribute to the decline in renal function, although there is little evidence that this operates in practice. Few data exist on renal haemodynamics in pregnancy in those with diabetes mellitus, let alone where complicated with nephropathy. Based on small numbers, pregnancy-induced increase in GFR of > 25% is seen in $\sim$ 30% of women with DN in the third trimester (35). A similar proportion showed a decline in GFR of > 15% in the same period. First trimester creatinine clearance did not predict subsequent third trimester change in GFR.

Lauszas et al (39) demonstrated that renal volume in women with nephropathy was not significantly different 4 months after delivery, compared to the third trimester, in contrast to those with less severe complications, where a significant post-partum reduction in volume occurred. Klebe et al (36) showed no increase in renal volume throughout pregnancy in a small group of women with White class F diabetes, unless nephrotic syndrome was present. Urinary tract infections are more common in pregnant women with diabetes than in those without, whilst dilatation of the collecting system may increase the risk of pyelonephritis.

PREGNANCY, INCIPIENT NEPHROPATHY AND PRE-ECLAMPSIA

The importance of microalbuminuria in pregnancy is difficult to gauge given the relatively few, and often conflicting, published studies. Albumin excretion has been shown to increase significantly by the third trimester and immediate post-partum period in most studies in non-diabetic pregnancy, and in both normo-albuminuric (41) and microalbuminuric subjects with diabetes (6, 44). McCance et al (41) observed a significantly greater rise in albumin excretion in the third trimester and immediate post-partum period in both diabetic and non-diabetic pregnancy, whereas Mogensen and Klebe (44) observed no increase in non-diabetic subjects. In the latter study, 14 of 31 (45%) normoalbuminuric subjects progressed to microalbuminuria by the later stages of pregnancy. Transient nephrotic syndrome (protein excretion > 3 g/24 h) developed in 4/12 subjects with established microalbuminuria studied by Biesenbach et al (6). All four had significantly higher systolic blood pressures. The rise in creatinine clearance in these individuals was only 10% compared to the mean increase of 22% in the non-microalbuminuric and 26% in the microalbuminuric group. The long-term significance for the mother of gestational microalbuminuria is not known.

The hope that an increase in UAE may herald pre-eclampsia, and so offer early detection of this complication of pregnancy, has so far proved unfounded. No difference in the frequency of pre-eclampsia has been observed in those developing microalbuminuria or with established microalbuminuria in both non-diabetic and diabetic pregnancy. Combs et al (10) did suggest that the level of early pregnancy proteinuria was linked to pre-eclampsia rates. In general, numbers studied are too few to draw significant conclusions, although Mogensen and Klebe (44) suggested that rising albumin excretion may forecast an adverse foetal outcome. Bar et al (3) have shown that the development of microalbuminuria in the second and third trimester is associated with high-risk hypertensive pregnancies and suggest poorer neonatal outcome in non-diabetic subjects. The role of microalbuminuria and pregnancy is thoroughly reviewed in Mogensen and Klebe (44).

Although pre-eclampsia may not be more common in diabetic subjects with microalbuminuria, paradoxically it may occur more often in diabetes. Early estimates of around 50% of pregnancies affected gradually fell to 25% in the 1960s and to about 10% in the 1980s (18). The latter observed pre-eclampsia in 33/334 of diabetic pregnancies, compared to 716/16 534 (4.3%) without diabetes. Pre-eclampsia was more common with increasing severity of diabetes. It is almost impossible to distinguish pre-eclampsia in subjects with diabetic nephropathy from the natural course of blood pressure change during pregnancy in these subjects. The presence of thrombocytopenia, disordered coagulation and rise in hepatic enzymes in the former may be the only certain way to distinguish these clinical entities.

MANAGEMENT OF PREGNANCY

Awareness of the risk of pregnancy on well-being and renal function with potential hazards for the foetus is especially desirable in women with diabetic nephropathy. A clear explanation of the long-term maternal and foetal prognosis is essential, particularly in women with impaired renal function. Unless a severe congenital malformation is detected, therapeutic termination for women with renal impairment is not generally advised, although advocated by some (16). Where severe renal impairment is present, women are recommended to wait until after transplantion, although for some this means postponing pregnancy for several years, possibly foregoing any hope of parenthood. Many chose to risk pregnancy. A definition of the grades of renal impairment is given in Table 14.1.

Table 14.2 outlines suggested guidelines for the management of pregnancy complicated with diabetic nephropathy. Pregnancy should be

Table 14.1 Definition of (pre-pregnancy) renal status, as given in (16). The equivalent values for μmol/l are approximated

Category	Serum creatinine	
	(mg/100 dl)	(μmol/l)
Preserved or mild renal impairment	< 1.4	< 125
Moderate renal impairment	1.4–2.5	125–220
Severe renal impairment	> 2.5	> 220

Reproduced from (16) by permission of WB Saunders Company.

Table 14.2   Recommendations for the management of pregnancy in women with diabetic nephropathy

---

Pre-pregnancy
- Optimize glycaemic control—check HbA_{1c}/review insulin regimen
- Optimize blood pressure—aim for 140/80/stop ACE inhibitor
- Examine for evidence of other micro- and macrovascular complications:
  - Dilated fundoscopy
  - Cardiac assessment—history, ECG
  - Consider autonomic function tests
  - Consider bladder ultrasound for post-micturition residue
- Determine renal function
  - Serum creatinine
  - Creatinine clearance
  - Urinary 24 h protein excretion
  - Consider isotope GFR measurement
- Advise of potential maternal and foetal complications

Intra-partum assessment
Booking visit
- As for pre-pregnancy if non-attender
- Renal function: serum creatinine, creatinine clearance, urinary 24 h protein
- Review diabetes control/insulin regimen
- Urine culture

Each visit
- Blood pressure
- HbA_{1c}
- Urine dipstick for protein
- Serum creatinine
- Review blood glucose monitoring

Each trimester
- Urinary 24 hour protein excretion and creatinine clearance
- Fundal examination

Foetal surveillance
- Booking visit—USS for dates
- 18–20 Weeks—detailed scan for congenital anomalies
- 28 Weeks on—USS for growth (performed fortnightly)
- Foetal movement chart/CTG

Frequency of visits is subject to personal preference, but usual practice is:

Up to 28 weeks	Monthly
28–32 weeks	Fortnightly
32 weeks on	Weekly

Post-partum
Mother
- Renal function—serum creatinine, creatinine clearance and urinary 24 h protein
- Blood pressure therapy—reintroduce ACE inhibitor at delivery (avoid whilst breast feeding)
- Review contraception and future plans for pregnancy
- Consider isotope GFR measurement after post-partum period

Infant
- Neonatal complications, e.g. hypoglycaemia/RDS/hyperbilirubinaemia
- Assessment of psychomotor development

---

managed jointly by obstetrician, diabetes physician and paediatrician. Where indicated, a nephrologist may be involved in the care, whilst the support of the diabetes nurse specialist, midwife and dietitian is essential. Early pregnancy visits should concentrate on optimizing glycaemic control and blood pressure, documenting renal function, excluding congenital malformations and preparing the mother for what is likely to prove a problematic pregnancy. Pre-and post-pregnancy isotopic GFR measurement may be helpful to determine renal function accurately.

The frequency with which renal function is assessed is, to a degree, a matter of personal preference; 24 h protein and creatinine clearance performed each trimester, with serum creatinine each visit, is advocated here, although others suggest monthly assessment (16). A rising serum creatinine should prompt more detailed assessment of renal function and a search for any remediable factor, such as a UTI, poor blood pressure control or a drug effect.

Throughout pregnancy blood pressure control is paramount, with the aim of achieving levels of 120–130/80–85 mmHg (40). Regular dose adjustment and introduction of additional agents are required. Evidence of specific class benefit is lacking in pregnancy in diabetic nephropathy. Some advocate β-blockers and calcium channel blockers as first line therapy (30), although many clinicians still use methyldopa. Only ACEIs are contraindicated. Their use has been associated with malformation of the skull and pulmonary hypoplasia if used in early pregnancy, and with oligohydramnios, neonatal renal failure and anaemia if prescribed in late gestation. Of interest is that ACEI therapy in the pre-conception period may confer benefit over disease progression within pregnancy. Hod et al (23) observed that protein excretion during pregnancy exceeded 1 g 24 h in only 2/8 individuals with nephropathy treated with captopril (maximum dose 75 mg/day) for at least 8 months prior to conception. In addition, overall renal function did not deteriorate during pregnancy.

Distinguishing pre-eclampsia superimposed upon chronic hypertension in DN from the exacerbations of chronic hypertension is difficult, although clinically important, as treatment for the former is delivery, whereas bed rest with improved BP control may suffice for the latter.

Regular fundal examination is essential to detect progressive disease that may require laser photocoagulation. Ten per cent of subjects (31/331) with background retinopathy at conception progressed to proliferation, whereas none occurred where fundal examination was normal (57). Rosenn et al (54) showed a doubling in progression rate of eye disease in subjects with chronic hypertension or pregnancy-induced hypertension. Anaemia is common in nephropathic pregnancy and may require treatment with erythropoietin in addition to iron and folic acid supplementation (27).

Regular foetal surveillance is performed using ultrasound examination throughout pregnancy. In early gestation, scanning confirms viability and exclude congenital malformation, whereas from the latter stages of the second trimester to term, serial examinations determine the adequacy of foetal growth. More invasive techniques to monitor foetal well-being are not routinely performed.

The decision to deliver the baby of a mother with diabetic nephropathy is a collective one, based upon gestation, the well-being of the mother and the fetus. Resistant severe hypertension, worsening renal function, nephrotic syndrome, severe pre-eclampsia and eclampsia are all indicators for delivery, some demanding greater immediacy than others. Nephrotic syndrome, developing late in gestation, need not be justification, alone, for early delivery, as Purdy et al (48) have shown no effect on maternal outcome where it develops after 34 weeks.

Where possible, gestation should exceed 34 weeks to improve neonatal outcome, although not to the degree where maternal safety is compromised.

MATERNAL OUTCOME—RENAL CHANGES DURING PREGNANCY

Increasing proteinuria during pregnancy is almost universal in diabetic nephropathy. In general the rise is two- to four-fold with the majority reverting to pre-pregnancy levels after delivery. Kimmerle et al (32) observed an average rise of 2.1–5 g from the first to the third trimesters, with the proportion excreting over 3 g increasing from 14% to 53%. Similar rises (and postpartum falls) have been observed (21,50). In a series of 26 women, protein excretion exceeded 6 g in 58% of cases in the third trimester (34), whereas Reece et al (50) recorded nephrotic range proteinuria in 71% of cases. Purdy et al (48) noted that heavy proteinuria, ($> 3 g/24 h$), in early pregnancy heralded a decline of GFR, whereas similar levels of protein excretion developing in the third trimester were more benign.

Blood pressure, too, rises with gestation and, as with protein excretion, almost invariably so in the third trimester, being responsible for delivery in many cases. Reece et al (50) observed a 15% increase in blood pressure in 19 of 31 subjects in their study throughout pregnancy. In a recent summary paper, 60% of 315 women with DN developed hypertension by the third trimester, with 41% deemed to have pre-eclampsia (52). However, it is frequently impossible to distinguish this entity from pregnancy-induced (or exacerbated) hypertension in nephropathy. The above figure needs to be viewed with caution. Without doubt, blood pressure plays a key role in pregnancy outcome in terms of both delivery date and maternal renal function.

Early studies suggested no acceleration of the rate of decline of GFR during pregnancy (34,50), although creatinine clearance did decrease in 39% of pregnancies in the latter study. More recently, Purdy et al (48) recorded a significant decline in five of 11 subjects, in whom the baseline GFR was < 45 ml/min. In three subjects renal function was stable, whereas in a further three a transient decline was noted. In addition, the acceleration in the five individuals was deemed to have led to a reduction of 36 months, on average, in the time (from pregnancy) to renal replacement therapy. Biesenbach et al (5) estimated the decline in GFR in five women with moderate renal impairment at 1.8 ml/min/month, almost twice that generally observed outwith pregnancy in untreated subjects and several-fold greater than now seen in many treated subjects. This marked decline may have been due to suboptimal blood pressure treatment during pregnancy. Pregnancy has been shown to accelerate the rate of decline of GFR in non-diabetic renal disease, including IgA nephropathy and membranoproliferative glomerulonephritis (31), albeit in only a few of those with established renal impairment (SCr > 160–180 µmol/1) and poorly controlled blood pressure at conception.

Retinopathy, too, may progress during pregnancy (37). Subjects with nephropathy may be at special risk of developing sight-threatening retinopathy and merit regular examination during pregnancy.

LONG-TERM OUTCOME

Until recently it was generally accepted that pregnancy did not accelerate the decline of GFR in nephropathic subjects (Table 14.3). This view has been challenged, at least in women with more advanced renal impairment (5,48). The latter considered pregnancy a contributory factor to the decline in 40% cases, and that decline during pregnancy rather than in the post-partum period was primarily responsible. These observations were not confirmed in a group of subjects with similar impairment of renal function (42).

On average, 25% of all women with diabetic nephropathy will commence RRT within 3 years of delivery. Reece et al (52) estimated that ~5% of women die within this time period. These data support the estimate of Hare and White (22), that 20% of children born to mothers with nephropathy will lose their mothers by age 10.

Gordon et al (20) observed a slower decline of GFR after delivery in nine women with first trimester proteinuria of < 1 g and creatinine clearance of > 90 ml/min, compared to those with more abnormal values, albeit the wide variation in the data precluded a significant difference. Miodovnik et al (43) estimate that the risk of developing ESRD in women with DN in pregnancy as 16% after 5 years, 30% after 10 years and 45% after 12 years from the start of nephropathy.

Table 14.3 Maternal outcome of pregnancy in women with diabetic nephropathy

Reference	(n)	Initial creatinine/creatinine clearance	Rate of fall of GFR (ml/min/month)	Follow-up (months) Mean or range	Outcome of ESRD	Time to ESRD (months)	Acceleration in decline of GFR
(34)	26	24–97 ml/min	0.81	6–35	3/23	24	No
(50)	31	25–245 ml/min (12 < 90 ml/min)	NS	6–108	6/27	36	No
(51)	11	53–203 μmol/l	NS	1–37	0/11	–	No
(21)	22	NS	NS	NS	1 Death 3 Deterioration	24 (6–120)	NS
(42)	6	≤ 75 ml/min	0.55	6–96	3/6	25 (10–36)	No
(5)	5	≤ 75 ml/min	1.40	13–42	5/5	29	Yes
(43)	46	94 ± 25 ml/min (11 < 80 ml/min)	0.67–0.83	36–190	12/46	72	No
(48)	11	159 ± 62 μmol/l	0.84*	35–138	7/11	23 (6–57)	Yes
(32)	33	50–214 μmol/l (10 < 80 ml/min)	0.65	5–120	8/29	36 (12–108)	No
(20)	46	120 ± 53 ml/min (11 < 90 ml/min)	1.30	34	3/34	21	Possible

ESRD, endstage renal disease (death or renal replacement therapy). NS, not stated. * Estimated.
Some of the duration follow-up results are interpolated from the data presented in the papers.

FETAL OUTCOME

Perinatal survival in children born to women with type I diabetes mellitus is comparable to that in women without diabetes (38). The principal series of reported pregnancies in subjects with diabetic nephropathy are summarized in Table 14.4. These studies are heterogeneous, with differing proportions of subjects having impaired renal function, as opposed to proteinuria with preserved renal function. Outcomes, therefore, may reflect these differences.

PERINATAL MORBIDITY

Perinatal outcome has improved significantly since the early 1970s, when around 70% survival could be expected (22). A decade later this had risen to 90% (34), with the majority of studies now reporting around 100% survival. A small series from Germany in women with impaired renal function (CrCl < 75 ml/min) at the outset of pregnancy, showed a much poorer outcome, with only 2/5 babies surviving.

Congenital anomalies are recorded in ~8% of pregnancies, ranging from 4–14.3%. Intra-uterine growth retardation (IUGR), defined as a birthweight below the 10th centile for the corresponding gestational age, occurs in 15% of pregnancies (Table 14.3). The risk increases with worsening maternal renal function (32). In a survey of 36 pregnancies, this group observed small-for-gestational-age cases in 30% (3/10) where creatinine clearance was < 80 ml/min, compared to 19% (5/26) where clearance was ≥ 80 ml/min. The rates of IUGR are comparable to those observed in non-diabetic renal disease (29).

Premature delivery before 34 weeks is observed in 20–30% of pregnancies (Table 14.4). It is probable that the majority of these are in women with renal impairment, rather than proteinuria alone (42). This group showed that women with moderately impaired renal function delivered, on average, 5 weeks earlier than those with proteinuria alone. Respiratory distress syndrome (RDS) complicated a significant proportion of pregnancies, occurring more frequently in mothers with renal impairment (50%) than in those without (15%) (32). Comparable data are found in non-diabetic renal disease (12), where a much higher incidence of pre-term delivery (< 37 weeks), 86% vs. 30%, respectively, in 11 women with severe renal insufficiency as compared to 26 with moderate impairment was observed. Over 50% of deliveries in nephropathic women occur before 37 weeks (35).

Table 14.4 Outcome in the offspring of women with diabetic nephropathy

Study	(n)	IUGR (%)	Preterm delivery* (%)	Perinatal survival (%)	Intensive care (days)	Complications		Children	
						Major congenital malformation (%)	RDS (%)	Follow-up (years)	Outcome (retardation) (%)
(34)	26	21	31	89	NS	11	23	1.8 (0.7–3.1)	5.5
(50)	31	16	23	94	NS	10	19	3 (0.5–9)	3.7
(51)	11	NS	NS	100	NS	NS	NS	NS	NS
(21)	22	15	27	100	NS	4	NS	NS	NS
(5)	5	100	100	40	NS	NS	80	NS	NS
(10)	62	NS	23	NS	NS	NS	NS	NS	NS
(32)	36	22	31	100	24 (2–122)	5.5	25	4.5 (0–10)	23
(20)	45	11	16	100	9.3 ± 13.6	4	22	NS	NS
(43)	46	9	22	91	NS	11	20	NS	NS
(42)	17	NS	41	100	15 (7–271)	5.8	NS	3.5	5.8
(48)	14	7	21 +	100	NS	14.3	64	NS	NS
Average	–	15	25	96	–	8	26	–	9.5

*< 34 weeks. Each paper should be consulted, as there are differences in case mix and level of assessment. IUGR, intrauterine growth retardation; NS, not stated.

LONG-TERM OUTCOME

There are few data on long-term outcome for children born to mothers with diabetic nephropathy. Rates of psychomotor retardation suggested by initial studies were surprisingly low at 3–6% (Table 14.4). The most detailed outcome data come from Düsseldorf (32), where systematic follow-up of 36 children for up to 11 years found that 25% of the children had varying degrees of psychomotor retardation, 11% (4/36) to a severe degree, albeit two had major congenital neurological malformations. Piecuch and Leonard (47), among others, have shown that outcome in non-diabetic pregnancies is related to gestational age. In their study infants born at 26 weeks had a 74% chance of survival with normal or borderline cognitive development, whereas among those at 24 weeks the comparable figure was 26%. In 88 children born to women with type I diabetes mellitus, no adverse effect of gestation on neurodevelopment outcome was documented, although for all gestation exceeded 28 weeks (46).

It must also be borne in mind that a number of these children, in infancy or early adolescence, will lose their mothers though premature death from renal failure or cardiovascular disease

PREDICTION OF FOETAL OUTCOME

The above discussion suggests that increasing prematurity is associated with more severe renal impairment, and this in turn may lead to psychomotor retardation. Gordon et al (20) identified a high-risk sub-group on the basis of protein excretion and serum creatinine from 45 women with diabetic nephropathy. The women were also subdivided on the basis of creatinine clearance into normal (< 90 ml/min), moderately decreased (60–89 ml/min) and severely decreased (< 60 ml/min). Outcome data on these women are presented in Table 14.5. Based on initial creatinine clearance, the data suggest that severe renal impairment was associated with a longer stay in neonatal intensive care (NICU), although the differences were not significant due to small numbers. High-risk babies spent twice as long in NICU, although again small numbers precluded a significant result. Women in the "high-risk" group delivered earlier and suffered more pre-eclampsia, whilst a 24 h protein excretion of < 1 g was associated with a more favourable outcome. Such outcomes are also observed in non-diabetic renal disease (28).

Reece et al (51) observed an inverse relationship between birthweight and blood pressure, pre-eclampsia and nephrotic syndrome, whilst no association was found with protein excretion.

Table 14.5 Predictors of perinatal outcome

	Number	Birth weight (g)	Gestational age (weeks)	NICU (days)	Pre-eclampsia (%)
Initial creatinine clearance (ml/min)					
> 90	34	2688 ± 868	34.5 ± 2.3	9.0 ± 14	47
60–90	7	2705 ± 250	36.4 ± 1.0	2.4 ± 2.3	57
< 60	4	2247 ± 903	34.5 ± 3.5	21.8 ± 13.7	75
High-risk criteria*					
Yes	12	2115 ± 727$^\phi$	34.3 ± 2.5$^{\phi\phi}$	15.7 ± 14.6	92$^\phi$
No	33	2847 ± 747	36.3 ± 2.0	7 ± 12.7	36.4

NICU, neonatal intensive care unit.
Data are given as mean ± SD or %.
*High-risk criteria: serum creatinine > 1.5 mg/dl or proteinuria > 3 g/24 h.
$^\phi p < 0.005$; $^{\phi\phi} p < 0.01$.
Adapted from (20), with permission of Elsevier Science.

PREGNANCY AND RENAL REPLACEMENT THERAPY

The resumption of normal renal function after transplantation is frequently associated with menstruation, ovulation and the return of fertility, whilst women on dialysis often present late when pregnant, partly due to the lack of awareness of the potential for conception. In 1975, Tagatz et al (60) reported the first successful pregnancy following a renal transplant in a patient with diabetes. Ogburn et al (45) summarized the data on three previously reported cases and added a further six. Live infants were delivered between 31 and 36 weeks in all pregnancies and birthweight, with one exception, was appropriate to gestational age.

Data on pregnancy in those on RRT are collated in Europe by the Europe by the European Dialysis and Transplantation Association (EDTA) and, in North America, by the National Transplant Patient Registry (NTPR). For the EDTA, Rizzoni et al (53) reported the outcome of 490 pregnancies (500 offspring) in women receiving RRT, 88.4% of which followed transplantation. Overall, the outcome was favourable, with a neonatal mortality rate of 1.8%. Approximately 35% of pregnancies delivered before 34 weeks and in 27 women congenital anomalies were reported. A case control study of 53 of the 490 pregnancies, the majority (94%) with serum creatinine ≤ 160 μmol/l, showed no adverse effect of pregnancy on renal function up to 36 months post-delivery. Graft failure was slightly less in the pregnant group. No data are given as to primary renal disease, although figures from the NTPR (1) suggest that diabetes may constitute 5–10% of cases. Overall, only 1% of women in the child-bearing years on the EDTA registry had a successful pregnancy.

Pregnancy has been recorded following combined renal and pancreas transplantation, although cases are few. Skannel et al (56) summarized five published cases with an additional case of their own. All delivered successfully at 35 weeks or later, with three babies small for gestation. Maternal renal function declined in two cases. The mean time from transplantation to conception was 18 months and all were maintained on cyclosporin and prednisolone through pregnancy. The largest series, to date, is reported from the International Pancreas Transplant Registry (4), with 19 live births in 17 women. Mean gestation was 35 weeks and birthweight 2150 g.

Nearly 20 years have elapsed since the first reported successful pregnancy in a woman with type 1 diabetes on CAPD (33). Pregnancies in dialysis patients, particularly with diabetes mellitus, remain rare. Of the 490 pregnancies cited above on the EDTA Registry, 11.2% were receiving haemodialysis and only 0.4% CAPD (53). Before 1990, only 20% of pregnancies in women conceiving on dialysis ended successfully (25), although recent data suggest that this has improved to around 50% (26). In a survey of dialysis units in the USA, most pregnancies occurred during the first year on dialysis, although over 20% were in women on dialysis for over 10 years (25). In general, babies born to women on dialysis show greater growth retardation than following transplantation and deliver earlier, on average around 32 weeks.

It is recommended that women wait at least 2 years after transplantation before embarking on a pregnancy (13). An increased risk of renal transplant rejection post-delivery has been reported, although there is no evidence that pregnancy compromises long-term renal allograft function (53).

CONCLUSION

Women who have mild renal impairment can be reassured that pregnancy does not accelerate the progression of their renal disease, neither should they anticipate an adverse outcome to their pregnancy. However, for women with more severe renal disease, the outcome for the mother and her offspring is less certain and success cannot be guaranteed. The literature and experience would suggest that a pregnancy progressing to 34 weeks or more is accompanied by a greater degree of foetal well-being. It is highly probable that women with increasingly severe renal disease will continue to become pregnant and that a successful outcome will depend, in large measure, on the combined skills of the physician, obstetrician and, above all, the neonatologist. Given the concern for the well-being of the child, such women may be better advised to postpone their decision to have a family until they have received a renal transplant, at which time a better outcome may be anticipated, although many will continue to become pregnant.

REFERENCES

1. Armenti VT, Ahlswede KM, Ahlswede BA et al. National Transplantation Pregnancy Registry-Outcomes of 154 pregnancies in cyclosporine-treated female kidney transplant recipients. *Transplantation* 1994; **57**: 502–6.
2. August P, Sealey JE. The renin–angiotensin system in normal and hypertensive pregnancy and in ovarian function. In *Hypertension: Pathophysiology, Diagnosis and Management*, Laragh JH, Brenner BM (eds). Raven: New York; 1761–78.
3. Bar J, Hod M, Erman A, Friedman S, Ovadia Y. Microalbuminuria: prognostic and therapeutic implications in diabetic and hypertensive pregnancy. *Diabet Med* 1995; **12**: 649–56.
4. Barrou BM, Gruessner AC, Sutherland DE, Gruessner RW. Pregnancy after pancreas transplantation in the cyclosporine era: report from the International Pancreas Transplant Registry. *Transplantation* 1998; **65**: 524–7.
5. Biesenbach G, Stoger H, Zazgornik J. Influence of pregnancy on progression of diabetic nephropathy and subsequent requirement of renal replacement therapy in female type 1 diabetic patients with impaired renal function. *Nephrol Dialysis Transpl* 1992; **7**: 105–9.
6. Biesenbach G., Zazgornick J, Stoger H et al. Abnormal increases in urinary albumin excretion during pregnancy in IDDM women with pre-existing microalbuminuria. *Diabetologia* 1994; **37**: 905–10.
7. Brown MA, Whitworth JA. The kidney in hypertensive pregnancies—victim and villain. *Am J Kidney Dis* 1992; **20**: 427–42.
8. Christiansen T, Stodkilde-Jorgensen H, Klebe JG, Flyvbjerg A. Changes in kidney volume during pregnancy in non-diabetic and diabetic rats measured by magnetic resonance imaging. *Exp Nephrol* 1998; **6**: 302–7.
9. Cietak KA, Newton JR. Serial quantitative maternal nephrosonography in pregnancy. *Br J Radiol* 1985; **58**: 405–13.
10. Combs CA., Rosenn B, Kitzmiller JL et al. Early pregnancy proteinuria in diabetes related to pre-eclampsia. *Obstet Gynecol* 1993; **82**: 802–7.
11. Connell FA, Vadheim C, Emanuel I. Diabetes in pregnancy: a population-based study of incidence, referral for care, and perinatal mortality. *Am J Obstet Gynecol* 1985; **151**: 598–603.
12. Cunningham FG, Cox SM, Harstad TW, Mason RA, Pritchard JA. Chronic renal disease and pregnancy outcome. *Am J Obstet Gynecol* 1990; **163**: 453–9.
13. Davison JM. Dialysis, transplantation and pregnancy. *Am J Kidney Dis* 1991; **27**: 127–32.
14. Davison JM, Lindheimer MD. Changes in renal haemodynamics and kidney weight during pregnancy in the unanaesthetized rat. *J. Physiol (Lond)* 1980; **301**: 129–36.
15. Davison JM, Noble MCB. Serial changes in 24 hour creatinine clearance during normal menstrual cycles and the first trimester of pregnancy. *Br J Obstet Gynaecol* 1981; **88**: 10–17.
16. Davison JM, Lindheimer MD. Renal disorders. In *Maternal–Fetal Medicine: Principles and Practice*, 3rd edn, Creasy RK, Resnik R (eds). Philadelphia: WB Saunders, 1994; 844–64.
17. Dunlop W. Serial changes in renal haemodynamics during normal human pregnancy. *Br J Obstet Gynecol* 1981; **88**: 1–9.
18. Garner PR, D'Alton ME, Dudley DK, Huard P, Hardie M. Pre-eclampsia in diabetic pregnancies. *Am J Obstet Gynecol* 1990; **163**: 505–8.
19. Garner P. Type 1 diabetes mellitus and pregnancy. *Lancet* 1995; **346**: 157–61.

20. Gordon M, Landon MB, Samuels P, Hissrich S, Gabbe SG. Perinatal outcome and long-term follow-up associated with modern management of diabetic nephropathy. *Obstet Gynecol* 1996; **87**: 401–9.

21. Grenfell A., Brudenell JM, Doddridge MC, Watkins PJ. Pregnancy in diabetic women who have proteinuria. *Q J Med* 1986; **59**: 379–86.

22. Hare JW, White P. Pregnancy in diabetes complicated by vascular disease. *Diabetes* 1977; **26**: 953–5.

23. Hod M, van Dijk DJ, Karp M et al. Diabetic nephropathy and pregnancy: the effect of ACE inhibitors prior to pregnancy on fetomaternal outcome. *Nephrol Dialysis Transpl* 1995; **10**: 2328–33.

24. Hostetter TH, Rennke HG, Brenner BM. The case for intrarenal hypertension in the initiation and progression of diabetic and other glomerulopathies. *Am J Med* 1982; **72**: 375–8.

25. Hou SH. Frequency and outcome in women on dialysis. *Am J Kidney Dis* 1994; **23**: 60–63.

26. Hou S. Pregnancy in chronic renal insufficiency and end-stage renal disease. *Am J Kidney Dis* 1999; **33**: 235–52.

27. Hou S, Orlowski J, Pahl M et al. Pregnancy in women with end-stage renal disease: treatment of anaemia and premature labor. *Am J Kidney Dis* 1993; **21**: 16–22.

28. Imbasciati E, Ponticelli C. Pregnancy and renal disease: predictors for fetal and maternal outcome. *Am J Nephrol* 1991; **11**: 353–62.

29. Jones DC, Hayslett JP. Outcome of pregnancy in women with moderate or severe renal insufficiency. *N Engl J Med* 1996; **335**: 226–32.

30. Jones DC. Pregnancy complicated by chronic renal disease. *Clin Perinatol* 1997; **24**: 483–96.

31. Jungers P, Houillier P, Forget D, Henry-Amar M. Specific controversies concerning the natural history of renal disease in pregnancy. *Am J Kidney Dis* 1991; **27**: 116–22.

32. Kimmerle R, Zass R-P, Cupisti S et al. Pregnancies in women with diabetic nephropathy: long-term outcome for mother and child. *Diabetologia* 1995; **38**: 227–35.

33. Kioko EM, Shaw KM, Clarke AD, Warren DJ. Successful pregnancy in a diabetic patient treated with continuous ambulatory peritoneal dialysis. *Diabet Care* 1983; **6**: 298–300.

34. Kitzmiller JL, Brown ER, Phillippe M et al. Diabetic nephropathy and perinatal outcome. *Am J Obstet Gynecol* 1981; **141**: 741–51.

35. Kitzmiller JL, Combs CA. Diabetic nephropathy and pregnancy. *Obstet Gynecol Clin N Am* 1996; **23**: 173–203.

36. Klebe JG, Mogensen CE, Christensen T. Nephropathy in pregnancy. In *Carbohydrate Metabolism in Pregnancy and the Newborn IV*, Sutherland HW, Stowers JM, Pearson DWM (eds). Springer-Verlag: London.

37. Klein BE, Moss SE, Klein R. Effect of pregnancy on progression of diabetic retinopathy. *Diabet Care* 1990; **13**: 34–40.

38. Landon MB. Diabetes mellitus and other endocrine diseases. In *Normal and Problem Pregnancies*, 2nd edn, Gabbe SG, Niebyl JR, Simpson JL (eds). New York: Churchill Livingstone, 1991; 1097–36.

39. Lauszus FF, Klebe LG, Rasmussen OW et al. Renal growth during pregnancy in insulin-dependent diabetic women. A prospective study of renal volume and clinical variables. *Acta Diabetologia* 1995; **32**: 225–9.

40. Lindheimer MD, Katz AI. Renal physiology and disease in pregnancy. In *The Kidney: Physiology and Pathophysiology*, 2nd edn. Seldin DW, Giebisch G (eds). New York: Raven, 1992; 3371–431.

41. McCance DR, Traub AI, Harley JMG, Hadden DR, Kennedy L. Urinary albumin excretion in diabetic pregnancy. *Diabetologia* 1989; **32**: 236–9.

42. Mackie ADR, Doddridge MC, Gamsu HR et al. Outcome of pregnancy in patients with insulin-dependent diabetes mellitus and nephropathy with moderate renal impairment. *Diabet Med* 1996; **13**: 90–96.

43. Miodovnik M, Rosenn BM. Khoury JC, Grigsby JL, Siddiqi TA. Does pregnancy increase the risk for development and progression of diabetic nephropathy? *Am J Obstet Gynecol* 1996; **174**: 1180–91.

44. Mogensen CE, Klebe JG. Microalbuminuria and diabetic pregnancy. In *The Kidney and Hypertension in Diabetes Mellitus*, Mogensen CE (ed.). Kluwer Academic: Boston, 1994; 381–8.

45. Ogburn PL, Kitzmiller JL, Hare JW et al. Pregnancy following renal transplantation in class T diabetes mellitus. *J Am Med Assoc* 1986; **255**: 911–15.

46. Persson B, Gentz J. Follow-up of children of insulin-dependent and gestational diabetic mothers. *Acta Paediatr Scand* 1984; **73**: 349–58.

47. Piecuch RE, Leonard CH. Outcome of very pre-term infants. *Contemp Rev Obstet Gynecol* 1998; **27**: 115–120.

48. Purdy LP, Hantsch CE, Molitch ME et al. Effect of pregnancy on renal function in patients with moderate-to-severe diabetic renal insufficiency. *Diabet Care* 1996; **19**: 1067–74.

49. Rasmussen PE, Nielsen FR. Hydronephrosis during pregnancy: a literature survey. *Eur J Obstet Gynecol Reprod Biol* 1988; **27**: 249–59.

50. Reece EA, Coustan DR, Hayslett JP et al. Diabetic nephropathy: pregnancy performance and feto-maternal outcome. *Am J Obstet Gynecol* 1988; **159**: 56–66.

51. Reece EA, Winn HN, Hayslett JP et al. Does pregnancy alter the rate of progression of diabetic nephropathy? *Am J Perinatol* 1990; **7**: 193–7.

52. Reece EA, Leguizamon G, Homko C. Pregnancy performance and outcomes associated with diabetic nephropathy. *Am J Perinatol* 1998; **15**: 413–21.

53. Rizzoni G, Ehrich JHH, Broyer M et al. Successful pregnancies in women on renal replacement therapy: Report from the EDTA Registry. *Nephrol Dialysis Transpl* 1992; **7**: 279–87.

54. Rosenn B, Miodovnik M, Kranias G et al. Progression of diabetic retinopathy in pregnancy: association with hypertension in pregnancy. *Am J Obstet Gynecol* 1992; **166**: 1214.

55. Rudolph JE, Schweizer RT, Bartws SA. Pregnancy in renal transplant patients. *Transplantation* 1976; **27**: 26–9.

56. Skannal DG, Miodovnik M, Dungy-Poythress LJ, Frost MR. Successful pregnancy after combined renal–pancreas transplantation: a case report and literature review. *Am J Perinatol* 1996; **13**: 383–7.

57. Star J, Carpenter MW. The effect of pregnancy on the natural history of diabetic retinopathy and nephropathy. *Clin Perinatol* 1998; **25**: 887–916.

58. Sturgiss SN, Wilkinson R, Davison JM. Renal haemodynamic reserve during normal pregnancy. *J Physiol* 1992; **452**: 317.

59. Sturgiss SN, Dunlop W, Davison JM. Renal haemodynamics and tubular function in human pregnancy. In *Renal Disease in Pregnancy*, Lindheimer MD, Davison JM (eds). Bailliére Tindall: London.

60. Tagatz GE, Arnold NI, Goetz FC, Najarian JS, Simmons RL. Pregnancy in a juvenile diabetic after transplantation (class T diabetes mellitus). *Diabetes* 1975; **24**: 497–501.

Part III

Treatment and Prognosis

15

Effect of Glycaemic Control on the Development and Progression of Diabetic Nephropathy

CHRISTOPH HASSLACHER

St Josefskrankenhaus, Heidelberg, Germany

In the last 10 years, several large-scale trials have clearly documented the important effect of glycaemic control on the *development* of diabetic nephropathy in patients with type 1 and type 2 diabetes. On the other hand, the interrelationships between glycaemic control and the *progression* of nephropathy have not been so intensively investigated. The role of glycaemic control in the primary and secondary prevention of diabetic nephropathy will therefore be considered separately.

EFFECT OF GLYCAEMIC CONTROL ON THE DEVELOPMENT OF NEPHROPATHY

In patients with type 1 diabetes, good glycaemic control leads to reduced incidence of microalbuminuria or macroalbuminuria. This correlation could already be shown by several trials in the 1980s. However, these mostly comprised a small number of patients observed for a short time. As shown by a meta-analysis of these studies, in consequence of more

Diabetic Nephropathy. Edited by C. Hasslacher.
© 2001 John Wiley & Sons, Ltd.

intensive insulin treatment compared to conventional therapy the improvement of the glycaemic control can significantly reduce the risk of nephropathy (1).

The DCCT Study was able to confirm and to extend these results in an impressive manner (2,3). In this study, 1441 patients were treated with either a more intensive form of insulin treatment (insulin pump or multiple injections of insulin) or conventional insulin treatment (1–2 insulin injections day). After comparable values of blood sugar and HbA_{1c} at the beginning of the study, the HbA_{1c} value fell from an initial 8.8% to an average of 7.0% in the intensively treated group, whereas it remained constant at 8.9% in the conventionally treated group. In the intensively treated group, 83.4% of patients had a mean HbA_{1c} of 8% or less. However, only 5% of patients attained sustained normal HbA_{1c} values, even in this group.

In the "primary prevention group", in which patients with a short duration of diabetes without retinopathy were observed, the cumulative incidence of microalbuminuria after 9 years of observation in the group receiving intensive treatment was 16% as compared to 27% in the conventionally treated group (Figure 15.1). This corresponded to a risk reduction of 34% in consequence of the more intensive therapy.

The "secondary prevention group" comprised patients with a longer duration of diabetes who already had retinopathy. Their albumin excretion was normal at the beginning of the study. The incidences of microalbuminuria in this group were 26% (intensive treatment) and 42% (conventional treatment), respectively. This corresponds to a risk reduction of 43% as a result of the improved glycaemic control.

Manifestation of an advanced stage of microalbuminuria (albumin excretion $> 70\,\mu g/min$) or occurrence of macroalbuminuria (albumin excretion $> 208\,\mu g/min$) was also significantly reduced under more intensive glycaemic control. There were risk reductions of 51% and 56%, respectively, for the combined cohorts.

Analysis of the data also showed that the favourable effect of intensive treatment was independent of age, duration of diabetes, smoking, neuropathy or retinopathy or the initial levels of HbA_{1c}, blood pressure, rate of albumin secretion, creatinine and LDL cholesterol.

A proportion of the patients of the DCCT Study ($n = 1375$) took part in a progress observation over a further 4 years (4). The treatment was now no longer carried out and monitored by study centres but by the patients' own doctors. In the intensively treated group, there was a slight deterioration of glycaemic control (mean HbA_{1c} value, 7.9%). The patient group that had previously received conventional treatment showed improvement of glycaemic control (mean HbA_{1c} value, 8.2%). This is possibly due to a change to a more intensive form of insulin treatment.

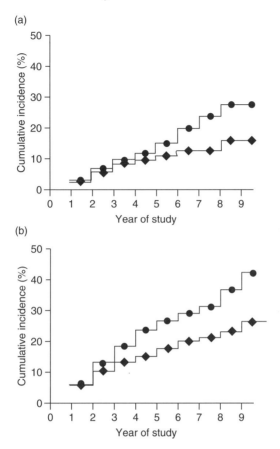

Figure 15.1 Cumulative incidence of development of microalbuminuria (AER > 28 µg/min) in the intensive (♦) and conventional (●) treatments groups. (A) primary prevention cohort ($p = 0.04$). (B) Secondary intervention cohort (among those with baseline AER < 28 µg/min, $p = 0.001$). From (3), with permission

Despite the change compared to the previous glycaemic control, the favourable effect of more intensive insulin treatment with regard to the occurrence of microangiopathy or macroangiopathy was sustained. The reduction of risk of microalbuminuria was now 53% and that for macro-albuminuria 86%. Similar effects were also shown with regard to the course of the retinopathy.

For patients with type 2 diabetes, there are two long-term studies comprising large numbers of patients which document the positive effect of improved glycaemic control on the manifestation of microalbuminuria and macroalbuminuria.

In the KUMAMOTO Study, the effect of a multiple daily insulin injection (MIT) was compared to that of conventional insulin treatment (CIT) over a period of 8 years in 55 patients with type 2 diabetes and normal albumin excretion (5,6). The HbA$_{1c}$ value averaged 7.2% in the trial group as compared to 9.4% in the conventionally treated group. The development of diabetic nephropathy was very much less (11.5%) in the group that received more intensive treatment than in the conventionally treated group (43.5%) (Figure 15.2).

In the UKPDS study (7), more than 4 000 patients with freshly diagnosed type 2 diabetes were observed over 15 years, either under a conventional or under a more intensive treatment with oral antidiabetics and/or insulin. In

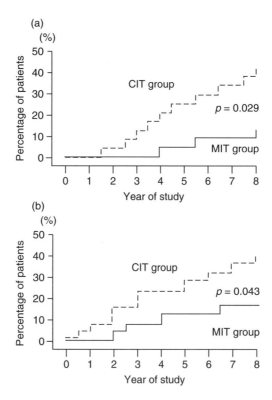

Figure 15.2 Cumulative incidences of change in nephropathy in patients with type 2 diabetes treated by intensive (−) and conventional (−−−) insulin injection therapy. A change in the severity of nephropathy was defined as one or more stages up among three stages (normoalbuminuria, microalbuminuria and albuminuria). The primary prevention (A) and secondary intervention (B) cohorts are shown. *p* Values were tested using the Mantel (log-rank) test. From (6), with permission

contrast to the DCCT study, glycaemic control did not remain constant but deteriorated with increasing observation time. However, the HbA_{1c} value of the group with intensified treatment was around 0.9% lower at all times. This led to a significant decrease of the risk of nephropathy, as is shown in Table 15.1 for various endpoint parameters. There was no difference with regard to the form of treatment chosen, i.e. oral anti-diabetics or insulin.

Table 15.1 Effect of intensive blood-glucose control on risk reduction of selected surrogate endpoints in UKPDS

	Duration of blood-glucose control (years)	Risk reduction (%)
Microalbuminuria	9	24
	12	33
Proteinuria	9	33
	12	34
Two-fold plasma creatinine increase	9	60
	12	74

From (7) by permission.

EFFECT OF GLYCAEMIC CONTROL ON THE PROGRESSION OF DIABETIC NEPHROPATHY

The influence of glycaemic control on the progression of nephropathy when microalbuminuria or macroalbuminuria is already present has not been investigated so intensively up to now. Nevertheless, the findings reported in the present studies indicate that glycaemic control as close as possible to normal should also be aimed for for at this stage of nephropathy.

In a combined evaluation of the STENO studies I and II, after 5 and 8 years of treatment with an insulin pump or conventional insulin therapy, 51 type 1 diabetics with incipient diabetic nephropathy were analysed with regard to the progression of the nephropathy (8). Progression in the stage of clinically manifest nephropathy was found in 3/26 patients in the insulin pump group (mean HBA_{1c} ca. 7.8%) as compared to 10/25 patients in the conventionally treated group (mean HbA_{1c} value ca. 8.8%). A multiple regression analysis of all patients showed that the initial urinary excretion of albumin and the mean HbA_{1c} value were the major factors influencing the result of this study.

These results are consistent in principle with the observation of the DCCT study, in which the occurrence of not only microalbuminuria but also macroalbuminuria was reduced by improved glycaemic control (2,3). The follow-up observation of the DCCT patients also clearly showed the positive effect of more intensive glycaemic control in secondary prevention (4). Of the patients who showed microalbuminuria of 29–203 μ g/min at the end of the DCCT Study, progression of nephropathy was found in 8% of the group with more intensive treatment, as compared to 31% in the group that received conventional treatment.

In further studies on adolescent patients with microalbuminuria, it could be demonstrated both histologically and by determining the albumin excretion that an improvement of the glycaemic control is associated with a delayed progression of the nephropathy (9,10).

In patients in an advanced stage of nephropathy, i.e. macroalbuminuria, the crucial effect of glycaemic control on progression decreases compared to that of other factors, e.g. hypertension. Nevertheless, various observation studies in type 1 diabetics could demonstrate the effect of glycaemic control on progression, even in this stage (11,12). It is of course not sufficient to treat only a single progression factor in these patients. The prognosis is only improved when an intensified multifactorial treatment concept is applied. It could thus be shown, in an Italian study (13), that an improvement of kidney function which is already restricted can be attained by maintaining blood sugar values close to normal (mean HbA$_{1c}$ 6.5%), intensified blood pressure therapy with ACE inhibitors and other substances (mean pressure 120/75 mm (Hg) and normalizing protein intake to 0.8 g/day. As shown in Figure 15.3, the creatinine clearance improved by an average of from 58 to 84 ml/min/year after 3 years of treatment.

Results were available from the KUMAMOTO Study, already mentioned above, for patients with type 2 diabetes and microalbuminuria (5,6). In 55 patients with microalbuminuria, the cumulative percentage of patients who

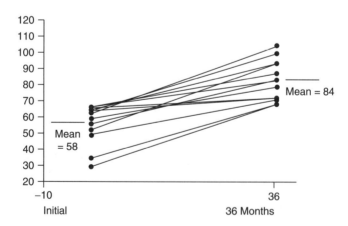

Figure 15.3 Means of glomerular filtration rate (GFR) in 13 patients at the start and end of the study. From (13), with permission

progressed to clinically manifest nephropathy was significantly lowered by improved glycaemic control with multiple insulin injections, as compared to conventional treatment (16% vs. 40%, respectively) (Figure 15.2). This corresponds to the results of the UKPDS study, in which a risk reduction, not only with regard to microalbuminuria but also to macroalbuminuria, could be demonstrated under intensified glycaemic control. Observation studies could also demonstrate an effect of glycaemic control in the stage of macroalbuminuria (14). Especially in patients with type 2 diabetes and nephropathy, it is not sufficient to treat only one progression factor because hypertension is often already present. This was impressively shown by the Steno type 2 Study (15). Progression of nephropathy was observed in only 11% of patients with intensive treatment of glycaemic control hypertension (ACE inhibitors) and hyperlipoproteinemia and administration of aspirin. Progression of nephropathy was observed in 25% of patients with conventional treatment. There were also similar findings with regard to retinopathy.

IS THERE A GLYCAEMIC THRESHOLD FOR THE DEVELOPMENT OF NEPHROPATHY?

In the DCCT Study, the improvement of metabolic control by intensive insulin treatment was associated with a three-fold rise in the risk of hypoglycaemia (2). The question therefore arises as to whether normoglycaemic control should really be aimed for in order to avoid nephropathy, or whether a less strict metabolic control is sufficient. According to an earlier study, in which albumin excretion and glycosylated haemoglobin were measured retrospectively, the risk of microalbuminuria was taken to be "almost flat" for HbA_{1c} values under 10.1% (estimated to be comparable to a HbA_{1c} value under 8.1%) (16). The authors concluded that only a slight clinical benefit could be attained from lowering this HbA_{1c} level and maintaining it at the lower level (16).

A threshold value could not be confirmed on the basis of the data of the DCCT study, which were obtained prospectively from a very much larger number of patients with a longer period of observation (more than 9000 patients/years) (17). As shown by Figure 15.4 for the combined intensive and the conventional treatment group, there is throughout an exponential correlation between the mean HbA_{1c} and the occurrence of microalbuminuria.

A calculation after logarithmic transformation of the data showed that a 10% reduction in HbA_{1c} is accompanied with a 25% reduction of the risk of microalbuminuria. On the other hand, the risk of severe hypoglycaemias

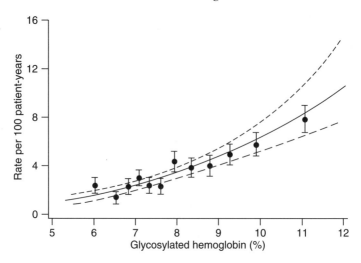

Figure 15.4 The absolute risk of microalbuminuria (hazard rate per 100 patient-years) in the combined treatment groups as a function of the updated mean HbA$_{1c}$ during follow-up in the DCCT; rate vs. HbA$_{1c}$ over the range observed in the trial. From (17), with permission

(coma) was very much less in the group with intensive metabolic control than in the group with conventional treatment. The risk of hypoglycaemia in the group with more intensive treatment rose by 18% per 10% HbA$_{1c}$ reduction and by 48% in the conventionally treated group. "Therefore, the DCCT continues to recommend implementation of intensive therapy with the goal of achieving normal glycaemia as early as possible in as many IDDM patients as is safely possible" (17).

For secondary prevention, i.e. for the progression from microalbuminuria to proteinuria, Warram et al (18) recently carried out a prospective investigation of the correlation with hyperglycaemia in microalbuminuric type 1 diabetics in a 4 year observation study. As shown by Figure 15.5, they found a non-linear dose–effect correlation. The risk of progression rose almost exponentially from normal HbA$_{1c}$ to a level of 8.5%, and remained fairly constant at higher HbA$_{1c}$ levels. This correlation was not affected by age, duration of diabetes, blood pressure or antihypertensive medication. It can be concluded from this that the risk of progression of microalbuminuria to proteinuria can only be reduced in diabetic patients when the HbA$_{1c}$ is lowered to less than 8.5% by more intensive metabolic control. This finding can also explain the unfavourable results of some studies, which have not found any benefit of more intensive insulin therapy for the progression of nephropathy (19,20).

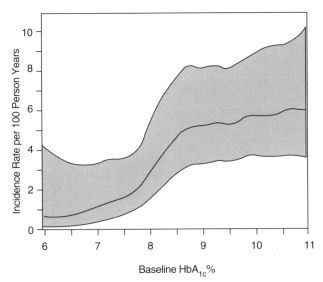

Figure 15.5 Predicted incidence rate of progression of microalbuminuria to proteinuria according to level of HbA_{1c} during the baseline period. The shaded region represents the pointwise = 2 SE band. From (18), with permission

PRACTICAL CONSEQUENCES OF RENAL FAILURE FOR ANTIDIABETIC THERAPY

Restricted kidney function has consequences for pharmacotherapy, since the kidney failure affects the pharmacokinetic profile of almost all oral antidiabetics and alters the insulin metabolism. In this context it should be mentioned that the serum creatinine value only reflects kidney function inadequately. In order to detect mild forms of kidney failure, the creatinine clearance should therefore be measured in patients with normal serum creatinine when they have macroalbuminuria.

Oral antidiabetics

Biguanides are contraindicated because of the danger of accumulation and development of lactacidosis in kidney failure. These substances should be discontinued early in such patients, i.e. creatinine clearance below 80 ml/ min.

Sulphonylureas of the first generation, such as chlorpropamide, acetohexamide or rolbutamide, are mainly excreted via the kidneys.

Prolonged elimination of these drugs in patients with renal insufficiency may result in drug accumulation and severe hypoglycaemic coma (21). These substances are therefore not recommended for treatment of patients with impaired renal function.

The pharmacokinetic profiles of the second-generation sulphonylureas are different and somewhat complex. For instant glyburide (glibenclamide) is primarily metabolized in the liver; only minor amounts are excreted unchanged by the kidneys. However, one of the main metabolites that has been found to exert hypoglycaemic action is excreted by the kidneys and might accumulate in patients with renal insufficiency (22). Severe hypoglycaemic episodes have been described, especially in older patients with impaired renal function (23). Glyburide should therefore be used with great caution in patients with renal dysfunction, i.e. creatinine clearance below 50–60 ml/min. Similar recommendations could be given for other second-generation substances, such as glisoxepide, glibonuride or gliclazide. Their dose must therefore be reduced in deteriorating kidney function. An exception is gliquidone, only 5% of which is eliminated via the kidneys, so that it can be administered even in restricted kidney function. The clearance of glimiperide, a new sulphonlyurea, is unexpectedly increased in patients with renal dysfunction, i.e. creatinine clearance below 50 ml/min (24). This finding is explicable on the basis of an altered protein binding of the drug in patients with renal insufficiency. There is an increase in unbound drug which can be eliminated faster. However, renal clearance of metabolites that partially exhibit hypoglycaemic effects is reduced in kidney dysfunction (24). Accumulation of metabolites may occur during long-term treatment and may cause hypoglycaemia. Therapy in these patients should be initiated with small doses, i.e. 0.5–1 mg daily, followed by a careful dose titration.

Repaglinide belongs to a new group of substances (meglinide) characterized by a rapid and short enhancement of insulin secretion. The agent is mainly degraded in the liver and only 8% is excreted via the kidneys. Pharmacokinetic investigations in type 2 diabetics with varying degrees of kidney failure have shown that repaglinide can be administered without reducing the dose up to a creatinine clearance of 40 ml/min. The plasma half-life is increased only in more severe kidney failure; the dose must therefore be reduced unless the patients are switched to insulin (25). In a study on 281 patients with type 2 diabetes and varying degrees of renal impairment, repaglinide showed a good efficacy and safety profile. When a careful dose titration was provided, risk of hypoglycaemic episodes was not increased in these patients (26).

With regard to the insulin sensitizer group, there are only a few published results on the pharmacokinetic properties in renal dysfunction. Based on studies with a small number of patients it could be shown that rosiglitazone and pioglitazone do not accumulate in severe kidney failure (creatinine clearance < 30 ml/min). Reduction of the dose seems to be not necessary (27,28). However, further investigations are needed in this field.

Insulin Treatment

Insulin kinetics are also changed on occurrence of renal failure. In individuals with healthy metabolism, the liver degrades about 80% of the insulin owing to the high concentration of insulin in the portal vein; the kidneys degrade about 20%. In insulin-dependent diabetics, the liver and kidneys are exposed to about the same concentration of insulin owing to peripheral insulin administration and thus each degrades about half of the hormone. In kidney failure (< 60 ml/min), there is protracted action of insulin due to reduced renal degradation, which must be taken into consideration in treatment. As a rule, the dose of insulin must hence be reduced. Owing to the better controllability, it is appropriate to use short-acting insulins. In general, patients with kidney failure or kidney replacement therapy should, if possible, be put on intensified insulin treatment. This requires special training (see Chapter 19).

SUMMARY

Several prospective studies in patients with type 1 and type 2 diabetes have shown that near-normal metabolic control is able to prevent or delay the manifestation of renal complications. There is no evidence for a glycaemic threshold for the development of diabetic nephropathy.

With the progress of nephropathy, glycaemic control becomes less important with regard to its effect on nephropathy. However, the present results indicate that good glycaemic control must also be aimed for in patients with advanced nephropathy. In the advanced stages of nephropathy, more intensive multifactorial interventions are absolutely necessary because of the multiplicity of factors affecting progression.

REFERENCES

1. Wang PH, Lau J, Chalmers TC. Meta-analysis of effects of intensive blood-glucose control on late complications of type 1 diabetes. *Lancet* 1993; **341**: 1306–9.
2. The Diabetes Control and Complications Trial Research Group. The effect of intensive treatment of diabetes of the development and progression of long-term

complications in insulin-dependent diabetes mellitus. *N Engl J Med* 1993; **329**: 977–86.

3. The Diabetes Control and Complications Trial Research Group. Effect of intensive therapy on the development and progression of diabetic nephropathy in the diabetes control and complications trial. *Kidney Int* 1995; **47**: 1703–20.

4. The Diabetes Control and Complications Trial/Epidemiology of Diabetes Interventions and Complications Research Group. Retinopathy and nephropathy in patients with type 1 diabetes four years after a trial of intensive therapy. *N Engl J Med* 2000; **342**: 381–9.

5. Ohkubo Y, Kishikawa H, Araki E et al. Intensive insulin therapy prevents the progression of diabetic microvascular complications in Japanese patients with non-insulin-dependent diabetes mellitus: a randomized prospective 6-year study. *Diabet Res Clin Pract* 1995; **28**: 103–17.

6. Shichiri M, Kishikawa H, Ohkubo Y, Wake N. Long-term results of the Kumamoto study on optimal diabetes control in type 2 diabetic patients, *Diabet Care* 2000; **23**(2): B21–9.

7. UK Prospective Diabetes Study Group. Intensive blood-glucose control with sulphonylureas or insulin compared with conventional treatment and risk of complications in patients with type 2 diabetes (UKPDS 33). *Lancet* 1998; **352**: 837–53.

8. Feld-Rasmussen B, Mathiesen ER, Jensen T, Lauritzen T, Deckert T. Effect of improved metabolic control on loss of kidney function in type 1 (insulin-dependent) diabetic patients: an update of the Steno studies. *Diabetologie* 1991; **34**: 164–70.

9. Bangstad HJ, Kofoed-Enevoldsen A, Dahl Jorgensen K, Hanssen KF. Glomerular charge selectivity and the influence of improved blood glucose control in type 1 (insulin-dependent) diabetic patients with microalbuminuria, *Diabetologia* 1992; **35**: 1165–9.

10. Bojesting M, Arnquist HJ, Karlberg BE, Ludwigsson J. Glycemic control and prognosis in type 1 diabetic patients with microalbuminuria. *Diabet Care* 1996; **19**: 313–17.

11. Hasslacher, C, Stech W, Wahl P, Ritz E. Blood pressure and metabolic control as risk factors for nephropathy in type 2 (insulin-dependent) diabetes. *Diabetologia* 1985; **28**: 6–11.

12. Nyberg G, Blohme G, Nordern G. Impact of metabolic control in progression of clinical diabetic nephropathy. *Diabetologia* 1987; **30**: 82–6.

13. Manto A, Cortroneo P, Marra G et al. Effect of intensive treatment in diabetic nephropathy in patients with type 1 diabetes. *Kidney Int* 1995; **47**: 231–5.

14. Hasslacher C, Bostedt-Kiesel A, Kempe H, Wahl P. Effect of metabolic factors and blood pressure on kidney function in proteinurie type 2 (non-insulin dependent) diabetic patients. *Diabetologia* 1993; **36**: 1051–6.

15. Gaede P, Vedel Pernille, Parving HH, Pedersen O. Intensified multifactorial intervention in patients with type 2 diabetes mellitus and microalbuminuria: the Steno type 2 randomised study. *Lancet* 1999; **353**: 617–22.

16. Krolewski AS, Laffel LMB, Krolewski M, Quinn M, Warram JH. Glycosylated hemoglobin and the risk of micralbuminuria in patients with insulin dependent diabetes mellitus. *N Eng J Med* 1995; **332**: 1251–5.

17. The Diabetes Control and Complications Trial Research Group. The absence of a glycemic threshold for the development of long term complications: the perspective of the diabetes control and complications trial. *Diabetes* 1996; **45**: 1289–98.

18. Warram JH, Scott LJ, Hanna LS et al. Progression of microalbuminuria to proteinuria in type 1 diabetes: nonlinear relationship with hyperglycemia. *Diabetes* 2000; **49**: 94–100.
19. Viberti GC, Bilous RW, Macintosh D, Bending JL, Keen H. Long-term correction of hyperglycaemia and progression of renal failure in insulin dependent diabetes. *Br Med J* 1983; **286**: 598–602.
20. Microalbuminuria Collaborative Study Group, UK. Intensive therapy and progression to clinical albuminuria in patients with insulin dependent diabetes mellitus and microalbuminuria. *Br Med J* 1995; **311**: 973–7.
21. Seltzer HS. Drug-induced hypoglycemia. A review based on 473 cases. *Diabetes* 1972; **21**: 955–66.
22. Rydberg T, Jönssen A, Roder M, Melander A. Hypoglycemic activity of glyburide (glibenclamide) metabolites in humans. *Diabet Care* 1994; **17** (9).
23. Asplund K, Wiholm BE, Lithner F. Glibenclamide-associated hypoglycaemia: a report on 57 cases. *Diabetologia* 1983; **24**: 412–17.
24. Rosenkranz B, Profozik V, Metelko Z et al. Pharmacokinetics and safety of glimepiride at clinically effective doses in diabetic patients with renal impairment. *Diabetologia* 1996; **39**: 1617–24.
25. Schuhmacher S, Abbasi I, Weise D et al. Single and multiple-dose pharmacokinetics of repaglinide in patients with type 2 diabetes and renal impairment. *Eur Clin Pharmacol* 2000; **57**: 147–52.
26. Hasslacher C, Koselj M, Gall MA, Sieber J, Leyck Dieken M. Safety and efficacy of repaglinide in 281 type 2 diabetic patients with and without renal impairment. *Diabetes* (in press).
27. Edwards G, Eckland DJ. Pharmakinetics of pioglitazone in patients with renal impairment. *Diabetologia* 1999; **42** (suppl 1): A230.
28. Chapelsky MC, Thompson K, Jorkasky D, Freed MI. Effect of renal impairment on the pharmacokinetics of rosiglitazone. *Clin Pharmacol Ther* 1999; **65**(2): 185.

16

Blood Pressure Control in Hypertensive Diabetic Patients with Proteinuria

RAFAEL F. SCHÄFERS, P. LÜTKES AND T. PHILIPP

Universitätsklinikum, Essen, Germany

EPIDEMIOLOGY OF HIGH BLOOD PRESSURE IN DIABETICS

The Risk of Hypertension

The prevalence of high blood pressure is markedly increased in patients with both type 1 and type 2 diabetes and high blood pressure considerably worsens the prognosis of the diabetic patient (38,58). The hypertensive (type 2) diabetic carries a risk of cardiovascular morbidity and mortality which is about four-fold increased compared with non-diabetic, non-hypertensive controls (59). Several recent placebo-controlled intervention trials that included both non-diabetic and diabetic patients with hypertension have clearly shown that the risk of fatal and non-fatal cardiovascular complications is considerably higher in hypertensive diabetics compared to hypertensives without diabetes (9,61). (Figure 16.1).

Diabetic nephropathy develops in about 40–50% of diabetics and the risk of developing diabetic nephropathy is clearly not confined to type 1 diabetics. The cumulative incidence of diabetic nephropathy in type 2 diabetics is comparable to that of type 1 diabetics (17). Diabetic nephropathy is now the leading cause of endstage renal failure in many Western societies (64).

Diabetic Nephropathy. Edited by C. Hasslacher.
© 2001 John Wiley & Sons, Ltd.

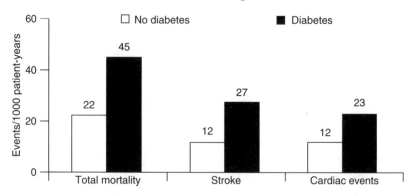

Figure 16.1 Comparison of mortality and morbidity between hypertensive patients with (black bars) and without (open bars) diabetes (type 2). Data are from the placebo group of the Syst-Eur trial (61) and are presented in events/1000 patient-years for total mortality and fatal and non-fatal stroke and cardiac events. It is evident that the hypertensive diabetic carries a higher risk than the hypertensive patient without diabetes

The presence of diabetic nephropathy is associated with a further decline of the prognosis of the diabetic patients: total mortality in type 1 diabetics with nephropathy is up to 100-fold higher relative to a non-diabetic controls (3), with 10 year mortality rates ranging between 50% and 80% (43). Many patients with diabetic nephropathy will die even before reaching the stage of terminal renal failure. Once on dialysis the prognosis of the diabetic patient remains grave, with mean survival times of about 5.5 years for type 1 and less than 3 years for type 2 diabetics (23). Hypertension is nearly invariably present in diabetic nephropathy, although the temporal relationship between the development of hypertension and nephropathy differs between type 1 and type 2 diabetes. While hypertension is found in the majority of type 2 diabetics when diabetes is first diagnosed independent of the presence of nephropathy, it is closely related to the development of nephropathy in type 1 diabetics (4). Therefore, the diagnosis of hypertension in a type 1 diabetic renders the diagnosis of nephropathy likely and should give rise to active screening for albuminuria if nephropathy has not yet been searched for.

ANTIHYPERTENSIVE THERAPY

What Is the Benefit of Antihypertensive Therapy in the Diabetic Patient?

There is no doubt that the hypertensive diabetic patient benefits from blood pressure lowering and that this benefit is at least comparable and may even exceed that observed in the non-diabetic patient. This is evident from large scale placebo-controlled intervention trials in hypertensives, which included both non-diabetic and diabetic patients without nephropathy. The placebo-controlled Systolic Hypertension in the Elderly Program (SHEP) studied the effects of blood pressure reduction by the diuretic chlorthalidone in elderly patients (> 60 years of age) with isolated, systolic hypertension (9). Total mortality was reduced by 26% in type 2 diabetic and by 15% in non-diabetic patients. The number of fatal and non-fatal strokes was lowered by 22% (diabetics) and 38% (non-diabetics), respectively, and the number of fatal and non-fatal myocardial infarctions by 54% (diabetics) and 23% (non-diabetics). These results were achieved *although* the fall in blood pressure in the diabetic group fell slightly short of that observed in the non-diabetic patients (mean fall in systolic/diastolic blood pressure: diabetics, 9.8/2.2 mmHg; non-diabetics, 12.4/4.1 mmHg). The Systolic Hypertension in Europe (Syst-Eur) trial was another study that examined the impact of antihypertensive treatment (by the calcium antagonist nitrendipine) on mortality and morbidity in elderly (> 60 years of age) patients with isolated systolic hypertension (61). Hypertensive diabetics profited more from effective blood pressure reduction than their non-diabetic counterparts. This was evident for total mortality as well as mortality and morbidity from both stroke and myocardial infarction. Similar to the results of the SHEP study, this superior efficacy in reducing mortality and morbidity in diabetics was attained despite an inferior blood pressure reduction in diabetics (8.6 vs. 10.3 mmHg mean reduction of systolic blood pressure).

These placebo-controlled studies in patients without nephropathy provide unequivocal evidence that the hypertensive type 2 diabetic benefits from effective blood pressure reduction and that the benefit is even superior than that observed in the non-diabetic hypertensive.

Although these studies have been performed in patients without nephropathy, the importance of effective reduction of blood pressure also holds true for patients with nephropathy, which is not surprising in view of the outstanding role of elevated blood pressure for the progression of diabetic nephropathy (cf. Chapter 2). Indeed, historically, the improvement of the prognosis of the diabetic patient by antihypertensive therapy has first been demonstrated in type 1 diabetic patients with overt nephropathy. Long-term and effective reduction of blood pressure by β-blockers and diuretics resulted in a 10 year mortality rate of 18% compared to mortality rates of 50–70% seen in historical control groups that had not received antihypertensive treatment (43) (Figure 16.2). Similar results have been reported by other investigators (16,30).

In summary, there is no doubt that effective reduction of blood pressure will improve the prognosis of the hypertensive diabetic with and without nephropathy.

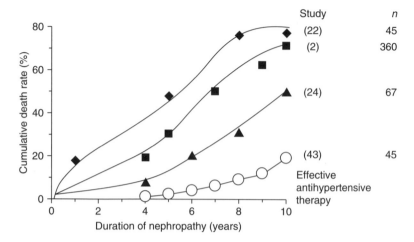

Figure 16.2 Impact of effective antihypertensive therapy on prognosis in proteinuric type 1 diabetics (adopted from Parving and Hommel (43). In the study by Parving and Hommel (43) (open circles), blood pressure reduction lowered the cumulative 10 years mortality rate to 18% compared to rates of 50–77% in historical control groups without effective therapy of elevated blood pressure (2, 22, 24) *n* Indicates the number of patients enrolled in these studies. In the study by Parving and Hommel (43), treatment of hypertension was mainly based on diuretics and β-blockers

What Is the Optimal Target Blood Pressure?

"Traditionally", a "target blood pressure" of below 140/90 mmHg has long been accepted as the treatment goal of antihypertensive therapy. Indeed, concerns have been raised that "aggressive" blood pressure reduction beyond this level may even again increase cardiovascular morbidity and mortality by compromising coronary perfusion especially in patients with pre-existing coronary artery disease (8), which is more prevalent in diabetic patients. However, recent evidence clearly suggests that hypertensive diabetic patients in particular benefit from lowering of blood pressure to levels even below 80 mmHg.

The Hypertension Detection and Follow-up Program (HDFP) (57) was one of the first trials that systematically compared the effects of the intensity of blood pressure reduction on morbidity and mortality. More intensive reduction of blood pressure resulted in an improved survival, both for the total cohort of patients studied and in the subgroup of patients with diabetes.

In the United Kindom Prospective Diabetes Study (UKPDS), the effects of tight blood pressure control were compared with less tight control in 1148 hypertensive patients with type 2 diabetes (63). Tight reduction of blood pressure to a mean level of 144/82 mmHg reduced total mortality compared with less tight control (mean blood pressure 154/87 mmHg) (22.4 vs. 27.2 deaths/1000 patient-years, $p = 0.17$). Furthermore, tight blood pressure control also impressively reduced the incidence of both macro- and microvascular diabetic complications; e.g. the risk of stroke and myocardial infarction was lowered by 44% and 21%, respectively ($p = 0.013$ and 0.13, respectively), and the risk of microvascular complications by 37% ($p = 0.009$).

The Hypertension Optimal Treatment study (HOT) is the largest study so far that specifically aimed to assess the optimal diastolic target blood pressure (15); a total of 18 790 hypertensive patients, of whom 1501 were type 2 diabetics, were randomly and prospectively assigned to three different levels of diastolic target blood pressures: < 80, < 85 and < 90 mmHg. While total mortality in the population as a whole was *not* different between patients assigned to a target blood pressure of 80 mmHg relative to those in the 90 mmHg group, there was a remarkable reduction in total mortality in the subgroup of diabetic patients who were most "aggressively" treated (target blood pressure < 80 mmHg: 9 deaths/1000 patient-years) compared to those randomized to the "conventional" target blood pressure of 90 mmHg (15.9 deaths/1000 patient-years, $p = 0.07$) (Figure 16.3). This reduction in total mortality was mainly attributable to a decrease in cardiovascular mortality, which went down from 11.1 cardiovascular deaths/1000 patient-years in the target group < 90 mmHg to 3.7 deaths/1000 patient-years ($p = 0.02$) in the "most agressively" treated patients, i.e. those assigned to a target blood pressure of below 80 mmHg.

In summary, these large-scale intervention studies demonstrate that lowering of blood pressure below the "traditional" target blood pressure of 90 mmHg diastolic is safe in the diabetic patient and should indeed be recommended, since it results in a reduction of mortality and morbidity superior to that seen with the "conventional" treatment goal of a reduction below 90 mmHg. This also holds true for patients with diabetic nephropathy. The Modification of Diet in Renal Disease (MDRD) study (21), which also included patients with diabetic nephropathy, demonstrated that tight blood pressure control to a level of 92 mmHg mean blood pressure (corresponding to a blood pressure of 125/75 mmHg) significantly slowed the deterioration of renal function relative to a less tight blood pressure reduction to 107 mmHg mean arterial pressure (corresponding to 140/90 mmHg). This benefit of a more intensive treatment of blood pressure was mainly seen in patients with a proteinuria of > 1 g/day, i.e. in those with more advanced renal disease. The finding that patients with more severe renal disease derive more benefit from blood pressure lowering therapy seems to be a generalized finding in both diabetic (26) and non-diabetic nephropathy (56). Therefore, in practical terms, the finding of gross proteinuria should

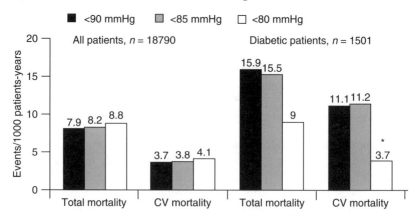

Figure 16.3   Defining the 'optimal' target blood pressure in the hypertensive
diabetic; results of the HOT trial (15). In this trial, a total of 18 790 patients were
prospectively randomized to three different target blood pressure groups: < 90, < 85
and < 80 mmHg diastolic. In these three target groups diastolic blood pressure was
actually reduced from a mean of 105 mmHg at baseline to a mean of 85.2, 83.2 and
81.1 mmHg during treatment. In the total study population there was no difference
in total mortality and cardiovascular (CV) mortality between the three different
groups; however, in the subgroup of 1501 type 2 diabetics, "most aggressive" blood
pressure reduction resulted in a marked reduction of total mortality ($p = 0.068$) and
of cardiovascular mortality ($p = 0.016^*$) in the target blood pressure group of
80 mmHg. Note that in diabetics "most aggressive" blood pressure reduction
resulted in a total and cardiovascular mortality similar to that seen in non-diabetics!
The results are presented as events/1000 patient-years

not result in therapeutic nihilism, but rather calls for immediate and
"aggressive" action to lower increased blood pressure levels. For type 2
diabetic patients the UKPDS Study provides evidence that tight control of
blood pressure reduces the development of nephropathy (63).

   Table 16.1 summarizes the target blood pressure values that should be
achieved in diabetic patients, as recommended by different societies. Unfortunately, the recommended target blood pressures vary somewhat between
the different societies. However, the recommendations agree that the conventional target of lowering blood pressure below 140/90 mmHg is no
longer sufficient; they also agree that the presence of nephropathy requires
an even more intensive lowering of blood pressure. In keeping with the
recommendations of the European Diabetes Policy Group (12) we recommend (51) that blood pressure be lowered below 135/85 mmHg in all
diabetics and to values even below 130/80 mmHg if there is evidence of
nephropathy. This recommendation is to be understood as a minimum
requirement; if tolerated, blood pressure should be lowered even beyond
these levels.

Table 16.1   Target blood pressure in the hypertensive diabetic as recommended by different societies

Target blood pressure	Recommending society
Without nephropathy: < 135/85 mmHg	European Diabetes Policy Group
Without nephropathy: < 130/85 mmHg	American Diabetes Association
	Joint National Committee
	World Health Organization – International
	Society of Hypertension
With nephropathy: < 130/80 mmHg	European Diabetes Policy Group
With nephropathy: < 125/75 mmHg	Joint National Committee
	National Kidney Foundation

Data from (1,12,18,60,67).

Effect of Antihypertensive Therapy on Diabetic Nephropathy

As explained above, effective reduction of blood pressure improves survival in patients with diabetic nephropathy (16,30,43). Equally important, it effectively slows the progression of diabetic renal disease. As a rule of thumb, in overt diabetic nephropathy in type 1 diabetics the glomerular filtration rate declines at a rate of approximately 10 ml/min/year; effective blood pressure lowering can nearly halve this rate to approximately 5 ml/min/year (45). Thus, even if the occurrence of terminal renal failure can often not be prevented, the need for dialysis will arise considerably later compared to the natural history of the disease. Thus, treatment of blood pressure will "present" to the patient up to several years off dialysis, which means a enormous improvement in the patient's quality of life (Figure 16.4).

Type 1 diabetics

In *overt nephropathy* (persistent albuminuria > 300 mg/24 h) lowering of blood pressure with both "conventional antihypertensives" like β-blockers and diuretics (34,45) and ACE inhibitors (26,44) consistently reduces the albumin/protein excretion rate and slows the progression of renal insufficiency. In *incipient nephropathy* (microalbuminuria 30–300 mg/24 h) therapy with ACE inhibitors retards the progression to overt nephropathy (28,55,65) and reduces microalbuminuria, even in patients whose blood pressure is still in the normotensive range (31,49,55).

Type 2 diabetics

Historically, the natural history and pathogenesis of diabetic nephropathy has first been studied in type 1 diabetics (35). Consequently, most studies on the effect of blood pressure reduction on mortality, morbidity and kidney

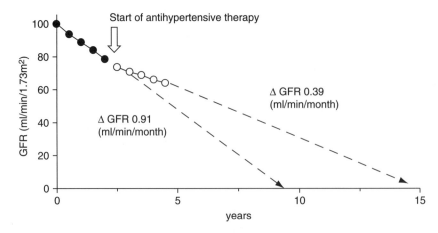

Figure 16.4 Retardation of the progression of renal failure by effective blood pressure reduction in type 1 diabetics with overt nephropathy. Before initiation of antihypertensive therapy, renal function declined at a rate of 0.91 ml/min/month (closed data points). Lowering of blood pressure slowed the decline of renal function to 0.39 ml/min/month (open data points). Data are from 10 type 1 diabetics with overt nephropathy (45). Extrapolation of the two sets of data before and after commencement of antihypertensive therapy demonstrates that terminal renal failure is expected to occur after approximately 9 years without, and after approximately 15 years with, effective antihypertensive therapy, thus saving the patients about 5–6 years off dialysis! Note that blood pressure therapy was based on combinations of β-blockers and diuretics with hydaralazine added if needed

function have been performed in type 1 diabetics and only more recently has the focus shifted to patients with type 2 diabetes. It must, however, strongly be emphasized that the long-held belief of diabetic nephropathy as a problem mainly affecting the type 1 diabetic is wrong: the cumulative incidence of nephropathy in type 2 diabetics is at least as high as in type 1 patients (17). Bearing in mind that type 2 diabetes is much more frequent than type 1, it is evident that most of the burden of diabetes-related renal complications will affect type 2 diabetics (27).

Although up until now relatively little data from adequately controlled studies are available for the type 2 diabetic with nephropathy, the available evidence suggests that control of blood pressure has similar beneficial effects on mortality, morbidity and preservation of renal function as in the type 1 diabetic. In a retrospective study using a "historical" control group, Hasslacher et al (16) found an improved survival by effective antihypertensive therapy, not only in type 1 but also in type 2 diabetics. In that study, antihypertensive therapy was mainly based on β-blockers and diuretics. In the placebo-controlled Systolic Hypertension in the Elderly Program (SHEP), the total study population of 4736 elderly patients with isolated systolic hypertension included a subgroup of 583 type 2 diabetics (9). Approximately 17% of these diabetic patients had evidence of nephropathy (1+ dipstick proteinuria) at baseline. Blood pressure was treated with a diuretic-based (chlorthalidone) regime. At 1 year follow-up, the incidence of proteinuria had decreased in the diuretic-treated group, but had increased in the placebo group. As already mentioned above, in the UKPDS trial tight control of blood pressure (with either the β-blocker atenolol or the ACE inhibitor captopril) reduced the occurence of micro-albuminuria relative to less tight control (63); this finding demonstrates that effective treatment of elevated blood pressure protects renal function in the type 2 diabetic patient, as it does in type 1 diabetics.

Choice of Antihypertensive Drugs for the Treatment of the Hypertensive Diabetic with Albuminuria/Proteinuria

The evidence presented so far demonstrates that first and foremost it is the effective lowering of elevated blood pressure that improves the prognosis and protects the kidney of the hypertensive diabetic with proteinuria. In order to achieve the recommended treatment goal of $< 130/80$ mmHg (see above), a combination therapy that will often comprise even more than two drugs will be required in the majority of patients, e.g. in the HOT study, 45% of the overall population (including diabetic and non-diabetics) patients in the target blood pressure group < 80 mmHg diastolic required combination therapy of two and 24% of three drugs (15). Set against this background, potential differences between the different classes of antihypertensive drugs regarding specific "nephroprotective" effects that go beyond those obtained by blood pressure reduction *per se* appear of secondary clinical relevance.

'Conventional' Antihypertensives: β-Blockers and Diuretics

As explained above, the first studies to demonstrate the benefit of antihypertensive therapy in proteinuric diabetics, in terms of both retarding renal functional impairment and improving survival, were almost exclusively based on a "conventional" regimen with β-blockers and diuretics, often given in combination. Therefore, the criticism that is often raised against the use of β-blockers and diuretics in diabetics, due to their potentially adverse metabolic effects, is not justified. These drugs do not do any harm to the proteinuric diabetic but protect his/her kidney and his/her life *despite* the small changes observed in serum lipids and electrolytes. Therefore, the changes in these surrogate parameters, which are indeed observed during therapy with these drugs, are of no or of only secondary clinical relevance [for review, see (7,32,52)].

In patients with nephropathy, *diuretics* will often be required for the symptomatic therapy of oedema and they can safely be combined with virtually all classes of antihypertensive drugs in order to increase antihypertensive efficacy. Thiazide-diuretics lose efficacy in patients with advanced renal insufficiency; therefore, they should be replaced by loop diuretics if serum creatinine exceeds 1.5–2.0 mg/dl. *β-Blockers* have an established role in both the treatment of angina pectoris and in secondary prevention following myocardial infarction. They effectively reduce mortality and cardiovascular morbidity, including recurrent infarction, in both diabetic and non-diabetic patients (20,68). Recently, they have been shown to reduce mortality in cardiac failure, even in patients who had already been treated with ACE inhibitors (6,33,40). In view of their proven benefit in the treatment of diabetic nephropathy (see above), and given the high prevalence of both coronary artery disease and heart failure in diabetic patients, there will be a clear-cut indication for the prescription of a β-blocking agent in many diabetic patients with proteinuria. Since glucose release in response to hypoglycaemia is controlled by β_2-adrenoceptors (25), only β_1-selective agents should be prescribed to diabetic patients (7). If β_1-selective agents are used, there is no evidence that these drugs precipitate hypoglycaemia. In the UKPDS trial, the frequency of hypoglycaemic episodes observed during treatment with atenolol was not increased compared to the ACE inhibitor captopril (62).

If β-blockers are prescribed to a patient with renal impairment, the different pharmacokinetic characteristics of different β-blockers should be remembered: while some β-blockers are mainly eliminated by hepatic metabolism (e.g. metoprolol), others are mainly cleared by the renal route (e.g. atenolol, sotalol) and others are eliminated by both hepatic metabolism and renal clearance (e.g. bisoprolol). Consequently, the dose should be adjusted to renal function if a β-blocker mainly cleared by the kidney is used. Measurement of heart rate is a simple method to monitor the pharmacodynamic action of β-blocking agents; therefore, heart rate provides a clinically useful parameter to guide dose selection and to exclude accumulation; conversely, it is also of help to assess patient compliance.

Taken together, and faced with the requirement for combination therapy in order to meet treatment goals, β-blockers and/or diuretics are indispensable drugs in the treatment of the hypertensive diabetic patient, both with and without proteinuria.

ACE Inhibitors

Evidence has accumulated during the last few years that ACE inhibitors convey a specific "nephroprotective" effect in addition to the beneficial effects of blood pressure reduction and therefore are even superior to the beneficial effects of "conventional" antihypertensives. The evidence is particularly convincing for type 1 diabetics.

A potential, specific "nephroprotective action" of ACE inhibitors was first suggested by three meta-analyses pooling studies investigating the effects of different antihypertensive drugs on proteinuria in hypertensive, diabetic patients (13,19,66). All three meta-analyses consistently found that for comparable reductions in blood pressure ACE inhibitors were superior to β-blockers, diuretics and calcium antagonists in reducing albuminuria/proteinuria. The indirect evidence from these meta-analyses was confirmed in a large, prospective, randomized trial that compared the effects of antihypertensive therapy between "conventional drugs" and the ACE inhibitor captopril on the progression of renal insufficiency, morbidity and mortality in 409 type 1 diabetics with overt nephropathy (proteinuria > 500 mg/day; serum-creatinine < 2.5 mg/dl) (26). During the median follow-up time of 3 years, the ACE inhibitor significantly slowed the decline in kidney function and reduced mortality (Figure 16.5). The rate of decline in creatinine clearance was 23%/year in the captopril group and 37% in the conventionally treated group in patients with a baseline serum-creatinine ≥ 1.5 mg/dl. It is noteworthy that patients with the worst kidney function benefited most from therapy with captopril. Based on these results, ACE inhibitors are the drugs of first choice in the type 1 diabetic with overt nephropathy. As

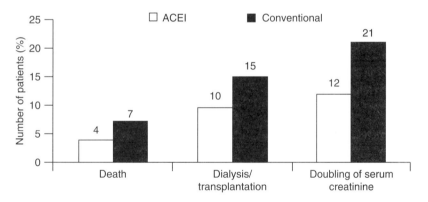

Figure 16.5 "Nephroprotective effect" of ACE inhibitor therapy in diabetic nephropathy. Influence of antihypertensive therapy based on the ACE inhibitor captopril (25 mg t.i.d.) (open bars) or on "conventional" drugs, mainly diuretic/β-blocker combinations. The bars indicate the percentage of patients in the captopril group (*n* = 207) (open bars) and in the "conventionally-treated" group (*n* = 202) (black bars) that reached the study end points of "death" or "need for dialysis or transplantation" and whose serum creatinine doubled during the study period (median follow-up of 3 years). Captopril therapy resulted in a significant reduction of all endpoints

explained in the section on type 1 diabetics (above), ACE inhibitors have also been shown to retard the progression from incipient to overt nephropathy, even if blood pressure is in the normotensive range.

Due to the lack of a comparable, large-scale study the evidence in favour of ACE inhibitors in type 2 diabetics with nephropathy is not quite as conclusive; taken together it does, however, also suggest a superiority of ACE inhibitors. In one study in a small number of type 2 diabetic patients with overt nephropathy, ACE inhibitor therapy was more effective in retarding the decline of glomerular filtration rate and reducing proteinuria than a β-blocker/diuretic combination (53). In a 5 year study in type 2 diabetics with microalbuminuria and *normal* blood pressure serum creatinine, albumin excretion rate and blood pressure remained stable with ACE inhibitor therapy; in the control group, microalbuminuria and serum-creatinine slightly increased, as did blood pressure (48). In a similar study in normotensive type 2 diabetics with albumin excretion rate in the *normal* range, the proportion of patients progressing to microalbuminuria over a 6 year period was significantly smaller with enalapril therapy, compared to patients in the placebo-group (47).

In summary, based on these results, ACE inhibitors are now regarded as the drugs of first choice for all diabetic patients with incipient or overt nephropathy. Blood pressure should be reduced to values of at least 130/80 mmHg or lower if tolerated; in order to meet this goal, monotherapy will not be sufficient in many patients. The ACE inhibitor should then be combined with low-dose diuretics, β_1-selective β-blockers or calcium antagonists. In order to postpone the occurrence of terminal renal failure as long as possible and thus save the patient as many years off dialysis as possible, it is essential to start therapy as early as possible, i.e. ACE inhibitors must not be withheld from any diabetic patient in whom overt nephropathy has been diagnosed and should also be given to patients with incipient nephropathy (see above). On the other hand, even in advanced renal insufficiency ACE inhibitors are of proven benefit; indeed, in the study by Lewis et al (26), reductions in proteinuria and the retardation of the progression of renal insufficiency was most pronounced in patients with more advanced disease, i.e. in those with the highest serum creatinine and largest proteinuria at baseline, respectively. Similar findings have been reported in non-diabetic nephropathy (21,56) (cf. section on Optimal Target Blood Pressure, above).

In practical terms, it is very important to remember the following if initiating ACE inhibitor therapy in a diabetic patient with nephropathy.

Since nearly all ACE inhibitors are eliminated by renal clearance, careful dose adjustment according to the degree of renal insufficiency is mandatory. It should be remembered that ACE inhibitors can precipitate acute renal failure and hyperkalaemia in patients with renal artery stenosis, a condition highly prevalent in diabetic patients (50). On the other hand, an initial decline in glomerular filtration rate with a corresponding increase in serum creatinine is usually observed during the first days of ACE inhibitor therapy (29). This reflects the renal pharmacodynamic mode of action of ACE inhibitors, which preferentially dilate the efferent glomerular arterioles, thus decreasing intraglomerular pressure; it is this mechanism that underlies the physiological basis of the specific "renoprotective" effect of the ACE inhibitors! Therefore, serum creatinine and potassium should be regularly monitored when ACE inhibitor therapy is initiated in order not to miss the development of acute renal failure and/or hyperkalaemia, which are rapidly reversible if the ACE inhibitor is immediately withdrawn. The occurrence of acute renal failure during ACE inhibitor therapy should give rise to active screening for the presence of renal artery stenosis.

Calcium Antagonists

Recently, the "calcium antagonist controversy" has raised concerns regarding the safety of calcium antagonists in the treatment of hypertension; specifically, it has been argued that calcium antagonists may increase cardiovascular mortality and morbidity (46). Studies on the use of calcium antagonists in hypertensive diabetics provide an inconclusive picture.

The Appropriate Blood Pressure Control in Diabetes (ABCD) trial compared the calcium antagonist nisoldipine and the ACE inhibitor enalapril as first-line antihypertensives in hypertensive type 2 diabetics, with and without renal insufficiency (11). Among patients treated with nisoldipin, there was a significantly higher incidence of fatal and non-fatal myocardial infarction. Similarly, the Fosinopril vs. Amlodipine Cardiovascular Events Randomized Trial (FACET) compared the calcium antagonist amlodipine with the ACE inhibitor fosinopril in hypertensive type 2 diabetics without nephropathy (54). Again, patients treated with the calcium antagonist had a significantly increased risk of major vascular events. Obviously, in both studies the ACE inhibitor was superior to the calcium antagonist in the prevention of cardiovascular events. However, it is impossible to conclude from these studies whether calcium antagonists actually increase the cardiovascular risk of the hypertensive diabetic, since neither study was placebo-controlled.

The Systolic Hypertension in Europe (Syst-Eur) trial suggests that this is indeed *not* the case, at least not in elderly diabetics (61). This *placebo-controlled* study investigated the effect of antihypertensive therapy on cardiovascular events in elderly patients ($\geq$ 60 years of age) with isolated systolic hypertension. The study enrolled mainly non-diabetic patients ($n = 4203$), but also included a subgroup of type 2 diabetics ($n = 492$). Therapy was based on the calcium antagonist nitrendipine and resulted in an impressive 55% reduction of overall mortality and a 76% lowering of cardiovascular mortality ($p < 0.05$) among diabetic patients.

In the HOT study, "aggressive" blood pressure reduction based on the calcium antagonist felodipine reduced mortality rates in diabetics to levels similar to those observed in non-diabetics (cf. Section on Optimal Target Blood Pressure, above, and Figure 16.3), providing additional evidence that calcium antagonists are not harmful to the hypertensive diabetic.

Non-pharmacological Measures

As for the non-diabetic hypertensive, non-pharmacological measures are an important and basic part of the management of the hypertensive diabetic with nephropathy. In type 2 diabetics, weight reduction and salt restriction *per se* are very effective in lowering blood pressure (10,41,59). In type 1 diabetics, salt restriction by itself appears to have little influence on blood pressure (36). It does, however, enhance responsiveness to antihypertensive drug therapy and is therefore recommended.

Smoking accelerates the development and progression of diabetic nephropathy (5,37,39) and should therefore be strongly discouraged. Normalization of increased serum lipids is another important part of general risk factor management (14).

SUMMARY

The optimal control of diabetes and of arterial hypertension determine the prognosis of the hypertensive diabetic patient. Cessation of smoking and lowering of elevated serum lipids are additional essential therapeutic goals. The normalization of blood pressure is the most important therapeutic measure in order to improve mortality and morbidity of the hypertensive diabetic patient and this holds particularly true for the diabetic with nephropathy. There is no doubt that early and "aggressive" lowering of blood pressure retards the progression of renal insufficiency in the diabetic patient with nephropathy, and thus postpones the occurrence of terminal renal failure, with the need for dialysis and transplantation, by several years! In the patient with nephropathy, blood pressure should be lowered to values *below 130/80 mmHg*, and even lower if there are no adverse effects. Reduction of blood pressure below these values should be the primary therapeutic goal in the hypertensive diabetic with nephropathy.

In the type 1 and type 2 diabetic with overt nephropathy, ACE inhibitors have been shown to convey a specific nephroprotective effect beyond the beneficial effect of blood pressure reduction and have also been shown to postpone the development of overt nephropathy in patients with microalbuminuria. Therefore, antihypertensive therapy should be started with an ACE inhibitor in diabetics with incipient and overt nephropathy. An ACE inhibitor should even be given if incipient or overt nephropathy has been diagnosed but blood pressure is still in the normotensive range. Combination therapy will be required in many patients in order to reach a target blood pressure of 130/80 mmHg. Low-dose diuretics, β-1 selective β-blockers and calcium antagonists would be the drugs of choice for combination therapy and additional coexisting diseases will usually guide the choice of the most appropriate drug to use.

In order to gain the maximum benefit and to postpone terminal renal failure as long as possible, it is essential to start therapy as early as possible, i.e. if incipient or overt nephropathy have been diagnosed, therapy with an ACE inhibitor should be initiated even if the blood pressure is still in the normotensive range. Conversely, even in advanced renal impairment, progression of renal disease will be retarded by effective blood pressure lowering.

REFERENCES

1. American Diabetes Association. ADA consensus statement. Treatment of hypertension in diabetes. *Diabet Care* 1996; **19**: S107–13.
2. Andersen AR, Sandahl Christiansen J, Andersen JK, Kreiner S, Deckert T. Diabetic nephropathy in type 1 (insulin-dependent) diabetes: an epidemiological study. *Diabetologia* 1983; **25**: 496–501.
3. Borch-Johnsen K, Andersen PK, Deckert T. The effect of proteinuria on relative mortality in type 1 (insulin-dependent) diabetes mellitus. *Diabetologia* 1985; **28**: 590–96.
4. Braun D, Unger H, Wagner A, Henrichs HR. Prävalenz der diabetischen Retinopathie und Nephropathie sowie der arteriellen Hypertonie in Abhängigkeit von der Diabetesdauer. *Diabet Stoffw* 1994; **3**: 333–8.
5. Chase HP, Garg SK, Marshall G et al. Cigarette smoking increases the risk of albuminuria among subjects with type I diabetes. *J Am Med Assoc* 1991; **265**: 614–17.
6. CIBIS-II Investigators and Committees. The Cardiac Insufficiency Bisoprolol Study II (CIBIS-II): a randomised trial. *Lancet* 1999; **353**: 9–13.
7. Cruickshank JM. Beta-blockers continue to surprise us. *Eur Heart J* 2000; **21**: 354–64.
8. Cruickshank JM, Thorp JM, Zacharias FJ. Benefits and potential harm of lowering high blood pressure. *Lancet* 1987; **1**: 581–4.
9. Curb JD, Pressel SL, Cutler JA et al. Effect of diuretic-based antihypertensive treatment on cardiovascular disease risk in older diabetic patients with isolated systolic hypertension. *J Am Med Assoc* 1996; **276**: 1886–92.
10. Dodson PM, Beevers M, Hallworth R et al. Sodium restriction and blood pressure in hypertensive type II diabetics: randomised blind controlled and crossover studies of moderate sodium restriction and sodium supplementation. *Br Med J* 1989; **298**: 227–30.

11. Estacio RO, Jeffers BW, Hiatt WR et al. The effect of nisoldipine as compared with enalapril on cardiovascular outcomes in patients with non-insulin-dependent diabetes and hypertension. *N Engl J Med* 1998; **338**: 645–52.

12. European Diabetes Policy Group 1998. Guidelines for diabetes care. A desktop guide to type 1 (insulin dependent) diabetes mellitus. *Diabet Nutr Metab* 1999; **12**: 345–78.

13. Gansevoort RT, Sluiter WJ, Hemmelder MH, de Zeeuw D, de Jong PE. Antiproteinuric effect of blood-pressure-lowering agents: a meta-analysis of comparative trials. *Nephrol Dialysis Transpl* 1995; **10**: 1963–74.

14. Haffner SM. The Scandinavian Simvastatin Survival Study (4S) subgroup analysis of diabetic subjects: implications for the prevention of coronary heart disease. *Diabet Care* 1997; **20**: 469–71.

15. Hansson L, Zanchetti A, Carruthers SG et al, for the HOT Study Group. Effects of intensive blood-pressure lowering and low-dose aspirin in patients with hypertension: principal results of the hypertension optimal treatment (HOT) randomised trial. *Lancet* 1998; **351**: 1755–62.

16. Hasslacher C, Borgholte G, Panradl U, Wahl P. Verbesserte Prognose von Typ-I- und Typ-II-Diabetikern mit Nephropathie. *Med Klin* 1990; **85**: 643–6.

17. Hasslacher C, Ritz E, Wahl P, Michael C. Similar risks of nephropathy in patients with type I or type II diabetes mellitus. *Nephrol Dialysis Transpl* 1989; **4**: 859–63.

18. Jacobson HR, Striker GE. Report on a workshop to develop management recommendations for the prevention of progression in chronic renal disease. *Am J Kidney Dis* 1995; **25**: 103–6.

19. Kasiske BL, Kalil RSN, Ma JZ, Liao M, Keane WF. Effect of antihypertensive therapy on the kidney in patients with diabetes: a meta-regression analysis. *Ann Int Med* 1993; **118**: 129–38.

20. Kjekshus J, Gilpin E, Cali G et al. Diabetic patients and beta-blockers after acute myocardial infarction. *Eur Heart J* 1990; **11**: 43–50.

21. Klahr S, Levey AS, Beck GJ et al, for the Modification of Diet in Renal Disease Study Group. The effects of dietary protein restriction and blood pressure control on the progression of chronic renal disease. *N Engl J Med* 1994; **330**: 877–84.

22. Knowles HC Jr. Long-term juvenile diabetes treated with unmeasured diet. *Trans Assoc Am Physicians* 1971; **84**: 95–101.

23. Koch M, Kutkuhn B, Grabensee B, Ritz E. Apolipoprotein A, fibrinogen, age, and history of stroke are predictors of death in dialysed diabetic patients: a prospective study in 412 subjects. *Nephrol Dialysis Transpl* 1997; **12**: 2603–11.

24. Krolewski AS, Warram JH, Christlieb AR, Busick EJ, Kahn CR. The changing natural history of nephropathy in type I diabetes. *Am J Med* 1985; **78**: 785–94.

25. Lager I, Blohme G, Smith U. Effect of cardioselective and non-selective β-blockade on the hypoglycaemic responses in insulin-dependent diabetics. *Lancet* 1979; **i**: 458–62.

26. Lewis EJ, Hunsicker LG, Bain RP, Rohde RD, for the Collaborative Study Group. The effect of angiotensin-converting-enzyme inhibition on diabetic nephropathy. *N Engl J Med* 1993; **329**: 1456–62.

27. Lippert J, Ritz E, Schwarzbeck A, Schneider P. The rising tide of endstage renal failure from diabetic nephropathy type II—an epidemiological analysis. *Nephrol Dialysis Transpl* 1995; **10**: 462–7.

28. Marre M, Chatellier G, Leblanc H et al. Prevention of diabetic nephropathy with enalapril in normotensive diabetics with microalbuminuria. *Br Med J* 1988; **297**: 1092–5.

29. Maschio G, Alberti D, Janin G et al, and the Angiotensin-converting-enzyme Inbibition in Progressive Renal Insufficiency Study Group. Effect of the angiotensin-converting-enzyme inhibitor benazepril on the progression of chronic renal insufficiency. *N Engl J Med* 1996; **334**: 939–45.
30. Mathiesen ER, Borch-Johnsen K, Jensen DV, Deckert T. Improved survival in patients with diabetic nephropathy. *Diabetologia* 1989; **32**: 884–6.
31. Mathiesen ER, Hommel E, Giese J, Parving HH. Efficacy of captopril in postponing nephropathy in normotensive insulin dependent diabetic patients with microalbuminuria. *Br Med J* 1991; **303**: 81–7.
32. McInnes GT, Yeo WW, Ramsay LE, Moser M. Cardiotoxicity and diuretics: much speculation—little substance. *J Hypertens* 1992; **10**: 317–35.
33. MERIT-HF Study Group. Effect of metoprolol CR/XL in chronic heart failure: Metoprolol CR/XL Randomised Intervention Trial in Congestive Heart Failure (MERIT-HF). *Lancet* 1999; **353**: 2001–7.
34. Mogensen CE. Long-term antihypertensive treatment inhibiting progression of diabetic nephropathy. *Br Med J* 1982; **285**: 685–8.
35. Mogensen CE, Christensen CK, Vittinghus E. The stages in diabetic renal disease—with emphasis on the stage of incipient diabetic nephropathy. *Diabetes* 1983; **32**: 64–78.
36. Mühlhauser I, Prange K, Sawicki PT et al. Effects of dietary sodium on blood pressure in IDDM patients with nephropathy. *Diabetologia* 1996; **39**: 212–19.
37. Mühlhauser I, Sawicki P, Berger M. Cigarette-smoking as a risk factor for macroproteinuria and proliferative retinopathy in type 1 (insulin-dependent) diabetes. *Diabetologia* 1986; **29**: 500–502.
38. Norgaard K, Feldt-Rasmussen B, Borch-Johnsen K, Saelan H, Deckert T. Prevalence of hypertension in type 1 (insulin-dependent) diabetes mellitus. *Diabetologia* 1990; **33**: 407–10.
39. Orth SR, Ritz E, Schrier RW. The renal risks of smoking. *Kidney Int* 1997; **51**: 1669–77.
40. Packer M, Bristow MR, Cohn JN et al, for the US Carvedilol Heart Failure Study Group. The effect of carvedilol on morbidity and mortality in patients with chronic heart failure. *N Engl J Med* 1996; **334**: 1349–55.
41. Pacy PJ, Dodson PM, Kubicki AJ, Fletcher RF, Taylor KG. Comparison of the hypotensive and metabolic effects of bendrofluazide therapy and a high fibre, low fat, low sodium diet in diabetic subjects with mild hypertension. *J Hypertens* 1984; **2**: 215–20.
42. Parving H-H, Andersen AR, Smidt UM et al. Effect of antihypertensive treatment on kidney function in diabetic nephropathy. *Br Med J* 1987; **294**: 1443–7.
43. Parving H-H, Hommel E. Prognosis in diabetic nephropathy. *Br Med J* 1989; **299**: 230–33.
44. Parving H-H, Hommel E, Smidt UM. Protection of kidney function and decrease in albuminuria by captopril in insulin dependent diabetics with nephropathy. *Br Med J* 1988; **297**: 1086–91.
45. Parving HH, Andersen AR, Smidt UM, Svendsen PA. Early aggressive antihypertensive treatment reduces rate of decline in kidney function in diabetic nephropathy. *Lancet* 1983; **1**: 1175–9.
46. Psaty BM, Heckbert SR, Koepsell TD et al. The risk of myocardial infarction associated with antihypertensive drug therapies. *J Am Med Assoc* 1995; **274**: 620–25.
47. Ravid M, Brosh D, Levi Z et al. Use of enalapril to attenuate decline in renal function in normotensive, normoalbuminuric patients with type 2

    diabetes mellitus. A randomized, controlled trial. *Ann Intern Med* 1998; **128**: 982–8.

48. Ravid M, Savin H, Jutrin I et al. Long-term stabilizing effect of angiotensin-converting enzyme inhibition on plasma creatinine and on proteinuria in normotensive type II diabetic patients. *Ann Intern Med* 1993; **118**: 577–81.

49. Rudberg S, Aperia A, Freyschuss U, Persson B. Enalapril reduces microalbuminuria in young normotensive type 1 (insulin-dependent) diabetic patients irrespective of its hypotensive effect. *Diabetologia* 1990; **33**: 470–76.

50. Sawicki PT, Kaiser S, Heinemann L, Frenzel H, Berger M. Prevalence of renal artery stenosis in diabetes mellitus: an autopsy study. *J Intern Med* 1991; **229**: 489–92.

51. Schäfers RF, Lütkes P, Ritz E, Philipp T. Leitlinie zur Behandlung der arteriellen Hypertonie bei Diabetes mellitus. Konsensus-Empfehlungen der Deutschen Liga zur Bekämpfung des hohen Blutdruckes e.V., der Deutschen Diabetes Gesellschaft und der Gesellschaft für Nephrologie. *Dtsch Med Wochenschr* 1999; **124**: 1356–72.

52. Schäfers RF, Philipp I, Lütkes P. Antihypertensive therapy with diuretics in type 2 diabetics—rational therapy or malpractice? *Ther Umsch* 2000; **57**: 368–73.

53. Slataper R, Vicknair N, Sadler R, Bakris GL. Comparative effects of different antihypertensive treatments on progression of diabetic renal disease. *Arch Intern Med* 1993; **153**: 973–80.

54. Tatti P, Pahor M, Byington RP et al. Outcome results of the fosinopril versus amlodipine cardiovascular events randomised trial (FACET) in patients with hypertension and NIDDM. *Diabet Care* 1998; **21**: 597–603.

55. The EUCLID Study Group. Randomised placebo-controlled trial of lisinopril in normotensive patients with insulin-dependent diabetes and normoalbuminuria or microalbuminuria. *Lancet* 1997; **349**: 1787–92.

56. The GISEN Group (Gruppo Italiano di Studi Epidemiologici in Nefrologia). Randomised placebo-controlled trial of effect of ramipril on decline in glomerular filtration rate and risk of terminal renal failure in proteinuric, non-diabetic nephropathy. *Lancet* 1997; **349**: 1857–63.

57. The Hypertension Detection and Follow-up Program Cooperative Research Group. Mortality findings for stepped-care and referred-care participants in the hypertension detection and follow-up program, stratified by other risk factors. *Prev Med* 1985; **14**: 312–35.

58. The Hypertension in Diabetes Study Group. Hypertension in diabetes study (HDS): I. Prevalence of hypertension in newly presenting type 2 diabetic patients and the association with risk factors for cardiovascular and diabetic complications. *J Hypertens* 1993a; **11**: 309–17.

59. The Hypertension in Diabetes Study Group. Hypertension in diabetes study (HDS): II. Increased risk of cardiovascular complications in hypertensive type 2 diabetic patients. *J Hypertens* 1993b; **11**: 319–25.

60. The Joint National Committee on Prevention, Detection, Evaluation and Treatment of High Blood Pressure. The Sixth Report of the Joint National Committee on Prevention, Detection, Evaluation, and Treatment of High Blood Pressure. *Arch Intern Med* 1997; **157**: 2413–46.

61. Tuomilehto J, Rastenyte D, Birkenhäger WH et al, for the systolic hypertension in Europe trial investigators. Effects of calcium-channel blockade in older patients with diabetes and systolic hypertension. *N Engl J Med* 1999; **340**: 677–84.

62. UK Prospective Diabetes Study Group. Efficacy of atenolol and captopril in reducing risk of macrovascular and microvascular complications in type 2 diabetes: UKPDS 39. *Br Med J* 1998a; **317**: 713–20.
63. UK Prospective Diabetes Study Group. Tight blood pressure control and risk of macrovascular and microvascular complications in type 2 diabetes: UKPDS 38. *Br Med J* 1998b; **317**: 703–13.
64. United States Renal Data System. Incidence and prevalence of ESRD. United States Renal Data System. *Am J Kidney Dis* 1998; **32**: S38–49.
65. Viberti G, Mogensen CE, Groop LC, Pauls JF. Effect of captopril on progression to clinical proteinuria in patients with insulin dependent diabetes mellitus and microalbuminuria. European microalbuminuria captopril study group. *J Am Med Assoc* 1994; **271**: 275–9.
66. Weidmann P, Boehlen LM, de Courten M, Ferrari P. Antihypertensive therapy in diabetic patients. *J Human Hypertens* 1992; **6**: S23–36.
67. WHO-ISH Guidelines Subcommittee. 1999 World Health Organization—International Society of Hypertension Guidelines for the Management of Hypertension. *J Hypertens* 1999; **17**: 905–18.
68. Yusuf S, Peto R, Lewis J, Collins R, Sleight P. Beta-blockade during and after myocardial infarction: an overview of the randomized trials. *Prog Cardiovasc Dis* 1985; **27**: 335–71.

17

Early Antihypertensive Intervention in Diabetic Patients with Incipient Nephropathy

MICHEL MARRE[1], BÉATRICE BOUHANICK[2]
AND SAMY HADJADJ[2]

[1]Hopital Bichat, Paris, and [2]Centre Hospitalier Universitaire, Angers, France

INTRODUCTION

Incipient diabetic nephropathy is defined as persistent microalbuminuria due to diabetes. It is a transition stage between supra-normal kidney function due to pressure disequilibrium within the diabetic glomeruli and established diabetic nephropathy with concomitant glomerulosclerosis. During this stage, morphological changes can already be observed (1). However, this is the precise period when interventions based on the haemodynamic changes characteristic of diabetes mellitus (see Chapter 4) allow prevention of ongoing sclerosis and renal failure, or reversion towards normal albumin excretion. Typically, incipient nephropathy is characteristic of type 1 diabetes, although this can be observed in type 2 diabetes. During this early stage, blood pressure remains within the normal range. However, there is a proportional increase of urinary albumin excretion (UAE) and of blood pressure during the course of diabetic nephropathy from the incipient stage (2). There may be two types of interventions based on pathophysiology: first, reducing blood glucose, as shown on occasion in

Diabetic Nephropathy. Edited by C. Hasslacher.
© 2001 John Wiley & Sons, Ltd.

several trials, including the DCCT; second, reducing pressure disequilibrium within the glomeruli, especially using angiotensin I-converting enzyme inhibitors (ACEIs). This latter intervention will be developed in this chapter.

EXPERIMENTAL STUDIES

Zatz et al (3,4) demonstrated, in streptozotocin-induced diabetic rats, that reducing pressure disequilibrium within the glomeruli prevents both albuminuria and glomerulosclerosis. This was especially efficient when angiotensin II (a promoter for post-glomerular vasoconstriction) was blocked with enalapril, and ACEI (4). However, systemic blood pressure was reduced by ACEIs in this first series of studies. Anderson et al (5) then demonstrated, by studying a control diabetic group on classical antihypertensive triple therapy, that the previously demonstrated benefit was attributable to the amelioration of the diabetes-related intra glomerular changes, and not only to blood pressure reduction.

ELIGIBILITY FOR STUDIES

Should subjects with incipient diabetic nephropathy be assigned to antihypertensive treatment on the basis of UAE, or of blood pressure values? Certainly on the basis of a persistent microalbuminuria, because definition of incipient diabetic nephropathy is based on this biological abnormality. Second, microalbuminuria is probably an early sign of, rather than a factor predictive for, diabetic nephropathy (6). In this connexion, UAE > 20 μg/min (or 30 mg/24 h) is clearly abnormal: more than 50% of healthy subjects excrete less than 5 mg/24 h. Finally, UAE reduction can be obtained independently of blood pressure reduction, as detailed below.

PILOT STUDIES

Follow-up studies indicated that early, aggressive antihypertensive treatment reduces effectively both albuminuria and the rate of GFR decline in patients with established diabetic nephropathy (7, 8). These were pragmatic studies in which classical antihypertensive drugs were used, including the β-blocker metoprolol. Then, Christensen and Mogensen reported a 6 year follow-up of six patients with incipient diabetic nephropathy before and during metoprolol treatment (9). UAE was reduced and GFR maintained unchanged with metoprolol. Taken together, these studies supported the concept that reducing blood pressure is an effective means of reducing microalbuminuria and protecting GFR in incipient diabetic nephropathy. However, clinical and experimental data supported that increased UAE results from increased glomerular capillary pressure, which is determined not only by systemic blood pressure but also by pre-/postglomerular vasoconstriction/dilation (10). This latter determinant is strongly regulated by the activity of the renin – angiotensin – aldosterone system. β-Blockers can modify glomerular hæmodynamics, because they reduce renin secretion, in addition to their actions on cardiac output and blood pressure (11). In the above-mentioned studies (7–9), changes in glomerular hæmodynamics were not studied in relation to those of renin secretion.

Similarly, we set up a double-blind, placebo-controlled trial demonstrating prevention or postponement of diabetic nephropathy with enalapril in normotensive diabetic subjects with microalbuminuria (12). However, blood pressure was reduced by enalapril compared to placebo, which made interpretation of this trial difficult, since reducing blood pressure reduces UAE in hypertensive subjects (13).

Thus, confusion rose from these observations, because alterations in systemic blood pressure and in glomerular hæmodynamics were not controlled simultaneously with changes in activity of the renin–angiotensin system. In a double-blind, double-dummy, 1-year parallel trial comparing enalapril to hydrochlorothiazide (two drugs with similar hypotensive effects but symmetrical actions on angiotensin II production) to reduce UAE of normotensive insulin-dependent subjects with microalbuminuria, we demonstrated that reducing systemic blood pressure reduces UAE in the long term only if the effectiveness of the renin – angiotensin system on glomerular hæmodynamics is simultaneously blocked (14).

Also, several studies indicated that microalbuminuria of normotensive type 1, insulin-dependent diabetic subjects could be reduced by ACEIs, while blood pressure was not modified significantly (15, 16). We reported in a short-term, double-blind study that small doses of ramipril can reduce microalbuminuria as effectively as hypotensive doses. This UAE reduction was obtained independently of blood pressure reduction, but it was related to the degree of ACE inhibition and to changes in the filtration fraction (17). Comparison of enalapril to hydrochlorothiazide to reduce microalbuminuria of normotensive type 1, insulin-dependent diabetic subjects led to similar conclusions: both drugs were similar in their hypotensive effects, but only enalapril reduced microalbuminuria; UAE changes were related to those of filtration fraction, not to those of blood pressure (14). Thus, dose – response curves for the renal and the hypotensive effects of ACEIs may not be superimposable.

COMPARISON OF ACEIS WITH OTHER ANTIHYPERTENSIVE DRUGS TO REDUCE UAE IN INCIPIENT NEPHROPATHY

As detailled above, we demonstrated that ACEIs are more effective than diuretics for reducing UAE in incipient nephropathy. The Melbourne Diabetic Nephropathy Study Group reported no difference between the ACEI perindopril and the calcium antagonist nifedipine in diabetic subjects with microalbuminuria (18); a type 2 error may account for this observed lack of difference. A recent, multicentre, 3 year, placebo-controlled, double-blind study confirmed that ACEIs (lisinopril) prevent progression to macroalbuminuria. In this study, the slope of UAE progression was higher on nifedipine than on lisinopril (19). These data obtained in incipient nephropathy are consistent with a meta-regression analysis supporting a preferential role for ACEIs to reduce UAE and to protect GFR of diabetic subjects (20).

BENEFITS OBTAINED WITH ACEIS

Several controlled studies were performed with ACEIs vs. placebo or standard treatment (12,15,21,17,22,23,19). A meta-analysis was performed recently, showing that ACEIs reduced progression from micro- to macroalbuminuria by 79% (odds ratio 0.31; 95% CI, 0.19–0.51) and provoked regression to normalbuminuria more often (odds ratio, 2.64; 95% CI, 1.74–3.09). After 1 year of treatment, UAE was 82% lower on ACEIs than on placebo (24).

Certainly GFR preservation is the only clinically significant outcome for intervention studies in diabetic nephropathy. Microalbuminuria is a surrogate end point. As outlined above, GFR is normal or still supranormal during incipient diabetic nephropathy, and GFR reduction is minimal at the time of clinical proteinuria onset. Also, clinical trials comparing captopril or enalapril to placebo or to metoprolol showed that GFR degradation was reduced by about 50% with ACEIs in type 1, insulin-dependent diabetic subjects with clinical proteinuria (25,26). The clinical usefulness of ACEIs given from the microalbuminuria stage was therefore questionable for type 1, insulin-dependent diabetic subjects with incipient nephropathy. Indeed, GFR evolution was not different between patients on captopril and those on placebo in 2–4 year clinical trials (15,21). Only a marginal difference was found by our group in a 1 year trial comparing enalapril to placebo (12). Laffel et al (22) reported that creatinine clearance was maintained by captopril over 2 years compared to placebo in type 1, insulin-dependent diabetic normotensive patients with microalbuminuria, and this was confirmed in a combined analysis of the two multicentre trials performed with captopril vs. placebo for 2 years (23). The median GFR slope was $6.4 \, \text{ml}/\text{min}/1.73 \, \text{m}^2/$ year in the placebo-treated patients. These data must be interpreted with caution for methodological reasons, because GFR was estimated from creatinine clearances: in the American trial, baseline GFR values were markedly low ($80 \, \text{ml}/\text{min}/1.73 \, \text{m}^2$); second, creatinine clearance can be altered by changes in tubular function provoked by renal vasodilator-like ACEIs. However, we found a comparable GFR decline in a recent 4 year follow-up study comparing two treatment strategies with enalapril. Patients' GFR were estimated with the ^{125}I-Iodothalamate constant infusion technique. Those normotensive type 1, insulin-dependent diabetic patients with microalbuminuria given enalapril from microalbuminuria identification kept their GFR unchanged (including those with initial hyperfiltration), while those given enalapril only if they progressed to macroalbuminuria reduced their GFR by $0.62 \, \text{ml}/\text{min}/1.73 \, \text{m}^2/\text{month}$. At follow-up, six of the 11 patients assigned to late enalapril treatment displayed GFR values $< 100 \, \text{ml}/\text{min}/1.73 \, \text{m}^2$ (the lower limit of normal values) (27). Taken together, these recent studies indicate that the GFR degradation slope is nearly as high in patients with incipient hephropathy as in patients with established nephropathy. These results support the current recommendation that ACEIs must be given from microalbuminuria identification in normotensive type 1, insulin-dependent diabetic patients.

PENDING QUESTIONS ON THE USE OF ACEIS IN INCIPIENT DIABETIC NEPHROPATHY

The above-mentioned data deal with normotensive type 1, insulin-dependent diabetic patients with microalbuminuria. The specific value of ACEIs vs. conventional antihypertensive treatment is not demonstrated for the kidney function of patients with essential hypertension (28), and this condition can sometimes, be associated with insulin-dependent diabetes.

The promising data obtained in type 1, insulin-dependent diabetic patients cannot be applied to type 2, non-insulin-dependent diabetic patients. Only one study reported a benefit for kidney function of normotensive type 2, non-insulin-dependent diabetic patients with microalbuminuria attributable to enalapril, compared to placebo (29, 30). However, the type 2, non-insulin-dependent diabetic patients in this study (29, 30) were relatively young and thin compared to those commonly encountered in clinical practice. Although such patients are identifiable and may share a renal prognosis similar to type 1, insulin-dependent diabetic patients (12), such results cannot be applied to the vast majority of type 2, non-insulin-dependent diabetic patients. Most of them are obese, with hypertension and mixed dyslipidaemia, and the prognostic value of micro-albuminuria deals with cardiovascular events (31). To date, no trial has established a clinical benefit from the preferential use of ACEIs in these patients (32).

ACKNOWLEDGEMENT

We thank Mrs Line Godiveau for excellent secretarial assistance.

REFERENCES

1. Osterby R. Glomerular structural changes in type 1 (insulin-dependent) diabetes mellitus: causes, consequences, and prevention. *Diabetologia* 1992; **35**: 803–12.
2. Mogensen CE, Osterby R, Hansen KW, Damsgaard EM. Blood pressure elevation versus abnormal albuminuria in the genesis and prediction of renal disease in diabetes. *Diabet Care* 1992; **15**: 1192–204.
3. Zatz R, Meyer TW, Rennke HG, Brenner BM. Predominance of hemodynamic rather than metabolic factors in the pathogenesis of diabetic glomerulopathy. *Proc Natl Acad Sci USA* 1985; **82**: 5963–7.
4. Zatz R, Dunn BR, Meyer TW, et al. Prevention of diabetic glomerulopathy by pharmacological amelioration of glomerular capillary hypertension. *J Clin Invest* 1986; **77**: 1925–30.
5. Anderson S, Rennke HG, Garcia DL, Brenner BM. Short and long-term effects of antihypertensive therapy in the diabetic rat. Kidney Int, 1989; **36**: 526–36.
6. Mogensen CE. Prediction of clinical diabetic nephropathy in IDDM patients: alternatives to microalbuminuria? *Diabetes* 1990; **39**: 761–7.
7. Mogensen CE. Long-term antihypertensive treatment inhibiting progression of diabetic nephropathy. *Br Med J* 1982; **285**: 685–8.
8. Parving HH, Andersen AR, Smidt UM, Svendsen PAA. Early aggressive antihypertensive treatment reduces the rate of decline in kidney function in diabetic nephropathy. *Lancet* 1983; **i**: 1175–9.
9. Christensen CK, Mogensen CE. Effect of antihypertensive treatment on progression of incipient diabetic nephropathy. *Hypertension* 1985; **7** (II): 109–13.
10. Brenner BM, Humes HD. Mechanisms of glomerular ultrafiltration. *N Engl J Med* 1977; **297**: 148–54.
11. Keeton T, Campbell WB. The pharmacological alterations of renin release. *Pharmacol Rev* 1980; **32**: 81–227.
12. Marre M, Chatellier G, Leblanc H et al. Prevention of diabetic nephropathy with enalapril in normotensive diabetics with microalbuminuria. *Br Med J* 1988; **297**: 1092–5.
13. Parving HH, Jensen HA, Mogensen CE, Evrin PE. Increased urinary albumin excretion rate in benign essential hypertension. *Lancet* 1974; **i**(15): 1190–92.
14. Hallab M, Gallois Y., Chatellier G et al. Comparison of reduction in microalbuminuria by enalapril and hydrochlorothiazide in normotensive patients with insulin dependent diabetes. *Br Med J* 1993; **306**: 175–82.

15. Mathiesen ER, Hommel E, Giese J, Parving HH. Efficacy of captopril in postponing nephropathy in normotensive insulin dependent diabetic patients with microalbuminuria. *Br Med J* 1991; **303**: 81–7.
16. Rudberg S, Aperia A, Freyschuss U, Persson B. Enalapril reduces microalbuminuria in young normotensive type 1 (insulin-dependent) diabetic patients irrespective of its hypotensive effect. *Diabetologia* 1990; **33**: 470–76.
17. Marre M, Hallab M, Billiard A. et al. Small doses of ramipril to reduce microalbuminuria in diabetic patients with incipient nephropathy independently of blood pressure changes. *J Cardiovasc Pharmacol* 1991; **18**: S165–8.
18. Melbourne Diabetic Nephropathy Study Group. Comparison between perindopril and nifedipine in hypertensive and normotensive diabetic patients with microalbuminuria. *Br Med J* 1991; **302**: 210–16.
19. Crepaldi G, Carta Q, Deferrari G, et al, the Italian Microalbuminuria Study Group in IDDM. Effects of lisinopril and nifedipine on the progression to overt albuminuria in IDDM patients with incipient nephropathy and normal blood pressure *Diabet Care* 1998; **21**: 104–10.
20. Kasiske BL, Kalil RS, Ma JZ, Liao M, Keane WF. Effect of antihypertensive therapy on the kidney in patients with diabetes: a meta-regression analysis. *Ann Int Med*, 1993; **118**: 129–38.
21. Viberti GC, Mogensen CE, Groop LC, Pauls JF, for the European Microalbuminuria Study Group. Effect of captopril on progression to clinical proteinuria in patients with insulin-dependent diabetes mellitus and microalbuminuria. *J Am Med Assoc* 1994; **271**: 275–9.
22. Laffel LBM, McGill JB, Gans DJ, on behalf of the North American Microalbuminuria Study Group. The beneficial effect of angiotension converting enzyme inhibition with captopril on diabetic nephropathy in normotensive IDDM patients with microalbuminuria. *Am J Med* 1995; **99**: 497–504.
23. The Microalbuminuria Captopril Study Group. Captopril reduces the risk of nephropathy in insulin-dependent diabetic patients with microalbuminuria. *Diabetologia* 1996; **39**: 587–93.
24. The ACE inhibitors in diabetic nephropathy trialist group: Should all patients with type 1 diabetes mellitus and microalbuminuria receive angiotensin-converting enzyme inhibitors? A meta-analysis of individual patient data. *Ann Intern Med* 2001; **134**: 370–9.
25. Björk S, Mulec H, Johnsen SA, Nyberg G, Aurell M. Renal protective effect of enalapril in diabetic nephropathy. *Br Med J* 1992; **304**: 339–43.
26. Lewis EJ, Hunsiker LG, Bain RP, Rohde RD, for the Collaborative Study Group. The effect of angiotensin-converting-enzyme inhibition on diabetic nephropathy. *N Engl J Med* 1993; **329**: 1456–62.
27. Marre M, Fabbri P, Bouhanick B, et al. Long-term follow-up of the glomerular filtration rate in normotensive type 1 diabetic subjects with microalbuminuria during angiotensin 1 converting enzyme inhibition. *Nephrol Dialysis Transplant* 1998; **13**: 1065–6.
28. Erley CM, Haefele U, Heyne N, Braun N, Risler T. Microalbuminuria in essential hypertension: reduction by different antihypertensive drugs. *Hypertension* 1993; **21**: 810–15.
29. Ravid M, Savin H, Jutrin et al. Long-term stabilizing effect of angiotensin converting enzyme inhibition on plasma creatinine and proteinuria in normotensive type II diabetic patients. *Ann Intern Med* 1993; **118**: 577–81.

30. Ravid M, Lang R, Rachmani R, Lishner M. Long-term renoprotective effect of angiotensin-converting enzyme inhibition in non-insulin-dependent diabetes mellitus. A 7-year follow-up study. *Arch Int Med* 1996; **156**: 286–9.
31. Mogensen CE. Microalbuminuria predicts clinical proteinuria and early mortality in maturity-onset diabetes. *N Engl J Med* 1984; **310**: 356–60.
32. UKPDS. Efficacy of atenolol and captopril in reducing risk of macrovascular and microvascular complications in type 2 diabetes: UKPDS 39. *Br Med J* 1998; **317**: 713–20.

18

Dietary Modifications in Patients with Diabetic Nephropathy

MONIKA TOELLER AND ANETTE E. BUYKEN

German Diabetes Research Institute at the Heinrich-Heine University,
Düsseldorf, Germany

This chapter deals with dietary modifications, particularly modifications of the protein intake, to retard the progression of diabetic renal disease. Specific nutritional aspects in persons requiring dialysis will not be covered.

MODIFICATION OF DIETARY PROTEIN INTAKE

Debates on the role of dietary protein intake for the onset or progression of diabetic renal disease commonly overlook the problem of high protein intake. Thus, before turning to protein restrictions, the practical relevance of high protein intake and its avoidance are addressed.

Avoidance of High Dietary Protein Intakes

High intakes of protein require increased renal excretory function and are associated with higher glomerular filtration rates (13, 18, 46). Clinical studies in persons with type 1 and type 2 diabetes reported adverse changes in renal function after the consumption of high-protein diets (1.4–3.5 g/kg body weight) for 1–4 weeks (22, 24, 26, 29). Furthermore, the Hoorn Study—a population-based, cross-sectional study conducted in persons

Diabetic Nephropathy. Edited by C. Hasslacher.
© 2001 John Wiley & Sons, Ltd.

with normal glucose tolerance, impaired glucose tolerance and people with type 2 diabetes—found an increased risk for microalbuminuria associated with higher protein intakes, independently of type 2 diabetes and hypertension (15). Similarly, in the EURODIAB Complications Study (10)—a clinic-based, cross-sectional study including 3250 European people with type 1 diabetes—higher protein intakes were related to higher levels of albumin excretion rate (AER) (37). The study demonstrated that mean AER remained < 20 µg/min in individuals with protein intakes up to 20% of total energy, while in those with a protein consumption > 20% of total energy, mean AER levels were in the microalbuminuric range (≥ 20 µg/min).

This finding confirmed the relevance of the current nutritional recommendation for people with diabetes not to exceed a protein intake of 20% of

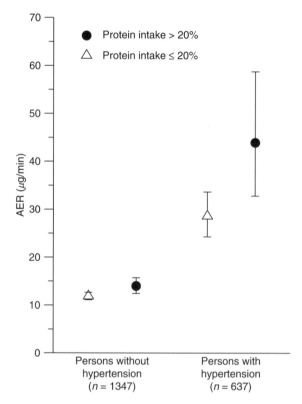

Figure 18.1 Geometric mean albumin excretion rate in individuals with protein intakes up to 20% of total energy (Δ) compared to subjects consuming more than 20% of protein (•): by strata of hypertension (< 135/85 mmHg vs. ≥ 135/85 mmHg or antihypertensive medication). Means are adjusted for energy intake, age, diabetes duration and HbA$_{1c}$ concentration.

total energy (8). In persons at specific risk for raised albuminuria, it appears particularly mandatory to direct more attention towards the avoidance of high protein intakes: results from the EURODIAB Complications Study suggest that protein intakes above 20% may be deleterious, specifically in those with hypertension ($\geq 160/95$ mmHg or antihypertensive medication) (37). When applying the recently proposed strict level for elevated blood pressure ($\geq 135/85$ mmHg) (11) to the EURODIAB cohort, AER was still markedly higher in hypertensive persons with type 1 diabetes who consumed more than 20% of protein (Figure 18.1).

Whereas high protein intakes are a common feature of affluent societies, persons with diabetes in Europe and North America generally consume even more protein than counterparts without diabetes (1, 7, 33, 35, 41). In the EURODIAB IDDM Complications Study, 22% of the European patients had a protein consumption above 20% of total energy (36). High protein intakes were observed in all European centres (Figure 18.2). Unanimously, about 70% of the protein was provided by animal sources. This animal protein intake corresponded to at least 10% of total energy (Figure 18.2), the lower level of the recommended range for total protein intake (8). However, specifically a higher consumption of animal protein appears to exert negative effects on renal function (9,17,21,37).

Generally, in routine visits, people with diabetes at risk for diabetic nephropathy and/or hypertension should be screened for high protein intakes (Table 18.2). Those individuals whose protein intake exceeds 20% of total energy should receive dietary advice from a dietician about how to avoid an undesirably high consumption of foods particularly rich in animal protein (Table 18.1).

Restriction of Dietary Protein Intake

Once renal function is disturbed, a restriction of dietary protein appears to retard the further progression of nephropathy. Such protective effects have been reported from virtually every animal model tested and were attributed to beneficial changes in renal haemodynamics, prevention of glomerular hypertrophy or reductions in further progression promoters of renal disease (proteinuria, hyperlipidaemia, eicosanoid production) (16).

However, evidence for persons with diabetes is less unequivocal. The long-term effect (≥ 6 months) of a low-protein diet on the progression of diabetic nephropathy has been investigated in a few small intervention studies, conducted predominantly in people with type 1 diabetes. Two cross-over studies in persons with type 1 diabetes suffering from clinically overt diabetic nephropathy reported beneficial effects on renal function after consuming a diet low (0.7 g protein/kg body weight) (42) or very low

Treatment and Prognosis

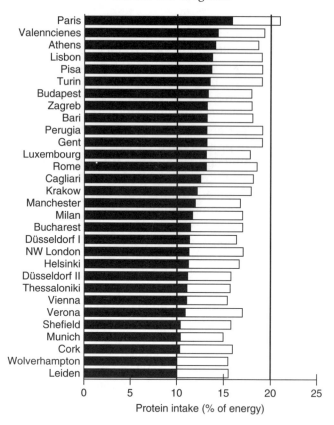

Figure 18.2 Animal protein (■) and vegetable protein (□) intake in 2868 persons with type 1 diabetes from 30 European centres. Solid vertical lines are upper and lower limits of dietary protein intake recommended for people with diabetes

(0.3–0.6 g protein/kg body weight) (2) in dietary protein (Table 18.3). However, concern has been raised that the long-term consumption of a diet with less than 0.6 g protein/kg body weight may cause protein undernutrition in persons with type 1 diabetes (4). Since malnutrition resembles a major predictor of mortality in those with end-stage renal disease (14), diets with 0.6 g protein/kg body weight or less are nowadays discouraged (8, 45).

Substantial benefits for the glomerular filtration rate or the urinary protein excretion after a long-term consumption of diets with 0.6 or 0.7 g protein/kg body weight were seen in three randomized controlled trials including macroalbuminuric persons with type 1 diabetes (5, 6, 46). In two further randomized controlled trials, a more moderate protein restriction (0.8 g/kg body weight) reduced the albuminuria of patients with micro- or macroalbuminuria (9, 30). Five of these studies (2, 6, 9, 42, 46) were included in a meta-analysis, from which Pedrini *et al* (25) concluded that a low-protein diet significantly slowed the progression of diabetic nephropathy (relative risk 0.56; 95% CI, 0.40–0.77). Results from a further meta-analysis

Table 18.1 Dietary modifications for prevention and treatment of diabetic nephropathy

---

When albumin excretion rate is still normal...
Avoid high protein intake, particularly high protein intake from animal sources
Keep protein intake within 10–20% of total energy
- Restrict the consumption of meat to one serving per day (~ 125 g)
- Consume cold meat and cheese in small amounts
- Two daily servings of milk or milk products are sufficient (e.g. one yoghurt and one glass of milk)
- Large amounts of curd should *not* be consumed
- Prefer consumption of protein from vegetable sources

When albumin excretion rate is raised and diabetic nephropathy suspected...
Reduce protein intake to target of 0.8 g/kg body weight/day (not below 0.6 g/kg body weight/day)
- Specific counselling by a trained dietitian based on individual needs and preferences is necessary

...and, in addition, blood pressure is elevated (≥ 130/80 mmHg)
If salt-sensitive, reduce salt intake to target of <6 g/day
- Avoid added salt
- Avoid obviously salted foods (particularly processed foods)
- Prefer meals cooked directly from natural ingredients
- Specific counselling by trained dietitian
- Monitoring of urinary sodium
If overweight, reduce body weight
- Avoid fasting and rapid or excessive weight loss
- Specific counselling by trained dietitian
Consume alcohol only in moderate quantities
- Women ≤ 15 g/day (one small glass of wine per day or equivalent of other drinks)
- Men ≤ 30 g/day (two small glasses of wine per day or equivalent of other drinks)
- For those on insulin or sulphonylureas: consume with a meal including carbohydrate

...and, in addition, serum cholesterol is elevated (total cholesterol > 185 mg/dl or LDL-cholesterol >115 mg/dl)
Restrict intakes of saturated fat and *trans*-fatty acids (< 10% of total energy) and dietary cholesterol intake (< 300 mg/day)
Substitute mono-unsaturated fat for saturated fat
Increase intake of fibre
- Choose meat, cold meat and sausage with a lower fat content
- Consume skimmed milk and fat-reduced milk products
- Restrict the consumption of high-fat snacks (potato chips, chocolate, etc.), cakes and cookies
- Prefer use of vegetable oils, particularly oils rich in mono-unsaturated fat
- Use fat and oils only in small quantities
- Consume five portions of vegetables or fruits per day
- Give preference to whole-meal or whole-grain cereals and cereal products

---

Based on recommendations from Diabetes and Nutrition Study Group (8), European Diabetes Policy Group (11, 12), WHO–International Society of Hypertension (44).

Table 18.2   Protein sources: how much dietary protein do they provide?

Protein source	Average protein content (g)
1 Serving of meat (120 g)	~ 25
1 Glass of milk (250 ml)	~ 8
1 Serving of yoghurt (150 g)	~ 5
2 Tablespoons of curd (60 g)	~ 8
1 Slice of cheese (Gouda, 45% fat) (30 g)	~ 8
1 Slice of pork sausage (30 g)	~ 5
1 Medium-sized slice of bread (60 g)	~ 4
2 Medium-sized potatoes (160 g)	~ 3
1 Serving vegetables (200 g)	~ 2

For a person with a (normal) body weight of 70 kg a protein restriction to 0.8 g protein per kg body weight corresponds to 55–60 g protein.

generally suggest only small benefits of low-protein diets for renal disease progression; however, the effect was found to be considerably greater in persons with type 1 diabetes as compared to people without diabetes (20).

Until now, in persons with type 2 diabetes, evidence for the effect of protein restriction on renal function is scarce. Two short-term intervention studies (4–5 weeks) suggested a beneficial role of protein restriction (0.6 or 0.7 g/kg body weight) in the treatment of overt nephropathy (32, 34). Only one recent randomized trial in persons with type 2 diabetes investigated the long-term effect of a protein restriction (0.8 g/kg body weight) on renal function in patients with microalbuminuria. However, the authors found it barely feasible to motivate persons with type 2 diabetes without overt nephropathy to substantially reduce their protein intake: on average, protein intake during the 28 months intervention was 1.10 g/kg body weight, as compared to 1.18 g/kg body weight at baseline. Nevertheless, after 12 months a 0.10 g/kg body weight change in the intake of protein was related to a 9% change in albuminuria (27); however, the effect was not sustained after 28 months of follow-up, neither was a beneficial influence on the course of the glomerular filtration rate observed (28).

Based on the current evidence, the European Diabetes Policy Group (11, 12) presently recommends a protein restriction with a target of 0.8 g/kg body weight (not below 0.6 g/kg body weight) for persons with type 1 diabetes when albumin excretion is raised and for people with type 2 diabetes when albumin excretion is raised and diabetic nephropathy is suspected.

For the clinical implementation of a protein consumption of 0.8 g/kg body weight, it should be recognized that in Europe and North America the vast majority of persons with both type 1 and type 2 diabetes consume more than twice as much dietary protein per day (1, 7, 33, 35, 36). Once persons with diabetes establish micro-or macroalbuminuria, protein intake remains simi-

Table 18.3 Clinical intervention studies in persons with type 1 diabetes investigating the effect of dietary protein on renal function

Reference	Design	Time period (months)	Patients	Protein intake	Assessment of protein intake	Effect on renal function
(2)	CO	CD: 17 LPD: 16	$n = 8$ (five men) Protein excretion: > 3.3 g/day Creatinine clearance: <45 ml/min	CD: 1.2–1.4 g/kg bw LPD: 0.3–0.6 g/kg bw	Urinary urea nitrogen measurements (daily)	CD: Creatinine clearance ⇓ LPD: Decline in creatinine clearance ⇓ Protein excretion ⇒
(42)	CO	CD: 12–39 LPD: 12–49	$n = 19$ Protein excretion: > 0.5 g/day GFR: >20 ml/min/ 1.73 m²	CD: 1.1 g/kg bw LPD: 0.7 g/kg bw	Dietary history and weighed food record (every 1–2 months) Urinary urea nitrogen measurements (every 3 months)	CD: GFR ⇒ AER ⇑ LPD: Decline in GFR ⇒ AER ⇓
(5)	RCT	CD: 12 LPD: 12	$n = 15$ AER: ≥ 30 µg/min Serum creatinine: ≤ 8 mg/dl	CD: 1.0 g/kg bw LPD: 0.6 g/kg bw	Dietary history Urinary urea nitrogen measurements (every 3 months)	CD: GFR ⇒ AER ⇑ Protein excretion ⇒ LPD: GFR ⇑ AER ⇒ Protein excretion ⇓
(6)	RCT	CD: 12 LPD: 5	$n = 16$ (9 men) Protein excretion: > 0.5 g/day Serum creatinine: < 1.9 mg/dl	CD: 1.4 g/kg bw LPD: 0.7 g/kg bw	Dietary interview (?) Urinary urea nitrogen measurements (periodically)	CD: GFR no difference AER ⇑ LPD: GFR no difference AER ⇓

continues

Table 18.3 (Continued)

Reference	Design	Time period (months)	Patients	Protein intake	Assessment of protein intake	Effect on renal function
(9)	RCT	CD: 24 LPD: 24	$n = 30$ (27 men) AER: 10–200 μg/min GFR: ≥ 90 ml/min/1.73 m^2	CD: 1.1 g/kg bw LPD: 0.8 g/kg bw	Diet history (every year) Urinary urea nitrogen measurements (every 4 months)	CD: GFR ⇓ AER no difference LPD: GFR ⇓ AER ⇓
(30)	RCT	CD: 6 LPD: 6	$n = 22$ (8 men) Protein excretion: > 0.3 g/day	CD: > 1.6 g/kg bw LPD: 0.8 g/kg bw	Diet history (every 3 months) Urinary urea nitrogen measurements (every 3 months)	CD: GFR ⇓ AER ⇑ LPD: GFR no difference AER ⇓
(46)	RCT	CD: > 12 LPD: > 12	$n = 35$ (21 men) Protein excretion: > 0.5 g/day	CD: ≥ 1.0 g/kg bw LPD: 0.6 g/kg bw	Diet history (every 3 months) Urinary urea nitrogen measurements (every 3 months)	CD: GFR ⇓ Protein excretion ⇑ LPD: decline in GFR ⇓ Protein excretion ⇓

CO, cross-over (non-randomized); RCT, randomized controlled trial; CD, control diet; LPD, low-protein diet; GFR, glomerular filtration rate; AER, albumin excretion rate.

larly high or increases even further (19, 23, 37, 38, 43). Therefore, people with raised albuminuria or overt nephropathy should first be screened by a trained dietitian for their protein intake (Table 18.2). If protein intake is undesirably high, the individual with diabetes should be advised to reduce protein intake towards the lower end of the recommended range (10–20% of total energy) (Table 18.2).

Specific dietary education is needed for a protein consumption of 0.8 g/kg body weight. Persons with nephropathy often find it difficult to maintain a low protein intake for a long time. Therefore, a protein restriction should be advised by skilled physicians and dietitians, seeking a balance between therapeutic needs and individual nutritional habits or preferences.

OTHER NUTRITIONAL MODIFICATIONS

The intake of dietary fat may also be related to diabetic nephropathy (3, 31, 45). In the EURODIAB Complications Study, albumin excretion rates of people with type 1 diabetes tended to decrease with higher intakes of mono-unsaturated fat (Figure 18.3). Hence, a modification of dietary fat

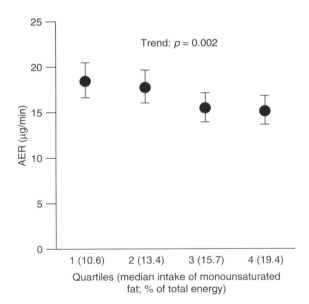

Figure 18.3 Geometric mean albumin excretion rate by quartiles of mono-unsaturated fat intake (% of energy). Means are adjusted for intakes of energy and protein (% of energy), age, diabetes duration, diastolic blood pressure and smoking habits (never, current, ex-)

intake, substituting mono-unsaturated fatty acids for saturated fatty acids, may directly contribute to a delayed progression of diabetic nephropathy. In addition, a modification and reduction of fat intake indirectly influences promoters of renal disease progression: a lower consumption of saturated fat and dietary cholesterol, together with an increased intake of dietary fibre, can beneficially affect the levels of both total and LDL-cholesterol and the risk for cardiovascular disease in people with diabetes (8, 39, 40). In practice, the substitution of vegetable protein for protein from animal sources also yields a desired modification of fat intake (Table 18.1).

As hypertension ranks among the most relevant progression promoters of nephropathy (16), people with diabetes who have an elevated blood pressure ($\geq 130/80$ mmHg) in addition to a raised albumin excretion rate should be encouraged to restrict their salt intake, reduce any overweight and consume alcohol only in moderate quantities (Table 18.1) (11, 12, 44).

REFERENCES

1. Alemzadeh R, Goldberg T, Fort P, Recker B, Lifshitz F. Reported dietary intakes of patients with insulin-dependent diabetes mellitus: limitations of dietary recall. *Nutrition* 1992; **8**: 87–93.
2. Barsotti G, Ciardella F, Morelli E et al. Nutritional treatment of renal failure in type 1 diabetic nephropathy. *Clin Nephrol* 1988; **29**: 280–87.
3. Bouhanick B, Suraniti S, Berrut G et al. Relationship between fat intake and glomerular filtration rate in normotensive insulin-dependent diabetic patients. *Diabet Metab* 1995; **21**: 168–72.
4. Brodsky IF, Robbins DC, Hiser E et al. Effects of low-protein diets on protein metabolism in insulin-dependent diabetes mellitus patients with early nephropathy. *J Clin Endocrinol Metab* 1992; **75**: 351–7.
5. Brouhard BH, LaGrone L. Effect of dietary protein restriction on functional renal reserve in diabetic nephropathy. *Am J Med* 1990; **89**: 427–31.
6. Ciavarella A, di Mizio G, Stefoni S, Borgnino LC, Vannini P. Reduced albuminuria after dietary protein restriction in insulin-dependent diabetic patients with clinical nephropathy. *Diabet Care* 1987; **10**: 407–13.
7. Close EJ, Wiles PG, Lockton JA et al. Diabetic diets and nutritional recommendations: what happens in real life? *Diabet Med* 1992; **9**: 181–8.
8. Diabetes and Nutrition Study Group of the European Association for the Study of Diabetes. Recommendations for the nutritional management of patients with diabetes mellitus. *Eur J Clin Nutr* 2000; **54**: 353–5.
9. Dullaart RP, Beusekamp BJ, Meijer S, van Doormaal JJ, Sluiter WJ. Long-term effects of protein-restricted diet on albuminuria and renal function in IDDM patients without clinical nephropathy and hypertension. *Diabet Care* 1993; **16**: 483–92.
10. EURODIAB Complications Study Group. Microvascular and acute complications in IDDM patients: the EURODIAB IDDM Complications Study. *Diabetologia* 1994; **37**: 278–85.

11. European Diabetes Policy Group 1998, International Diabetes Federation, European Region. A desktop guide to type 1 (insulin-dependent) diabetes mellitus. *Exp Clin Endocrinol Diabet* 1998; **106**: 240–69.
12. European Diabetes Policy Group 1999, International Diabetes Federation, European Region. A desktop guide to type 2 diabetes mellitus. *Diabet Med* 1999; **16**: 716–30.
13. Fioretto P, Trevisan R, Giorato C et al. Type I insulin-dependent diabetic patients show an impaired renal hemodynamic response to protein intake. *J Diabet Complic* 1988; **2**: 27–9.
14. Held PJ, Port FK, Turenne MN et al. Continous ambulatory peritoneal dialysis and hemodialysis: comparison of patient mortality with adjustment for comorbid conditions. *Kidney Int* 1994; **45**: 1163–9.
15. Hoogeveen EK, Kostense PJ, Jager A et al. Serum homocysteine level and protein intake are related to risk of microalbuminuria: the Hoorn Study. *Kidney Int* 1998; **54**: 203–9.
16. Jacobson HR (1991). Chronic renal failure: pathophysiology. *Lancet* **338**: 419–27.
17. Jibani MM, Bloodworth LL, Foden E, Griffiths KD, Galpin OP. Predominantly vegetarian diet in patients with incipient and early clinical diabetic nephropathy: effects on albumin excretion rate and nutritional status. *Diabet Med* 1991; **8**: 49–53.
18. Jones SL, Kontessis P, Wiseman M et al. Protein intake and blood glucose as modulators of GFR in hyperfiltering diabetic patients. *Kidney Int* 1992; **41**: 1620–28.
19. Kalk WJ, Osler C, Constable J, Kruger M, Panz V. Influence of dietary protein on glomerular filtration and urinary albumin excretion in insulin dependent diabetes. *Am J Clin Nutr* 1992; **56**: 169–73.
20. Kasiske BL, Lakatua JDA, Ma JZ, Louis TA. A meta-analysis of the effects of dietary protein restriction on the rate of decline in renal function. *Am J Kidney Dis* 1998; **31**: 954–61.
21. Kontessis PS, Bossinakaou I, Sarika L et al. Renal, metabolic and hormonal responses to proteins of different origin in normotensive, nonproteinuric type I diabetic patients. *Diabet Care* 1995; **18**: 1233–40.
22. Kupin W, Cortes P, Dumler F et al. Effect on renal function of change from high to moderate protein intake in type I diabetic patients. *Diabetes* 1987; **36**: 73–9.
23. Nyberg G, Norden G, Attman PO et al. Diabetic nephropathy: is dietary protein harmful? *J Diabet Compl* 1987; **1**: 37–40.
24. Pedersen MM, Mogensen CE, Jorgensen FS et al. Renal effects from limitation of high dietary protein in normoalbuminuric diabetic patients. *Kidney Int* 1989; **27**: 115–21S.
25. Pedrini MT, Levey AS, Lau J et al. The effect of dietary protein restriction on the progression of diabetic and nondiabetic renal diseases: a meta-analysis. *Ann Intern Med* 1996; **124**: 627–32.
26. Percheron C, Colette C, Astre C, Monnier L. Effects of moderate changes in protein intake on urinary albumin excretion in type I diabetic patients. *Nutrition* 1995; **11**: 345–9.
27. Pijls LTJ, de Vries H, Donker AJM, van Eijk JTM. The effect of protein restriction on albuminuria in patients with type 2 diabetes mellitus: a randomized trial. *Nephrol Dialysis Transpl* 1999; **14**: 1445–53.
28. Pijls LTJ, de Vries H, Donker AJM, van Eijk JTM. The effect of protein restriction on glomerular filtration rate and albuminuria; a randomised trial with 28 months follow-up. *Diabetologia* 1998; **41**: A46 (abstr).

29. Pomerleau J, Verdy M, Garrel DR, Houde Nadeau M. Effect of protein intake on glycaemic control and renal function in type 2 (non-insulin-dependent) diabetes mellitus. *Diabetologia* 1993; **36**: 829–34.
30. Raal FJ, Kalk WJ, Lawson M et al. Effect of moderate dietary protein restriction on the progression of overt diabetic nephropathy: a 6 month prospective study. *Am J Clin Nutr* 1994; **60**: 579–85.
31. Riley MD, Dwyer T. Microalbuminuria is positively associated with usual dietary saturated fat intake and negatively associated with usual dietary protein intake in people with insulin-dependent diabetes mellitus. *Am J Clin Nutr* 1998; **67**: 50–57.
32. Shichiri M, Nishio Y, Ogura M, Marumo F. Effect of low-protein, very-low-phosphorus diet on diabetic renal insufficiency with proteinuria. *Am J Kidney Dis* 1991; **18**: 26–32.
33. Shimakawa T, Herrera-Acena MG, Colditz GA et al. Comparison of diets of diabetic and nondiabetic women. *Diabet Care* 1993; **16**: 1356–62.
34. Sugimoto T, Kikkawa R, Haneda M, Shigeta Y. Effect of dietary protein restriction on proteinuria in non-insulin diabetic patients with nephropathy. *J Nutr Sci Vitaminol* 1991; **37**: S87–92.
35. Toeller M. Diet and Diabetes. *Diabet Metab Rev* 1993; **9**: 93–108.
36. Toeller M, Klischan A, Heitkamp G et al, and the EURODIAB IDDM Complications Study Group Nutritional intake of 2868 IDDM patients from 30 centres in Europe. *Diabetologia* 1996; **39**: 929–39.
37. Toeller M, Buyken A, Heitkamp G et al, and the EURODIAB IDDM Complications Study Group. Protein intake and urinary albumin excretion rates in the EURODIAB IDDM Complications Study. *Diabetologia* 1997; **40**: 1219–26.
38. Toeller M, Buyken AE. Protein intake—new evidence for its role in diabetic nephropathy. *Nephrol Dialysis Transpl* 1998; **13**: 1926–7.
39. Toeller M, Buyken AE, Heitkamp G et al, and the EURODIAB IDDM Complications Study Group. Fiber intake, serum cholesterol and cardiovascular disease in European individuals with type 1 diabetes. *Diabet Care* 1999a; **22** (2): B21–8.
40. Toeller M, Buyken AE, Heitkamp G et al, and the EURODIAB IDDM Complications Study Group. Associations of fat and cholesterol intake with serum lipid levels and cardiovascular disease: The EURODIAB IDDM Complications Study. *Exp Clin Endocrinol Diabet* 1999b; **107**: 512–21.
41. Virtanen SM, Räsänen L, Mäenpää J, Akerblom HK. Dietary survey of Finnish adolescent diabetics and non-diabetic controls. *Acta Paediatr Scand* 1987; **76**: 801–8.
42. Walker JD, Bending JJ, Dodds RA et al. Restriction of dietary protein and progression of renal failure in diabetic nephropathy. *Lancet* 1989; **2**: 1411–15.
43. Watts GF, Gregory L, Naoumova R, Kubal C, Shaw KM. Nutrient intake in insulin dependent diabetic patients with incipient nephropathy. *Eur J Clin Nutr* 1988; **42**: 697–702.
44. World Health Organization-International Society of Hypertension. World Health Organization—International Society of Hypertension guidelines for the management of hypertension. *J Hypertens* 1999; **17**: 151–83.
45. World Health Organization. Report of a Joint FAO/WHO/UNU Expert Consultation. Energy and protein requirements. *WHO Tech Rep Ser* 1985; **724**.
46. Zeller K, Whittaker E, Sullivan L, Raskin P, Jacobson HR. Effect of restricting dietary protein on the progression of renal failure in patients with insulin dependent diabetes mellitus. *N Engl J Med* 1991; **324**: 78–84.

19

Training of Patients with Diabetic Nephropathy

BIRGIT ADAM AND CHRISTOPH HASSLACHER

St Josefskrankenhaus, Heidelberg, Germany

INTRODUCTION

The patient plays a crucial role in the management of chronic illnesses, since carrying out the treatment instituted by the physician becomes part of his/her everyday life. The patient him/herself should thus become active in the treatment process with a self-determined role. As shown by diabetes mellitus throughout the world, this leads to better results of treatment, more patient satisfaction and therefore to an overall improvement in the prognosis and the quality of life.

By intensive training, the patient acquires the necessary competence and assurance in self-treatment. This is an absolute prerequisite, not only in primary prevention, but also in preventing the secondary illnesses typical of diabetes. Training the nephropathy patient makes high demands not only on the patient but also on the training team. The reasons for this are multifarious:

1. Special features in the metabolic situation in progressive stage of nephropathy: there is a major rise in the risk of hypoglycaemia in consequence of the reduced renal excretion of numerous substances that lower blood glucose or as a result of reduced insulin catabolism. Disorders of lipid metabolism also occur. In addition, the protein intake must be normalized or indeed reduced.

Diabetic Nephropathy. Edited by C. Hasslacher.
© 2001 John Wiley & Sons, Ltd.

2. As a rule, a hypertension develops that is often difficult to control. This requires regular self-checks of blood pressure and possibly self-medication by the patient.
3. There is increasing mental stress resulting from the spectre of impending dialysis and from the often serious complications contingent on macro-angiopathy (coronary heart disease, arterial occlusive disease), retino-pathy and/or neuropathy (gastroparesis, orthostatic hypertension).

Outlines of potential training programmes, as well as their structure and contents, will be set out below. The contents relate specifically to diabetic nephropathy. The general topics imparted in basic training will not be dealt with here.

TRAINING STRUCTURE

Both individual and group training are feasible alternatives. Experience from general diabetes training indicates that a combination of both is more likely to be successful. In patients with kidney diseases passing through various stages, additional training attuned to the individual course of the disease and personal factors is therefore especially appropriate. Group training is advantageous to impart generally relevant knowledge. It is also less time-consuming and less staff-intensive in relation to the individual patient. Furthermore, it generates the desired group-dynamic effects.

Since such intensive management is required, the group size should not exceed eight patients. Participation of family members or friends of the patients is an advantage, because they are in an especially good position to support or carry out the necessary health-related activities (e.g. measure-ment of blood pressure) or behavioural changes (nutrition) in the patient's home.

The time scale of a training programme should comprise a maximum of two to three units of instruction per day (theory and practice).

TRAINING PROGRAMMES AND TOPICS

Since the clinical picture of diabetic nephropathy changes in the course, different priorities are required in the training programmes. An appropriate classification is:

1. *Training programme for patients with incipient or clinically manifest nephropathy (microalbuminuria and macroalbuminuria).* The topics of the training programme in these patients are listed in Table 19.1. It is important not only that the topics are discussed in theory, but also that the everyday relevance of the topics treated is brought home to the patient as often as possible by practical exercises. The practical knowledge imparted includes:
   - Learning methods of self-observation (nutrition, exercise, amount of fluid drunk, smoking, etc.).
   - Introduction and practice of self-checks of blood pressure.
   - Drawing up of a diet plan that takes individual lifestyle into consideration.
   - Practical exercises and demonstrations, illustrated with meals and examples of foods.
   - Chiropody and foot gymnastics.

   In patients with preterminal renal failure, the special aspects of nutrition (calorie intake, protein intake, electrolyte and fluid intake) and the various possibilities of renal replacement therapy (different dialysis techniques, transplantation) should be discussed beyond the context of the training topics in Table 19.1.

2. *Training programme for patients with renal replacement therapy.* Table 19.2 lists the training topics in diabetic patients already carrying out a form of renal replacement therapy. Imparting practical knowledge is also of very great importance, facilitating its implementation in the patients' everyday life (see above).

Besides acquiring knowledge and practical skills by training, special attention should also be paid to psychosocial counselling on coping with the illness. As a rule, realizing that one has a chronic illness is a dramatic insight for every person afflicted. It entails a crisis in the individual life history that affects the way the rest of life is planned.

Besides the inherent difficulties of having diabetes, acknowledgement of a life-long dependence on one of the forms of kidney replacement therapy is an additional factor in chronic renal failure. Psychological problems in tackling and coping with this situation are frequent. Relationship crises in couples and within the family, as well as social isolation, interfere with effective performance. Such crises thus also affect the trainability of chronically ill patients. Long-term psychosocial care is often required in order to enable diabetics to deal with the stress and mostly increasing secondary problems of the disease.

Table 19.1 Training programme in diabetes mellitus with incipient and clinically manifest nephropathy

---

- *Structure and function of the kidneys*
- *Signs and diagnosis of diabetic nephropathy*: Excretion of albumin, serum creatinine, creatinine clearance, blood pressure characteristics, 24 h urine, serum urea, etc.
- *Individual stages of nephropathy*: induction of damage, stages of diabetic nephropathy, additional risk factors (smoking, disorders of lipid metabolism)
- *Possibilities of therapy in incipient or clinically manifest nephropathy*: pharmacotherapy and non-pharmacotherapy
- *Hypertension*: influence, therapy, self-measurement, target values
- *Nutrition in diabetic nephropathy (microalbuminuria, macroalbuminuria)*: healthy nutrition according to the International Nutrition Societies' advice with regard to nutrition in the various stages of nephropathy
- *Special features in diabetic nephropathy*: hypoglycaemic episodes, contrast media, nephrotoxic medication, urinary tract infections, etc.
- *Diagnosis and possibilities of treatment in secondary diseases*: treatment of neuropathy, retinopathy, AOD, diabetic foot syndrome
- *Dealing with secondary illnesses*: experience of the illness, motivation for treatment, self-responsibility. Formulation and evaluation of the patient's own treatment aspirations

---

Table 19.2 Training programme in diabetes with renal replacement therapy

---

- *Possible treatments in renal replacement therapy*: methods in renal replacement therapy, advantages, disadvantages
- *Dietary treatment in renal failure*: energy and nutrient intake, electrolyte intake, fluid intake, vitamins
- *Hypertension*: influence, therapy, self-measurement, target values
- *Diabetes and dialysis*: diabetes therapy in various methods of dialysis
- *Special features in renal replacement techniques*: shunt care, dialysis and travel, medication, etc.
- *Living with dialysis*: coping with chronic illnesses, living with the "machine", self-help groups
- *Perspectives with regard to kidney transplantation*: indication, type of transplant, rejection, medication
- *Treatment of other secondary illnesses*: diabetes-specific secondary illnesses, complications resulting from chronic renal failure (anemia, hyperparathyroidism, etc.)
- *Dialysis and social matters*: severe handicap identity card, sickness benefit, reimbursement of travel costs, occupational retraining, financial assistance, etc.

THE TRAINING TEAM

The diversity of the individual topics described requires a well-trained team of instructors. The team should comprise participants from the following fields: physicians, diabetes counsellors/dietary assistants, psychologists, special nurses (dialysis nurses). Social counsellors, physiotherapists and chiropodists are important for additional support.

SUMMARY

Diabetologists and nephrologists have discussed and drawn up interdisciplinary concepts and cooperation models for treating diabetic nephropathy. The need to train patients has been acknowledged. However, there has been no general practical implementation of this up to now. It will be an important task in the future to achieve further optimization of treatment in kidney patients.

20

Endstage Renal Failure in Diabetes Mellitus: Special Problems of Treatment and Monitoring

MARTIN ZEIER

University of Heidelberg, Heidelberg, Germany

INTRODUCTION

There has been a remarkable increase in the number of diabetic patients, mostly of type 2, admitted to renal replacement therapy. Significant differences in frequencies of uraemic diabetic patients between European countries are observed. In some regions of Germany the numbers of newly admitted diabetic patients to renal replacement therapy are as high as those reported for Caucausians in the USA, whereas in Southern Europe (e.g. Italy, France) these figures are markedly less (13,25). It is of great practical importance to distinguish the insulin-dependent type 1 diabetic patient (who could benefit from pancreas or islet transplantation) and the diabetic patient with normal or high circulating insulin levels to which their tissues, are resistant. Because type 2 diabetes is much more prevalent in the general population (85–90%) the high prevalence of type 2 diabetes in patients admitted in endstage renal failure is not surprising. The renal risk, however, is equivalent in both type 1 and type 2 diabetes. The cumulative prevalence of proteinuria and, in proteinuric patients, the prevalence of renal failure, is similar in both type 1 and type 2 diabetes (14).

Diabetic Nephropathy. Edited by C. Hasslacher.
© 2001 John Wiley & Sons, Ltd.

EVALUATION OF THE DIABETIC PATIENT WITH PRETERMINAL RENAL FAILURE

The evaluation of the diabetic patient with preterminal renal failure has several assignments to estimate the progression rate of renal failure. The natural history of progression of diabetic nephropathy is described in detail elsewhere in this volume but concomitant renal diseases may influence the history of diabetic nephropathy. Some of this coincident kidney diseases are listed below.

Ischaemic Renal Disease

In addition, a minority of patients suffer from specific renal problems together with the coexisting diabetic nephropathy. Renal ischaemia or atherosclerotic renal atery stenosis is much more common in diabetics than was previously assumed (32). In this case one should be cautious regarding ACE-inhibitors or angiotensin receptor blocking antihypertensives. Frequent control of s-creatinine, s-potassium and bodyweight is mandatory. A two-fold increase in s-creatinine should prompt the physician to stop this type of medication.

Urinary Tract Infection

Urinary tract infection frequently led to renal parychematous infection with purulent papillary necrosis and intrarenal abscess formation. This is now rare due to the frequent use of antibiotics and the better management of urinary tract infection. Urinary tract infection may be frequent in diabetics, especially when residual urine is present.

Glomerulonephritis

Glomerulonephritis, particularly membranous glomerulonephritis, is thought to be more frequent in diabetics, but this has not been not supported by other studies.

Acute Renal Failure

Diabetic patients with nephropathy are exceptionally susceptible for acute renal failure after administration of radiocontrast media (36), the risk being similar with ionic and non-ionic materials. The risk may be reduced by fluid administration and a temporary stop of diuretics. In patients with severly elevated serum-creatinine a dialysis procedure immediately after the radiographic procedure is warranted, without any delay in time.

Hydroxyethyl starch and ACE inhibitors also cause deterioration of renal function in diabetic patients, especially in those with congestive heart failure (28).

RENAL REPLACEMENT THERAPY IN DIABETIC PATIENTS WITH ENDSTAGE RENAL FAILURE

Haemodialysis: Optimal Start of Dialysis in the Patient with Diabetic Nephropathy

It is generally accepted that renal replacement therapy should be considered at a creatinine-clearance of approximately 9–14 ml/min in non-diabetic uraemic patients (15). It is now accepted that in the patient with diabetic nephropathy, dialysis should be started at a higher residual renal function than in non-diabtetic patients with renal insufficiency (30). In any case, dialysis should be started before the clinical status deteriorates, secondary to fluid overload, malnutrition, hyperkalaemia and infection. This is usually the case when the GFR declines below 20 ml/min. Diabetic patients with progression to endstage renal failure must be seen on a regular basis by a nephrologist. Repeated control of residual renal function by creatinine-clearance (24 h specimen collection) and 24 h urine for urea excretion to determine the magnitude of malnutrition are of great importance. Vascular access surgery (usually arteriovenous fistula) some months before the initiation of the dialysis treatment helps to avoid central venous lines and its concomitant complications. Blood drawing for regular serum chemistry is restricted to the dorsal hand veins only. If these guidelines are accepted, vascular grafts (e.g. PTFE) are inevitable.

Prognosis of Patients with Diabetic Nephropathy on Haemodialysis and Assessing the Adequacy of Haemodialysis

In the past, the prognosis for diabetic nephropathy was discouraging, with 77% of patients dying within 10 years after the onset of persistent proteinuria. Despite some improvement, diabetics do fare worse on renal replacement therapy than non-diabetics, athough patient survival has continously increased in recent years. In a matched control study, actuarial 5 year survival in diabetics is worse than in matched non-diabetic dialysis patients and this difference has not diminished in recent years (31). According to the EDTA report of 1991, the actuarial 5 year survival between 1985 and 1990 was 38% in 45–54 year old type 1 diabetics vs. 70% in age-matched non-diabetic patients. Similar figures were noted for type 2 diabetics in the age group 55–64 years with an actuarial 5 year survival of 31% vs. 58% in age matched non-diabetic dialysis patients (29).

This is in agreement with the data of the Collaborative Transplant Study (courtesy of Professor Opelz), where overall patient and graft survival is worse in diabetic renal transplant recipients than in non-diabetics. This, however, contrasts the experience of some major centres with particular experience in diabetic patients who currently find no difference (23).

Cardiovascular disease and serious infections are the major causes of death in haemodialysed and transplanted diabetics. Despite recent improvement, rehabilitation of haemodialysed diabetics continues to be inferior to that of non-diabetics. Improvement of survival is a matter of reduction of cardiovascular death and infection.

Cardiovascular Death and Adequacy of Dialysis

Cardiac death is strongly predicted by a history of vascular disease (peripheral vascular and/or carotid), myocardial infarction and angina pectoris. Proliferative retinopathy and polyneuropathy were associated with an increased cardiac risk, in the latter possibly due to an imbalance of autonomic cardiac innervation. Hypotensive cardiac episodes during dialysis are also predictive for cardiac death.

This has major implications for hemodialysis procedures with low ultrafiltration rates and prolonged duration of dialysis sessions (24). In practice, ultrafiltration in diabetics should not exceed more than 500–600 ml/h on haemodialysis. This means dialysis session of more than 4 h and in larger patients of more than 5 h hemodialysis three times per week.

The intensity of dialysis is an issue which is currently under discussion. Guidelines have been created to assure adequate dialysis. Although the measurement of the "dose of dialysis" is difficult, the DOQI (8) (Dialysis Outcomes Quality Initiative) for adequate dialysis are summarized. According to DOQI, a Kt/V (indicator for adequacy of dialysis, where K is the dialyser clearance rate, t the net duration of dialysis and V the corrected body volume) of above 1.2 (e.g. a 70 kg patient dialysed for 5 h) is adequate. Lower Kt/V, especially below 1, is associated with a higher mortality rate and this is particularly true for the patient with diabetic nephropathy. Besides adequate dialysis the following factors must be considered to improve the survival of diabetics on dialysis.

Special Problems of Diabetic Patients on Haemodialysis

Vascular Access

It is often more difficult to establish vascular access in a diabetic patient because of poor arterial inflow (atherosclerosis, media calcification of the artery) and venous run-off (hypoplasia or thrombosed veins) in chronically ill patients, with numerous stays in hospital. Arterio-venous anastomosis should be placed in the upper forearm to maintain adequate shunt blood flow. It is therefore advisable to establish vascular access early, when creatinine clearance is above 20–25 ml/min. In malnourished, older individuals, this level of GFR impairment can be reached even at a serum-creatinine of 2 mg/dl.

One should patiently wait for maturing of the fistula: early puncture tends to be associated with haematoma formation, scarring, stenosis and thrombosis and should be avoided, even if dialysis has to be performed by a central venous catheter. Some authors have reported poor functioning of the vascular access in diabetics, with only 64% of fistula functioning after 1 year compared to 83% in non-diabetics (1).

Metabolic Control on Renal Replacement Therapy

In clinical practice, the need for insulin decreases upon the institution of maintenance haemodialysis. The insulin supplementation remains complex because of the prolongation of the insulin half-life in uraemic patients and the confounding effects of reduced food intake (anorexia of renal failure) and of refeeding (during the haemodialysis session). Most nephrologists prefer to dialyse against glucose (200 mg/dl) to achieve better stabilization of plasma glucose concentrations. One must consider, however, that glucose-containing dialysate does not guarantee normoglycaemia if the prescribed insulin dose is too high. Oral sulphonylurea must be avoided, in fact is strictly forbidden, because of prolonged hypoglycaemia in endstage renal failure (22). If glucose-free dialysate is used, glucose loss (amounting to 80–100 g per dialysis session) may occur. It has been argued that the glucose loss into the dialysate contributes to catabolism but no convincing evidence for this was produced in a control trial (9).

Diabetic control is occasionally rendered difficult by diabetic gastroparesis and the tendency of gastric motility to deteriorate acutely during dialysis sessions.

Adequate control of glycaemia is important: hyperglycaemia causes intense thirst and subsequent increased fluid intake, as well as osmotic water shift and shift of potassium from the intracellular to the extracellular space, with the attending risk of circulatory and pulmonary congestion and hyperkalaemia. Poorly controlled diabetics are also more susceptible to infection.

Intradialytic and Interdialytic Blood Pressure

Blood pressure in the diabetic is primarily volume-dependent. Consequently, hypertension tends to be more common in dialysed diabetics, who have higher predialytic blood pressures, are more frequently on antihypertensive drugs and more often require multidrug therapy than non-diabetic uraemic patients. The problem is compounded by the fact that intradialytic hypotension is more frequent in diabetics; as a consequence it is often difficult to reach the target dry weight. On the other hand, interdialytic weight by excessive fluid intake is associated with survival on dialysis (20).

Intradialytic hypotension is a multifactorial problem; inadequate circulatory adjustment to volume subtraction (as a consequence of autonomous polyneuropathy) and left ventricular diastolic malfunction (necessitating higher left ventricular filling pressures) have both been implicated in its genesis. Hypotensive episodes have been associated with an increased risk of sudden cardiac death, acute myocardial ischaemia, deterioraton of maculopathy and non-thrombotic mesenteric ischaemia.

Treatment of Lipid Abnormalities in Diabetic Patients with Renal Failure

In diabetic patients, prospective studies have shown that hypercholesterolaemia and hypertriglyceridaemia are strong predictors of coronary heart disease (12). Major dyslipidaemia is seen only in untreated type 1 diabetic patients. A strong correlation exists between HbA_{1c} and plasma cholesterol, triglyceride and high density lipoproteins (34). In type 2 diabetes, dyslipidaemia persists even when glycosaemia is well controlled, presumably due to an underlying genetic defect which predisposes to both diabetes and disturbed lipid metabolism (21).

In a prospective study (37), a relationship between coronary risk and cholesterol concentrations in diabetics admitted for hemodialysis has been established. Non-accumulating fibrates or HMG-Co-reductase inhibitors are indicated for the treatment of dyslipidaemia which does not respond to dietary manipulation. Regular control of creatinine kinase (rhabdomyolysis) is recommended.

Erythropoietin and Iron Substitution in Uraemic Diabetic Patients

Left ventricular hypertrophy (LVH) is more prevalent in diabetics compared to non-diabetics with endstage renal disease, and it is possible that the beneficial effects of erythropoietin on LVH could be particularly relevant for diabetic patients (18).

To date, the effects of erythropoietin on peripheral vascular disease and microangiopathic complications associated with diabetes have not been systematically assessed. The possible benefits of an improved oxygen supply to target areas require further study. Several case reports indicate that anaemia may develop in diabetic patients prior to preterminal renal failure.

Currently, there is no reason to recommend a different target haemaglobin for diabetic and non-diabetic patients; a haemoglobin of 11–12 g/dl is therefore also appropriate for diabetic patients.

Attention must be paid to the rate at which the haemoglobin is increased in diabetic patients. These patients are particularly at risk of adverse effects related to rapid expansion of the red cell mass and the impact of such expansion on blood volume and viscosity. Furthermore, glycosylation of erythropoietin can modify the erythropoietin clearance rate.

Increases in blood pressure, vascular access clotting and even seizures have been observed more frequently in diabetic dialysis patients when haemoglobin was increased too rapidly. A suggested mode of correction of anaemia in diabetic patients is as follows: a cautious dosage of erythropoietin (initial dose of 2000 IU three times weekly, followed by increments of 2000 IU at monthly intervals) and careful adjustment of heparinization during dialysis. If haemoglobin increases by > 1.3 g/dl over 2 weeks, the erythropoietin dose should be reduced. Once the target haemoglobin has been reached, the weekly dosage should be reduced and haemoglobin monitored at regular intervals.

It is important to establish adequate iron substitution in erythropoietin-treated dialysed diabetic patients. Gastrointestinal blood loss must be excluded, particularly in diabetic patients who receive anticoagulants for vascular complications. Anorexia and malnutrition are further factors for low plasma iron levels. In clinical practice intravenous iron substitution, at the end of the dialysis procedure, is safe and effective. A target ferritin level of above 250 mg/dl is advisable. During infection episodes, however, iron substitution should temporarily be stopped.

Malnutrition in Dialysis-dependent Diabetics

It is important that diabetic patients on dialysis maintain adequate energy (35–40 kcal/kg/day). In addition, protein intake should not be below 1.3 g/kg day because of the known higher protein requirements of dialysis patients. Anorexia and prolonged habituation to dietary restrictions are important reasons for malnutrition of the diabetic patient on dialysis. Malnutrition is a common concern in dialysed diabetic patients.

Infections in Uraemic Diabetic Patients

Bacterial infections are common complications in uraemic diabetic patients (19), in whom polymorphnuclear leukocyte function is depressed, particularly when acidosis is present. Leukocyte adherence, chemotaxis and phagocytosis may be affected. Antioxidant systems involved in bactericidal activity may also be impaired. Cutaneous responses to antigen challenges and measures of T cell function may be depressed. There is evidence that improving glycaemic control in diabetic patients improves immune function, e.g. the efficiency of intracellular killing of microorganisms may improve with better glycaemic control. Blood glucose levels should be closely controlled in diabetic patients with infections.

Uraemic diabetics have several particular sites where infections can occur: arteriovenous fistula and central venous catheters, CAPD catheter, urinary tract, sinus and diabetic foot ulcer. Infections of the dialysis access, either haemodialysis or CAPD, are mostly caused by *Staphylococcus* and need specific therapy. Diabetic patients with prolonged hospital stay should be screened for methicillin-resistant *Staphylococcus*, an emerging problem.

Urinary tract infections are common in diabetic dialysis patients due to diminishing residual diuresis, imcomplete bladder emptying from autonomic neuropathy and following diagnostic or therapeutical instrumentation of the urethra or bladder.

Chronic sinus infections may be detected by X-ray and should be treated by antibiotics and if necessary drainage. Diabetic foot infection is detected by routine foot inspection and should be avoided by appropriate prophylaxis.

Diabetic Retinopathy in Uraemic Diabetic Patients

Diabetic retinopathy is the leading cause of blindness in patients 25–74 years of age, and current estimates suggest it is responsible for 12 000–24 000 new cases of blindness in the USA each year (7). It is subdivided into non-proliferative retinopathy and proliferative retinopathy. Proliferative retinopathy is associated with haemorrhagic activity of retinal neovascularization. The presence of and severity of neovascularization are the factors with the strongest association with visual loss. Anticoagulation (heparin) during the haemodialysis procedure and the application of platelet aggregation inhibitors (e.g. aspirin) can cause severe retinal bleeding and blindness.

Diabetic uraemic patients need regular ophthalmologic controls at a frequency of 3–6 months.

In the past, visual prognosis in the dialysed diabetic was extremely poor. Diabetic patients beginning dialysis between 1966 and 1971 had a 29% risk of becoming blind and vision was lost in 41% of eyes at risk. These figures have improved in parallel with improvement of dialysis procedures and better control of blood pressure: patients admitted between 1976 and 1979 had only a 1% risk of amaurosis. This documents the overriding roles of blood pressure control and prophylactic laser treatment.

Bone Disease and the Importance of Serum-phosphate Control

Bone formation and turnover are generally diminished and osteopenia is common in patients with type 1 diabetes without nephropathy, but not in the type 2 diabetic patients (38). In the uraemic diabetic, serum parathyroid hormone levels tend to be low. Relative hyposecretion of parathyroid hormone may therefore account for the common observation of low trabecular volume and low cellular activity on the bone trabecules. This low bone turnover may explain the fact that diabetics are more likely to accumulate aluminium in their bones (2).

The diabetic uraemic should be treated with calcium-containing phosphate binders, which are ingested with every meal (500–1000 mg according to the amount of food). Aluminium-containing phosphate binders should be avoided because of possible aluminium intoxication. Vitamin D supplementation (e.g. 10 000 U 25-(OH) vitamin D_3 once weekly) is recommended.

Serum-phosphate control is important not only to prevent renal bone disease, but to prevent stiffness of the large arterial vessels. Increased stiffness of the aorta (4) is associated with reduced survival in endstage renal disease and vascular stiffness is correlated with the increase in serum-phosphate.

Continuous Ambulatory Peritoneal Dialysis (CAPD) in Diabetic Patients

CAPD has both medical and social benefits and most patients with diabetes are eligible for it. This technique enables patients to stay at home, where they can rapidly be taught the home dialysis regime and allows flexibility in treatment. The medical benefits of CAPD include slow and sustained ultrafiltration and a relative absence of rapid fluid and electrolyte changes and preservation of residual renal function. The choice of the dialysis therapy depends on such factors as nephrologist's bias, existence of extrarenal disease (visual capacity which enables the patient to perform the bag exchanges properly), treatment availability and other medical and social factors.

In CAPD the major osmotic agent for water removal is glucose. It is therefore of note to consider an extra amount of glucose (approximately

600–800 kcal) per treatment-day in the uraemic diabetic. Insulin dosage has to be adjusted. Some authors propose that insulin be administered via the CAPD fluid. This route of application is not without difficulties, because adsorption of insulin into the CAPD bag and possible infection by instillation of insulin into the bag are possible.

Assessing the Quality of Dialysis in CAPD

Adequacy of dialysis is an important issue in CAPD as well as in haemodialysis. In the past years several studies were undertaken to correlate the dose of dialysis (e.g. adequacy of dialysis) and survival in the CAPD patient population. According to the DOQI guidelines, which are based on numerous studies (6), a weekly *k t/V* of 2 or even more (weekly peritoneal creatinine clearance of more than 70 l) is nowadays considered an adequate dose of dialysis. In most patients this is only achievable when a certain amount of peritoneal fluid (more than 50 l/week) and a considerable residual renal function are combined. This has two implications: (a) CAPD in diabetic patients should be started early (as in haemodialysis, at a creatinine clearance of approximately 20 ml/min); and (b) residual renal function has to be monitored vigorously. If there is a substantial fall in residual renal function (below 5 ml/min), in many cases adequate peritoneal dialysis is impossible. Inadequate peritoneal dialysis has a high mortality rate (6) and patients must be taken off peritoneal dialysis and either transfered to haemodialysis or, if possible, transplanted.

RENAL AND PANCREAS TRANSPLANTATION

In the meantime, studies have shown that besides the improvement in quality of life, there is also better survival in uraemic patients post-transplantation (5,26,33). Despite these encouraging data, acturarial patient survival post-transplant is less favourable in diabetes compared to other primary renal diseases. It is indispensable to examine a diabetic uraemic thoroughly for vascular complications and infectious foci before the patient qualifies for the transplant waiting list.

Pretransplant Evalulation of the Uraemic Diabetic Patient

In the pretransplant evaluation of a diabetic patient, several aspects should be considered. Most important is the vascular tree, the Achilles' heel of every successful transplantation procedure.

Careful evaluation of pelvic and lower extremity arteries must be performed. Non-invasive methods (e.g. Doppler and Duplex techniques) as well as invasive procedures (e.g. angiography) may be applied. If the patient has a considerable residual renal function, CO_2 angiography or magnetic resonance angiography are the procedures of choice. Plain radiography of the pelvis documents the magnitude of media calcification in the uraemic diabetic (4).

Coronary artery disease is an important issue in diabetic patients on dialysis. Non-invasive testing is often not substantial (16) and coronary angiography is still the most helpful procedure to rule out severe coronary stenosis in this patient population. Additional information on cardiac valves are no less important, since aortic stenosis is a common problem in dialysis patients.

Before transplantation, peripheral vascular surgery is mandatory, particularly on the ipsilateral side of the graft, to avoid circulatory complications of the lower extremities post-transplant.

Cardiac surgery (bypass or valve replacement) is nowadays a common procedure in non-diabetic and diabetic patients with an in-hospital mortality rate of 5.4% (17), which is roughly comparable to those of non-uraemic cardiac patients.

Chronic infections are common in diabetic patients and several sites of infection in diabetic patients have to be considered (see above). Infection of the native kidneys may be due to renal calculi or papillary necrosis and secondary obstruction, and infection of the bladder is often due to multiresistant bacteria.

Cholecystolithiasis is common in diabetics and recurrent cholecystitis should be an indication for cholecystectomy. Uraemic patients often suffer from chronic constipation and colonic diverticula are common. In female diabetic patients, gynaecological infections or tumours must be excluded by bacteriological work-up and cytology.

RESULTS

Since the introduction of cyclosporin, graft survival has improved continously for diabetic and non-diabetic transplant recipients. Thorough pretransplant work-up of the diabetic patient, as mentioned above, has led to an almost identical 1 year patient survival post-transplant in specialized centres (23).

The effect of glucose control is important for patient and transplant long-term function. Mesangial expansion has been shown in transplanted kidneys in type 1 diabetics but several studies have documented beneficial effects of combined pancreas transplantation on the renal allograft (3). The transplantation of a pancreas with normalization of glucose metabolism makes lesions of diabetic nephropathy in native kidneys reversible (10,11). Glucose control for the prevention of extrarenal diabetic lesions (vascular, neuropathic) by successful pancreas transplantation is documented by several studies (27, 35).

In the future, new techniques such as insulin gene manipulation in autologous cells (e.g. myoblasts, hepatocytes or fibroblasts) or islet cell transplantation will be the procedure of choice. Such grafts are currently technically feasible in patients who are recipients of other, usually renal, grafts. Another possibility is to graft encapsulated xeno-islets, protected against immune attack by encapsulation in a biocompatible membrane.

REFERENCES

1. Martin LC, Lewin NW, Smith DW. Hemodialysis access site morbidity. *Proc Clin Dialysis Transpl Forum* **10**: 277–82.
2. Andres DL, Kopp JB, Maloney NA, Coburn JW, Sherrard DJ. Early deposition of aluminium in bone in diabetic patients on hemodialysis. *New Engl J Med* 1987; **316**: 292–6.
3. Bilous RW, Mauer SM, Sutherland DER et al. The effects of pancreas transplantation on the glomerular structure of renal allografts in patients with insulin-dependent diabetes. *N Engl J Med* 1989; **321**: 80–85.
4. Blacher J, Guerin AP, Pannier B et al. Impact of aortic stiffness on survival in endstage renal disease. *Circulation* 1999; **99**: 2434–9.
5. Bonal J, Cleries M, Vela E. Transplantation versus hemodialysis in elderly patients. Renal Registry Committee. *Nephrol Dialysis Transpl* 1997; **12**: 261.
6. Churchill DN. Implications of the Canada–USA (CANUSA) study of the adequacy of dialysis on peritoneal dialysis schedule. *Nephrol Dialysis Transpl* 1998; **13** (6): 158–63.
7. D'Amico DJ. Diseases of the retina. *N Engl J Med* **331**: 95–110.
8. *DOQI: Clinical Practice Guidelines: Executive Summaries*. National Kidney Foundation; 17.
9. Farrel PC, Hone PW. Dialysis induced catabolism. *Am J Clinic Nutr* 1980; **33**: 1417–22.
10. Fioretto P, Mauer SM, Bilous RW et al. Effects of pancreas transplantation on glomerular structure in insulin-dependent diabetic patients with their own kidneys. *Lancet* 1993; **342**: 1193–6.
11. Fioretto P, Steffes MW, Sutherland DE, Goetz FC, Mauer SM. Reversal of lesions of diabetic nephropathy after pancreas transplantation. *N Engl J Med* 1998; **339**: 69–75.
12. Fontbonne A. Hypertriglyceridaemia as a risk factor of coronary artery disease mortality in subjects with impaired glucose tolerance. *Diabetologia* 1989; **32**: 300–304.
13. Geberth S, Lippert J, Ritz E. The apparent epidemic increase in the incidence of renal failure from diabetic nephropathy. *Nephron* 1993; **65**: 160.
14. Hasslacher C, Borholte G, Ritz E, Wahl P. Impact of hypertension on prognosis in IDDM. *Diabet Metab* 1989; **15**: 338–42.

15. Hakim RM, Lazarus JM. Initiation of dialysis. *J Am Soc Nephrol* 1995; **6**: 1319–28.

16. Herzog CA, Marwick TH, Pheley AM et al. Dobutamine stress echocardiography for the detection of significant coronary artery disease in renal transplant candidates. *Am J Kidney Dis* 1999; **33**: 1080–90.

17. Herzog CA, Ma JZ, Collins AJ. Long-term outcome of dialysis patients in the United States with coronary revascularization procedures. *Kidney Int* 1999; **56**: 324–32.

18. Isamail N. Use of erythropoietin, active vitamin D3 metabolites and alkali agents in predialysis patients. *Semin Nephrol* 1997; **17**: 270–84.

19. Joshi N, Caputo GM, Weitekamp MR, Karchmer AW. Infections in patients with diabetes mellitus. *Engl J Med* 1999; **341**: 1906–11.

20. Kimmel PL, Varela MP, Peterson RA et al. Interdialytic weight gain and survival in hemodialysis patients: effects of duration of ESRD and diabetes mellitus. *Kidney Int* 2000; **57**: 1141–51.

21. Kostner GM, Karadi I. Lipoprotein alterations in diabetes mellitus. *Diabetologia* 1988; **36**: 1113–17.

22. Krepinsky J, Ingram AJ, Clase CM. Prolonged sulfonylurea-induced hypoglycaemia in diabetic patients with endstage renal disease. *Am J Kidney Dis* (2000); **35**: 500–505.

23. Larrson O, Attman PO, Blohme I, Nyberg G, Brynger H. Morbidity and mortality in diabetic and non-diabetic patients of living related kidney donors. *Nephrol Dialysis Transpl* 1987; **2**: 109–16.

24. Laurent G, Calemard E, Charra B. Haemodialysis for French diabetic patients. *Nephrol Dialysis Transpl* 1999; **14**: 2044–5.

25. Lippert J, Ritz E, Schwarzbeck A, Schneider P. The rising tide of endstage renal failure from diabetic nephropathy type II—an epidemiological analysis. *Nephrol Dialysis Transpl* 1995; **10**: 462–5.

26. Lufft V, Kliem V, Tusch G, Dannenberg B, Brunkhorst R. Renal transplantation in older patients: is graft survival affected by age? A case control study. *Transplantation* 2000; **15**: 790–94.

27. Navarro X, Kennedy WR, Loewenson RB, Sutherland DER. Influence of pancreas transplantation on cardiorespiratory reflexes, nerve conduction and mortality in diabetes mellitus. *Diabetes* 1990; **39**: 802–6.

28. Packer M, Lee WH, Medina N, Yushak M, Kessler PD. Functional renal insufficiency during long-term therapy with captopril and enalapril in severe chronic heart failure. *Ann Intern Med* 1987; **106**: 346–54.

29. Raine AE. Epidemiology, development and treatment of endstage renal failure in type 2 (non-insulin-dependent) diabetic patients in Europe. *Diabetologia* 1993; **36**: 1099–104.

30. Ritz E, Koch M, Fliser D, Schwenger V. How can we improve prognosis in diabetic patients with end-stage renal disease? *Diabetes Care* **22** (Suppl 2) B80–B83.

31. Ritz E, Strumpf C, Katz F, Wing AJ, Quellhorst E. Hypertension and cardiovascular risk factors in hemodialysed diabetic patients. *Hypertension* 1985; **7**: 118–25.

32. Sawicki PT, Kaiser S, Heinemann L, Frenzel H, Berger M. Prevalence of renal artery stenosis in diabetes mellitus-an autopsy study. *J Intern Med* 1991; **229**: 489–92.

33. Schnuelle P, Lorenz D, Trede M, van der Woude FJ. Impact of renal cadaveric transplantation on survival in endstage renal failure: evidence for reduced

mortality risk compared with hemodialysis during long-term follow-up. *J Am Soc Nephrol* 1998; **9**: 2135–41.

34. Semenkovic CF, Ostlund RE, Schechtman KB. Plasma lipids in patients with type I diabetes mellitus: influence of race, gender and plasma glucose control. *Arch Intern Med* 1989; **149**: 51–6.

35. Smets YF, Westendorp RG, van der Pijl JW et al. Effect of simultaneous pancreas-kidney transplantation on mortality of patients with type-1 diabetes and end-stage renal failure. *Lancet* 1999; **353**: 1915–19.

36. Spinosa DJ, Angle JF, Hagspiel KD, et al. Lower extremity arteriography with use of iodinated contrast material or gadodiamide to supplement CO_2 angiography in patients with renal insufficiency. *J Vasc Interv Radiol* 2000; **11**: 35–43.

37. Tschöpe W, Koch M, Thomas B, Ritz E. Serum lipids predict cardiac death in diabetic patients on maintenance hemodialysis. *Nephron* 1993; **64**: 354–8.

38. Van Daele PLA, Stolk RP, Burger H. Bone density in non-insulin-dependent diabetes mellitus. *Ann Intern Med* 1995; **122**: 409–14.

21

Prognosis of Patients with Diabetic Nephropathy

GEORG BIESENBACH

General Hospital, Linz, Austria

INTRODUCTION

Diabetes mellitus is the most common cause of new end-stage renal disease in North America and Europe (63). The poor prognosis of patients with diabetic nephropathy is well known in both in type 1 and type 2 diabetes. The high mortality and morbidity, especially in type 2 diabetic patients with nephropathy, are mainly caused by coronary artery, cerebrovascular and peripheral vascular disease (20). The survival of type 1 diabetic patients requiring renal replacement therapy has been dramatically improved during the last decade; however, prognosis for type 2 diabetic patients with endstage renal disease continues to be extremely poor (3).

PROGNOSIS IN TYPE 1 DIABETIC PATIENTS WITH NEPHROPATHY

About 35% of type 1 diabetic patients develop microalbuminuria, which is a strong predictor for persistent macroproteinuria (29), and one-third of the patients acquire clinical nephropathy leading to end-stage renal disease. The risk of this complication peaks during the second decade of diabetes and declines thereafter (1).

Diabetic Nephropathy. Edited by C. Hasslacher.
© 2001 John Wiley & Sons, Ltd.

Prognosis of Type 1 Diabetic Patients with Microalbuminuria and Overt Proteinuria

The main risk factors for the progression of diabetic nephropathy are poor metabolic control and elevated blood pressure; hypercholesterolaemia and smoking are also well-known risk factors (10). The Diabetes Control and Complications Trial (DCCT) demonstrated impressively that intensive insulin therapy with good blood glucose control delays the onset and slows the progression of diabetic nephropathy. In this study, intensive therapy reduced the occurrence of microalbuminuria by 39% and that of albuminuria by 54% (13). Early aggressive antihypertensive therapy can prevent the progression of each stage of diabetic nephropathy, and is associated with improved survival in type 1 diabetic patients (16,31,42,49). In the early 1980s Parving et al (41) showed that the fall in glomerular filtration rate (GFR) in type 1 diabetics with overt nephropathy could be reduced to 2 ml/min/year after 3 years of effective antihypertensive treatment. In a recent study (48), stabilization of GFR rate was achieved in type 1 diabetic patients with overt nephropathy, who reached the goal of intensified antihypertensive treatment even in the presence of impaired renal function. It has also been shown that, when antihypertensive care is based on blood pressure self-monitoring and subsequent adaption of antihypertensive drugs treatment, blood pressure can be normalized in the majority of hypertensive patients (48,49).

During the 1980s the prognosis of type 1 diabetic patients with nephropathy improved when compared with the decade before, mainly due to more effective antihypertensive treatment (36). In a prospective study of Parving and Hommel (42), type 1 diabetic patients who developed persistent macroproteinuria during 1974–1978 were followed until death or for at least 10 years. The cumulative death rate was 18% (10 years after the onset of clinical nephropathy), in contrast to previous studies which reported death rates of 50% and 77%, respectively, 10 years after the onset of nephropathy. Uraemia and myocardial infarction were the main causes of death. In a WHO multinational study of vascular disease, diabetes type 1 diabetic patients with proteinuria and hypertension had a significantly increased mortality risk: 11-fold for diabetic men and 18-fold for diabetic women when compared with type 1 diabetics without nephropathy (65). The excessive risk of cardiovascular disease and stroke was a major contribution to the excess all-cause mortality in these diabetic patients. The relative excess mortality was found to diminish with increasing age but to increase with increasing duration of diabetes. The mortality of type 1 diabetic patients with nephropathy is similar in Europe and North America but considerably higher in Japan than in the USA (13,14,37).

Prognosis of Type 1 Diabetic Patients with Endstage Renal Disease

Until the early 1980s the prognosis of type 1 diabetic patients with renal failure was extremely poor; the 3 year survival rate of diabetic patients on dialysis therapy was less than 50% (19). Renal transplantation was successful in rare cases (28). A single-centre study of 100 patients, published in 1986, reported a 5-year survival of only 19% (31). The prognosis of these patients was much poorer than for non-diabetic patients of similar age and sex, mainly due to macrovascular complications (20). The overwhelming cause of death of diabetic patients with renal failure was myocardial ischaemia (28). In a German study, the cardiovascular mortality of type 1 diabetic patients receiving haemodialysis treatment was 4.8 times higher than that of non-diabetic haemodialysis patients (45). Sudden death (80%), myocardial infarction (13%) and stroke (7%) were the main causes of cardiovascular death. Systolic blood pressure over 166 mmHg at the start of dialysis and left ventricular hypertrophy, and especially left ventricular dilatation, were the best predictors of cardiovascular death.

During the 1980s, data from a national survey in the USA suggested a better survival of up to 3 years after kidney transplantation, particularly when grafts from live donors were used (35). The large series of renal transplants reported in 1985 from Minneapolis showed even better results (55). In contrast, the prognosis of type 1 diabetic patients treated with haemodialysis or CAPD is significantly poorer than that of kidney-transplanted patients, although the prognosis has been improved under each kind of renal replacement therapy. However, changes in patient survival over the last two decades are difficult to assess, because type 1 and type 2 diabetic patients were not accurately differentiated in earlier studies. According to the US Report Data System (USRDS), the 1 year survival of diabetics on dialysis increased from 65% in 1980 to 74% in 1990, but this Annual Data Report also did not make a careful distinction between the two types of diabetes (21). Today it is generally accepted that all type 1 diabetic patients with renal disease should be transplanted.

The results of kidney transplantation alone in type 1 diabetic patients have been dramatically improved during the last years. Meanwhile, the graft survival rates in type 1 diabetics are similar to those of non-diabetic patients (56). Simultaneous pancreas–kidney transplantation has become the method of choice for these patients, and has been highly successful over the past decade (57). Pancreas transplantation is the only modality that is able to induce a euglycaemic state in insulin-dependent diabetic patients. In a recent study it has been demonstrated that pancreas transplantation can reverse the lesions of diabetic nephropathy in type 1 diabetic patients, but reversal requires more than 5 years of normoglycaemia, and transplantation must be performed in an early stage without uraemia. (18).

Out of nearly 10 000 pancreas transplants that have been reported to the International Pancreas Transplant Registry 1997, more than 7400 were performed in the USA (57). The majority of patients (90%) received simultaneous pancreas–kidney grafts. The improvement in results during the last years was associated with the introduction of FK506 (tacrolimus) and mycophenolate mofetil for immunosuppression (54). In the USA the 1 year pancreas graft survival rate after simultaneous cadaver pancreas–kidney transplantation improved from 74% during 1987–1989 to 82% during 1994–1996, and the 3 year patient survival rate increased to more than 90% during recent years (57). In a recent study, Tyden et al (59) reported a significantly higher 10 year survival in type 1 diabetics with combined pancreas–kidney transplantation than in patients with kidney graft alone.

In an own single-center study (9), the 5-year survival rate of all new type 1 diabetic patients starting renal replacement therapy during 1991–1997 was 83% in comparison to 88% overall survival in age-matched non-diabetic patients (age < 40 years) during the same period (Figure 21.1). However, the majority of type 1 diabetic patients received a simultaneous pancreas and kidney transplant (75%) and a kidney transplant alone (18%), respectively. In contrast, kidney transplantation was performed in only 65% of the non-diabetic individuals during the same period of observation.

In conclusion, mortality in type 1 diabetic patients with nephropathy has been significantly reduced, and the survival of kidney or pancreas–kidney-transplanted diabetic patients dramatically increased during the last decade.

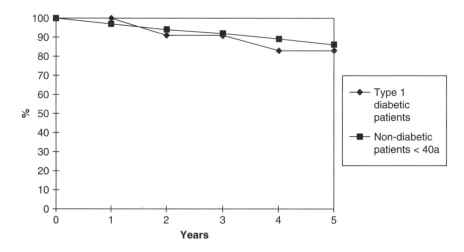

Figure 21.1 Five-year survival of type 1 diabetic patients and age-matched non-diabetic patients (age < 40 years) who started renal replacement therapy in a single dialysis centre during the years 1991–1997 (9). From (67), with permission

PROGNOSIS IN TYPE 2 DIABETIC PATIENTS WITH NEPHROPATHY

The earlier opinion that renal prognosis is less adverse in type 2 diabetic patients as compared with type 1 diabetes has been revised during recent years. It is now established that the development of diabetic nephropathy is similar in both types of diabetes (46). In the course of type 2 diabetes, 20–40% of patients have an elevated urinary albumin excretion (52); 20–25% of patients develop overt proteinuria in the subsequent years.

Prognosis of Type 2 Diabetic Patients with Microalbuminuria and Overt Proteinuria

Microalbuminuria in type 2 diabetes is related not only to subsequent diabetic macroproteinuria, but even more strongly to increased mortality, mainly due to cardiovascular disease (12,38). Several arteriosclerosis-related risk factors are more frequently seen in microalbuminuric patients, especially lipid abnormalities, elevated lipoprotein(a) concentrations, increased arterial pressure and haemostatic disturbances with increased serum fibrinogen levels (30,50). Moreover, it is well known that microalbuminuria is also a significant risk factor for early death in non-diabetic subjects (66) and it can been assumed that microalbuminuria is a marker for endothelial cell injury and reflects widespread vascular disease. In type 2 diabetic patients with microalbuminuria, the percentage increase in mortality depends on the range of albumin concentrations in urine. Although micro-albuminuria was also a predictor for subsequent proteinuria in a 10 year follow-up study, only a few of the microalbuminuric type 2 diabetic patients died from renal disease; the main cause of death was cardiac infarction or cardiac insufficiency (51). The predictive value of microalbuminuria for subsequent clinical nephropathy appears to be lower in type 2 diabetic patients but there are no exact data in the literature, as many of the micro-albuminuric patients died during follow-up studies (39).

The prevalence of risk factors for nephropathy and cardiovascular disease are very high in genetically predisposed peoples. Especially in diabetic blacks and native Americans the overall prevalence of proteinuria is more than 40%, depending on the duration of diabetes. In addition, the incidence of macrovascular complications is higher in black and native Americans than in the Caucasian population with diabetes (26, 44, 53). This can be explained by a genetic predisposition and a higher incidence of prediabetic hypertension.

The course of renal function in type 2 diabetic patients with diabetic nephropathy has been described controversially in the literature (40). Earlier studies reported a slower decline of GFR in proteinuric type 2 diabetic patients than in type 1 diabetic subjects. In the study of Gall et al (21), the mean decline in GFR of proteinuric type 2 diabetic patients was only 5.7 ml/ min/year, but the fall of GFR varied considerably between patients. In contrast, Nielsen et al (40) described a similar progression to overt protein-uria in microalbuminuric type 2 diabetic patients, and Hasslacher et al (25) found an identical risk for renal failure after 5 years of macroproteinuria in both types of diabetes. These results have been confirmed by other authors, who observed a similar rate of progression in the predialysis phase in type 1 and type 2 diabetic patients with overt proteinuria (4).

In all studies concerning type 2 diabetic patients, hypertension had the same impact on the progression of diabetic nephropathy as that observed in type 1 diabetes (2, 43, 46). However, poor metabolic control was also shown to be a risk factor for the progression of nephropathy in type 2 diabetic patients, as known for type 1 diabetes (26). The recently published results of the UK Prospective Diabetes Study Group (UKPDS) have shown that aggregate, intensive therapy of diabetes improves the health-care status of type 2 diabetic patients (60). Additionally, in a superimposed hypertension study, a tight blood pressure control (mean systolic blood pressure 144 vs. 154 mmHg) reduced the risk of macrovascular and microvascular complic-tions (61). In the same study, the efficacy of atenolol and captopril in reducing the risk of macrovascular and microvascular complications was not significantly different (62). There is good evidence that in type 2 dia-betic patients with nephropathy the same preventive measures are effective as in type 1 diabetes, including glycaemic control, blood pressure control, protein restriction and avoiding smoking (6, 27, 47). In addition, patients with coronary heart disease should be treated with β-blockers, and ACE inhibitors should be administered in cases of cardiac insufficiency (17, 58).

Prognosis of Type 2 Diabetic Patients with Endstage Renal Disease

Due to the rising prevalence of type 2 diabetes and better patient survival, the incidence of uraemia in type 2 diabetic patients has dramatically increased in Europe and North America (46). The well-known poor prog-nosis of type 2 diabetic patients requiring dialysis therapy has been docu-mented in several studies (23). During the 1980s the 5 year survival rate of patients on renal replacement therapy was 25%, according to data from the EDTA Registry (11). However, earlier studies concerning the outcome of endstage renal disease in diabetic patients were characterized by a lack of precision in the classification of diabetes. Meanwhile, some authors have reported an improved survival in proteinuric patients with type 2 diabetes

(24), probably a result of better antihypertensive treatment and improved management of patients with coronary heart disease. However, a significant improvement in the survival rate of type 2 diabetic patients on haemodialysis could not be confirmed by other authors. In our dialysis centre the 1 year and 5 year survival rates were 55% and 17% respectively, among type 2 diabetic patients who were dialysed during the years 1980–1986. In patients who were started on dialysis in 1987–1993, the 1 year and 5 year survival increased to 78% and 23%, respectively (3). In the USA the first-year mortality decreased consistently for diabetic patients, from 46% in 1985 to 27% in 1995 (64). There is a well-known rapid progression of macrovascular disease with a high incidence of cardiovascular complications in type 2 diabetic patients requiring haemodialysis therapy. It has been shown that the survival prognosis of diabetics on dialysis is poorly predicted by elevated admission blood pressure, left ventricular hypertrophy and other factors, but is strongly predicted by the presence of lipidaemia (34). Diabetic patients requiring dialysis therapy have a higher prevalence of left ventricular hypertrophy and a higher incidence of haemodialysis-associated hypotension (8, 15). Moreover, the survival rate s significantly decreased among smoking patients on haemodialysis (7). In recent studies, an improvement of the 5 year survival rate of diabetic patients on haemodialysis as well as CAPD had been reported (46). Nevertheless, 40–50% of patients with diabetic nephropathy will die within the first 3 years of maintenance dialysis, mostly from cardiovascular cases (11).

The prognosis of type 2 diabetic patients with endstage renal disease can be improved by kidney transplantation. However, for the large majority, maintanance haemodialysis and for a smaller group CAPD are the only renal replacement regimens that will be employed. In the USA, only 8% of type 2 diabetic patients received a kidney transplant. The prognosis of the diabetic patients appears to be better on haemodialysis than on CAPD, although this questio is an open matter of discussion. According to the USRDS, the survival rate of diabetic patients treated by CAPD was significantly lower than for those on haemodialysis (57). In our single-centre study (9), the 5 year survival of type 2 diabetic patients starting dialysis therapy during 1991–1997 was 29% vs. 39% in the age-matched non-diabetic subjects (age $\geq$ 40 years), as shown in Figure 21.2. Only a minority of the diabetic (6%) and non-diabetic patients (11%) received a kidney graft during the period of observation.

There are only few data in the literature concerning the prognosis of type 2 diabetic patients in the pre-dialysis phase. In a prospective study over a period of 7 years 40% of nephropathic type 2 diabetic patients died before the start of dialysis treatment (5). There is also a dramatically rapid progression of macrovascular disease during the pre-dialysis phase (8). There is no doubt that the management of diabetic patients with renal disease in the predialysis phase requires furthe improvement (33).

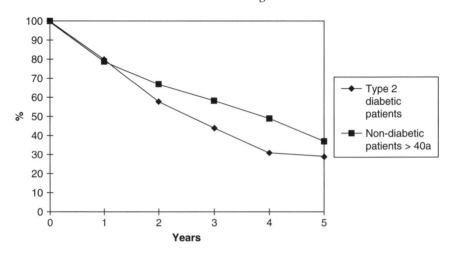

Figure 21.2　Five-year survival of type 2 diabetic patients and age-matched non-diabetic patients (age ≥ 40 years) who started renal replacement therapy in a single dialysis centre during the years 1991–1997 (9). From (67), with permission

In conclusion, the mortality of type 2 diabetic patients is very high due to concomitant macrovascular diseases. Therefore, the main goal in the future must be the prevention of endstage renal disease in patients with type 2 diabetes.

REFERENCES

1. Anderson AR, Christiansen JS, Andersen JK, kreiner S, Deckert T. Diabetic nephropathy in Type I (insulin-dependent) diabetes: an epidemiologic study. *Diabetologia* 1983; **25**: 496–501.
2. Baba T, Murabayashi S, Tomiyama T, Takebe K. Uncontrolled hypertension is associated with a rapid progression of nephropathy in type 2 diabetic patients with proteinuria and preserved renal function. *Tohoku J Exp Med* 1990; **161**: 311–18.
3. Biesenbach G, Grafinger P, Hubmann R et al. Changes in the survival rates and causes of death in type II diabetic patients requiring dialysis treatment during the years 1980 to 1986 and 1987 to 1993. *Nieren- und Hochdruckkr* 1996; **25**: 45–9.
4. Biesenbach G, Janko O, Zazgornik J. Similar rate of progression of the predialysis phase in type I and type II diabetic patients. *Nephrol Dialysis Transpl* 1994; **9**: 1097–102.
5. Biesenbach G, Zazgornik J. High mortality and poor quality of life during predialysis period in type II diabetic patients with diabetic nephropathy. *Renal Failure* 1994; **6**: 263–72.
6. Biesenbach g, Grafinger P, Janko O, Zazgornik J. Influence of cigarette-smoking on the progression of clinical diabetic nephropathy in type 2 diabetic patients. *Clin Nephrol* 1997; **48**: 146–50.

7. Biesenbach G, Zazgornik J. Influence of smoking on the survival rate of diabetic patients requiring hemodialsis. *Diabet Care* 1996; **19**: 625–8.

8. Biesenbach G, Zazgornik J. Vascular disease in type II diabetes: progression before and after commencing haemodialysis. *Nephrology* 1997; **3**: 195–8.

9. Biesenbach G, Hubmann R, Janko O. Percentage of type I- and type II-diabetic patients with end-stage renal disease, renal replacement therapy and patient survival in a single dialysis center, 1991–1999. *Kidney Blood Press Res* 1999; **22**(abstr): 218–19.

10. Bretzel RG. Can we further slow down the progression to end-stage renal disease in diabetic hypertensive patients? *J Hypertension* 1997; **15**(2): 83–8.

11. Brunner FP, Selwood N. Profile of patients on RRT in Europe and death rates due to major causes of death groups. *Kidney Int* 1992; **36**(38): 1113–17.

12. Damsgaard EM, Froland A, Jorgensen OD, Mogensen CE. Eight-to nine-year mortality in known non-insulin-dependent diabetics and controls. A prospective study. *Kidney Int* 1992; **41**: 731–5.

13. DCCT Research Group. The Diabetes Control and Complications Trial Research Group. The effect of intensive treatment of diabetes on the development and progression of long-term complications in insulin-dependent diabetes mellitus. *N Engl J Med* 1993; **329**: 977–86.

14. Diabetes Epidemiology Research International Group. Major cross-country differences in risk of dying for people with IDDM. *Diabet Care* 1991; **14**: 49–54.

15. Dorhout Mess EJ, Özbasli C, Akcicek F. Cardiovascular disturbances in hemodialysis patients: the importance of volume overload. *J Nephrol* 1995; **8**: 71–8.

16. Earle KA, Morocutti A, Viberti GC. Permissive role of hypertension in the development of proteinuria and progression of renal disease in insulin-dependent diabetic patients. *J Hypertens* 1997; **15**: 191–6.

17. Estacio R, Jeffers BW, Hiatt WR et al. The effect of nisoldipine as compared with enalapril on cardiovascular outcomes in patients with non-insulin-dependent diabetes and hypertension. *N Engl J Med* 1998; **338**: 645–52.

18. Fioretto P, Steffes MW, Sutherland DER, Goetz FC, Mauer MD. Reversal of lesions of diabetic nephropathy after pancreas transplantation. *N Engl J Med* 1998; **339**: 69–75.

19. Flynn CT. Why blind diabetics with renal failure should be offered treatment. *Br Med. J* 1983; **287**: 1177–8.

20. Friedman EA, Beyer MM. Uremia in diabetics: the prognosis improves. *Klin Wochenschr* 1980; **58**: 1023–8.

21. Friedman R, Gross J. Evolution of glomerular filtration rate in proteinuric NIDDM patients. *Diabet Care* 1991; **14**: 355–9.

22. Gall MA, Nielsen FS, Smidt UM, Parving HH. The course of kidney function in type 2 (non-insulin-dependent) disbetic patients with diabetic nephropathy. *Diabetologia* 1993; **36**: 1071–8.

23. Grenfell A, Bewick M, Parsons V et al. Non-insulin-dependent diabetes and renal replacement therapy. *Diabet Med* 1988; **5**: 172–6.

24. Hasslacher C, Borgholte G, Panradl U, Wahl P. Improved diagnosis of type I and type II diabetes with nephropathy. *Med Klinik* 1990; **85**: 643–6.

25. Hasslacher C, Ritz E, Wahland P, Michael C. Similar risks of nephropathy in patients with type I or type II diabetes mellitus. *Nephrol Dialysis Transp* 1984; **4**: 859–69.

26. Hasslacher C, Bostedt-Kiesel A, Kempe HP, Wahl P. Effect of metabolic factors and blood pressure on kidney function in proteinuric type 2 (non-insulin-dependent) diabetic patients. *Diabetologia* 1993; **36**: 1051–6.

26. Hirata-Dulas CAI, Rith-Najarian SJ, McIntyre MC et al. Risk factors for nephropathy and cardiovascular disease in diabetic Northern Minnesota American Indians. *Clin Nephrol* 1996; **46**: 92–8.
27. Hung-Hsiang Liou, Tung-po Huang, Vito m Campese. Effect of long-term therapy with coptopril on proteinuria and renal function in patients with non-insulin-dependent diabetes and with non-diabetic renal diseases. *Nephron* 1995; **69**: 41–8.
28. Jacobs C, Brunner FP, Brynger H et al. The first five thousand diabetics treated by dialysis and transplantation in Europe. *Diabet Nephrop* 1984; **2**: 12–16.
29. Jones RH, Mackay JD, Hayakawa H, Parsons V. Progression of diabetic nephropathy. *Lancet* 1979; **26**: 1105–6.
30. Jones SL, Close CF, Mattock MB et al. Plasma lipid and coagulation factor concentrations in insulin dependent diabetes with microalbuminuria. *Br Med J* 1989; **298**: 487–90.
31. Kasiske BL, Kalil RS, Ma JZ, Liao M, Keane WF. Effect of antihypertensive therapy on the kidney in patients with diabetes: a meta-regression analysis. *Ann Intern Med* 1993; **118**: 29–138.
32. Khalil RB, Steinmüller DR, Novick AC et al. A critical look at survival of diabetics with end-stage renal disese. *Transplantation* 1986; **41**: 598–602.
33. Koch M, Tschöpe W, Ritz E. Must the care of diabetics with renal failure in the predialysis phase be improved? *Dtsch Med Wochenschr* 1991; **116**: 1543–8.
34. Koch M, Thomas B, Tschöpe W, Ritz E. Survival and predictors of death in dialysed patients. *Diabetologia* 1993; **36**: 1113–17.
35. Krakauer H, Grauman JS, McMullan MR, Creede CC. The recent US experience in the treatment of end-stage renal disease by dialysis and transplantation. *N Engl J Med* 1983; **306**: 1558–63.
36. Lewis EJ, Hunsicker LG, Bain RP, Rhode RD. The effect of angiotensin-converting enzyme inhibition on diabetic nephropathy. *N Engl J Med* 1993; **329**: 1456–62.
37. Matsushima M, Tijima N, LaPorte RE et al, for the Diabetes Epidemiology Research International (DERI) US–Japan Mortality Study Group. Markedly increased renal disease mortality and incidence of renal replacement therapy among IDDM patients in Japan in contrast to Allegheny County, Pennsylvania, USA. *Diabetologia* 1995; **38**: 236–43.
38. Mogensen CE, Damsgaard EM, Froland A et al. Microalbuminuria in non-insulin-dependent diabetes. *Clin Nephrol* 1992; **38** (I): 28–38.
39. Mogensen CE. Microalbuminuria predicts clinical proteinuria and early mortality in maturity-onset diabetes. *N Engl J Med* 1984; **310**: 365–70.
40. Nielsen S, Schmitz A, Mogensen CE. Rate of progression of nephropathy in normo- and microalbuminuric type 2 diabetic patients. *Diabetologia* 1991; **34** (2A), 144–9.
41. Parving HH, Smidt UM, Andersen AR, Svendsen A. Early aggressive anti-hypertensive treatment reduces rate of decline in kidney function in diabetic nephropathy. *Lancet* 1983; **I**: 1175–9.
42. Parving HH, Hommel E, Damkjaer Nielsen M, Giese J. Effect of captopril on blood pressure and kidney function in normotensive insulin dependent diabetics with nephropathy. *Br Med J* 1989; **299**: 533–6.
43. Ravid M, Savin H, Lang R et al. Proteinuria, renal impairment, metabolic control and blood pressure in type 2 diabetes mellitus. *Arch Intern Med* 1992; **152**: 1225–9.

44. Rith-Najarian SJ, Valway SE, Gohdes DM. Diabetes in Northern Minnesota Chippewa tribe: prevalence and incidence of diabetes and and incidence of major complications, 1986–1988. *Diabet Care* 1993; **16**(I): 266–9.
45. Ritz E, Strumpf C, Katz F, Wing AJ, Quellhorst E. Hypertension and cardiovascular risk factors in hemodialyzed diabetic patients. *Hypertension* 1985; **7** (II): 118–24.
46. Ritz E, Keller Ch, Bergis K, Strojek K. Pathogenesis and course of renal disease in IDDM/NIDDM. *Am J Hypertens* 1997; **10**: 202–7.
47. Ritz E, Stefanski A. Diabetic nephropathy in type II diabetes. *Am J Kidney Dis* 1996; **27**: 167–94.
48. Sawicki PT. Stabilization of glomerular filtration rate over 2 years in patients with diabetic nephropathy under intensified therapy regimes. *Nephrol Dialysis Transpl* 1997; **12**: 1890–99.
49. Sawicki PT, Mühlhauser I, Didjurgeit U et al. Intensified antihypertensive therapy is associated with improved survival in type 1 diabetic patients with nephropathy. *J Hypertens* 1995; **13**: 26–9.
50. Seghieri G, Alviggi I, Caselli P et al. Serum lipids and lipoproteins in type 2 diabetic patients with persistent microalbuminuria. *Diabet Med* 1990; **7**: 810–14.
51. Schmith A, Väth M. Microalbuminuria: a major risk factor in non-insulin-dependent diabetes. A 10-year follow-up study of 503 patients. *Diabet Med* 1988; **5**: 126–34.
52. Schnack C, Scheithauer W, Winkler J, Gisinger CH, Schernthaner G. Prevalence of microalbuminuria in non-insulin-dependent diabetes mellitus. Effect of disease duration, glycemic control and blood pressure. *Diabet Metab (Paris)* 1988; **14**: 184–8.
53. Stephens GW, Gillaspy JA, Clyne D, Mejia A, Pollak VE. Racial differences in the incidence of end-stage renal disease in types I and II diabetes mellitus. *Am J Kidney Dis* 1990; **15**: 562–7.
54. Stratta RJ. Simultaneous use of tacrolimus and mycophenolate mofetil in combined pancreas–kidney transplant recipients: a multi-center report. *Transpl Proc* 1997; **29**: 654–5.
55. Sutherland DER, Fryd DS, Payne WD, Ascher N, Simmons RL, Najarian JS. Renal transplantation in diabetics at the University of Minnesota. *Diabet Nephrop* 1985; **4**: 123–6.
56. Sutherland DER, Gruessner RWG. Current status of pancreas transplantation for the treatment of type 1 diabetes mellitus. *Clin Diabet* 1997; **15**: 152–6.
57. Sutherland DER, Gruessner RWG. Current status of pancreas transplantation in diabetic renal allograft recipients (abstract). *Semin Dialysis* 1997; **10**: 231–3.
58. Tse WY, Kendall M. Is there a role for beta-blockers in hypertensive diabetic patients? *Diabet Med* 1994; **11**: 137–44.
59. Tyden G, Bolinder I, Solders G, Brattström C, Ibell A, Groth CG. Improved survival in patients with insulin-dependent diabetes mellitus and end-stage diabeic nephropathy 10 years after combined pancreas and kidney transplantation. *Transplantation* 1999; **67**: 645–8.
60. UK Prospective Diabetes Study (UKPDS) Group. Intensive blood-glucose control with sulfonylureas or insulin compared with conventional treatment and risk of complications in patients with type 2 diabetes. *Lancet* 1998; **352**: 837–54.
61. UK Prospective Diabetes Study Group. Tight blood pressure control and risk of macrovascular and microvascular complications in type 2 diabetes (UKPDS 38): *Br Med J* 1998; **317**: 703–13.

62. UK Prospective Diabetes Study Group. Efficacy of atenolol and captopril in reducing risk of macrovascular and microvascular complications in type 2 diabetes (UKPDS 39). *Br Med J* 1998; **317**: 713–20.

63. US Renal Data System. *USRDS 1994 Annual Data Report.* The National Institutes of Health, National Institute of Diabetes and Digestive and Kidney Diseases: Bethesda, MD, June, 1994.

64. US Renal Data System. USRDS 1998 Annual Data Report. *Am J Kidney Dis* 1988; **32**(1): 69–80.

65. Wang S-L, Head J, Stevens L. Excess mortality and 1st relation to hypertension and proteinuria in diabetic patients. *Diabet Care* 1990; **19**: 305–12.

66. Yudkin JS, Forrest RD, Jackson CA. Microalbuminuria as predictor of vascular disease in non-diabetic subjects. Islington diabetes survey. *Lancet* 1988; **II**: 530–33.

67. Biesenbach G, Hubmann R, Grafinger P et al. 5-year overall survival rates of uremic type 1 and type 2 diabetic patients in comparison with age-matched nondiabetic patients with end-stage renal disease from a single dialysis center from 1991 to 1997. *Diabetes Care* 2000; **23**: 1860–2.

Index

Index compiled by A. C. Purton

THE DIABETES IN PRACTICE SERIES .....

DIABETIC NEPHROPATHY
Edited by: C.Hasslacher, St Josefkrankenhauses, Heidelberg, Germany

This Volume focuses on the clinical relevance of diabetic nephropathy, which is a leading cause of end-stage renal failure and renal replacement treatments, while providing a solid grounding in current and basic clinical research.

047148992 1   336pp   2001

PSYCHOLOGY IN DIABETES CARE
Edited by: FJ Snoek and TC Skinner

Bridging the gap between psychological research on self-care and management of diabetes, and the delivery of care and services provided by the diabetes care team, this book provides a background and practical guidelines on behavioural issues much needed by health care professionals.

0471 97703 9   294pp   2000

EXERCISE AND SPORT IN DIABETES
Edited by: Bill Burr and Dinesh Nagi

A rare look at the benefits and risks of strenuous and easy exercise for people with diabetes. Accessible to all diabetes patient carers, it allow the reader to fully understand the issues, and brief patients accordingly:
- accumulating the most up-to-date information
- exploring issues with a practical outlook

0471 98496 5   194pp   1999

HYPOGLYCAEMIA IN CLINICAL DIABETES
Edited by: Brian M Frier and B Miles Fisher

An up-to-date and accessible publication, covering a very common problem in the clinical management of diabetes. It discusses risk factors and treatment regimes, while concentrating on the clinical and practical aspects of hypoglycaemia.

0471 98264 4   301pp   1999

CHILDHOOD AND ADOLESCENT DIABETES
Edited by: Simon Court and Bill Lamb

The management of diabetes in children and young people continues to develop in important areas, including self-monitoring, insulin delivery, dietary prescription, concept of control and the early identification of complications. This book is practical and invaluable to all members of the diabetes specialist team working with children.

0471 97003 4   384pp   1997

DIABETES AND PREGNANCY
An International Approach to Diagnosis and Management
Edited by: Anne Dornhorst and David R Hadden

A comprehensive and practical guide to the present state of knowledge regarding diabetic pregnancy. It summarises published literature, and offers clear and valuable information on the practicalities of providing special care, before, during and after pregnancy.

0471 96204 x   424pp   1996

PREDICTION, PREVENTION AND GENETIC COUNSELING IN IDDM
Edited by: Jerry P Palmer

A summary of the latest developments, examining and analysing how diabetes can be predicted through genetic, immune and cell markers, metabolic assessment, environmental factors and animal models.

0 471 95525 6   462pp   1996

DIABETIC COMPLICATIONS
Edited by: Ken M Shaw

A comprehensive review of diabetes care; outlining the nature of the complication, how susceptibility and risk can be identified, the importance of screening during the early stages and the manner in which appropriate investigation and management should be undertaken.

0 471 96678 9   244pp   1996

JOURNALS

DIABETES METABOLISM RESEARCH AND REVIEW

A print and electronic journal that publishes original articles and state-of-the-art reviews in diabetes and related areas of metabolism. This journal is dedicated to publishing papers within the shortest achievable lead times. It offers immediate publication of original papers after editorial acceptance, as pre-print on-line. It also includes a current-awareness section that cites papers published.

Diabetes Metabolism Research and Review provides a unique perspective on a wide range of topics.

PRACTICAL DIABETES INTERNATIONAL

Explores all aspects of the world wide clinical science and practice of diabetes medicine. The journal recognises the importance of each member of the healthcare team in the delivery of diabetes care and reflects the diversity of professional interest in its editorial contents.

To receive further information on any of these books or Journals, please tick the relevant boxes and return this card, stating your address, to:

Life and Medical Sciences
John Wiley & Sons Ltd
Baffins Lane, Chichester
West Sussex
PO19 1UD, UK

Fax: ++ 44 (0) 1243 770154
Visit the Wiley Home Page at
http://www.wiley.co.uk

 WILEY

1418